Essentials of Neurology

Fifth Edition

Sir John Walton

TD, MD, DSc, Dr de l'Univ (Hon, Aix-Marseille) DSc (Hon, Leeds), DSc
(Hon, Leicester), FRCP, FACP(Hon), FRCP (Edin.) (Hon)
Professor of Neurology, University of Newcastle upon Tyne,
Neurologist, Newcastle General Hospital, and Newcastle Health Authority

Pitman

PITMAN PUBLISHING LIMITED
128 Long Acre, London WC2E 9AN

Associated Companies
Pitman Publishing Pty Ltd, Melbourne
Pitman Publishing New Zealand Ltd, Wellington

Distributed in the United States of America and
Canada by Urban & Schwarzenberg Inc., 7 East Redwood
Street, Baltimore, MD 21202

First published 1961
Fifth edition 1982
Reprinted 1984

Library of Congress Cataloging in Publication Data

Walton, John Nicholas.
  Essentials of neurology.

  Includes bibliographies and index
  1. Nervous system—Diseases. I. Title. [DNLM:
1. Nervous system diseases. WL 100 W239e]
RC346.W25 1982   616.8   82-3817
ISBN 0-272-79673-5   AACR2

British Library Cataloguing in Publication Data

Walton, *Sir* John, *1922–*
  Essentials of neurology.—5th ed.
  1. Nervous system—Diseases
  I. Title
  616.8   RC346
ISBN 0–272–79673–5

Text set in 10/12pt Linotron 202 Times,
printed and bound in Great Britain
at The Pitman Press, Bath

Contents

Plates

Preface to the Fifth Edition

Developments in neurology during the last five years, together with the comments and advice of those who read and reviewed the first four editions, have necessitated substantial changes in the text, although the general structure of the book remains the same. Each chapter has been carefully revised, some sections have been rewritten, and there have been numerous additions but since redundant and outdated material has been deleted the book is very little longer. Several new illustrations, including examples of CAT scans, have been included, and especially extensive changes have been made in the chapters on investigations in neurology, aphasia and the special senses and on neuromuscular and metabolic diseases. Numerous cross-references and several tables have also been included. The chapter on treatment has been revised extensively bearing in mind the major advances in pharmacology which have occurred in recent years. The references at the end of each chapter have also been brought up to date but, as in previous editions, those given have been selected in order to bring to the attention of the reader other books which he may consult in order to widen his knowledge of neurology and related disciplines and in which he will find references to original sources of information. In a text-book of this size and scope, it is still my view that references to scientific papers would be inappropriate; it would be difficult to select a suitable short list which would cover adequately all of the topics which are discussed, while comprehensive lists of references to journals would be too weighty in a short commentary of this nature.

In the face of rising costs and in an attempt to keep the price of the book within limits which will not put it beyond the pocket of the average medical student, only one new plate and several diagrams and line drawings have been added in this edition. In the fourth edition Plate I was prepared from a series of plates reproduced from *Aids to the Examination of the Peripheral Nervous System* published in 1975 by Her Majesty's Stationery Office on behalf of the Medical Research Council. I am grateful to the MRC and to HMSO for permission to reproduce these illustrations. I also wish to thank Professor R. W. Gilliatt and Dr R. G. Willison of the National Hospital, Queen Square, who were responsible for the preparation of some of these illustrations in the Department of Medical Illustration of the Institute of Neurology, and Dr M. J. McArdle and Dr M. D.

O'Brien who prepared others in the Department of Medical Illustration and Photography, Guy's Hospital Medical School. The CAT scans now reproduced in Plate III were kindly made available by Dr Arnold Appleby. Figures 2, 3, 4 and 5 are taken from the third edition of 'A Physiological Approach to Clinical Neurology' by Professors J. W. Lance and J. G. McLeod and I am grateful to them and to Butterworth and Co. for permission to reproduce them. Figures 7, 9 and 10 come from *Introduction to Basic Neurology* by Professor H. D. Patton, J. W. Sundsten, W. E. Crill and P. D. Swanson published by Saunders and here again I am indebted to the authors and publishers. I have also drawn upon some material, especially in the section on ocular movement, previously published in the section on Neurology contributed by myself to the volume entitled *Pathophysiology* (Volume 1 of the *International Textbook of Medicine*), edited by Drs Lloyd H. Smith and Samuel O. Thier and published by Saunders (Philadelphia). I have also included two tables on the composition of the cerebrospinal fluid modified from the chapter written by Dr R. H. Johnson in the book *Scientific Foundations of Neurology*, edited by Dr Macdonald Critchley, Dr J. L. O'Leary and Professor W. B. Jennett and published by Heinemann. Figure 8 is reproduced from the eighth edition of *Brain's Diseases of the Nervous System* edited by myself and I am grateful to Oxford Medical Publications for permission to include this diagram too. As in the third edition, I am glad to express my gratitude to Dr G. L. Gryspeerdt for the reproductions of radiographs and gammaencephalograms, and to Dr D. D. Barwick and Miss B. P. Longley for the composite illustration of the electroencephalogram; photographic reproductions have been made in the Department of Photography, the University of Newcastle upon Tyne. As always, I am deeply indebted to my secretary, Miss Rosemary Allan, for her invaluable assistance in the preparation of this fifth edition, and to Mr Stephen Neal, Miss Katherine Watts and the staff of Pitman Medical for all their help and co-operation.

John Walton

Newcastle upon Tyne
July 1981

Preface to the First Edition

Although there can be no absolute distinction between diseases of the nervous system and those which affect other organs or systems of the human body, by convention the clinical science of neurology embraces those many disorders which affect the functioning of the central and peripheral nervous system. This book has been written in order to help the undergraduate or postgraduate student to learn the principles of neurological diagnosis and treatment. It is hoped that it will also assist the practising physician in his management of patients suffering from this variety of illness.

The first ten chapters of the book are devoted to a consideration of the cardinal symptoms and signs of neurological disease, to the mechanism of their production and the various pathological changes which may produce these clinical manifestations. In this review of the principles of neurological diagnosis, brief mention is made of investigative methods, some simple and others highly specialised, but only in sufficient detail to indicate to the student or practitioner the indications for employing these methods, their failings and their dangers, and the information which they are likely to divulge. The ensuing chapters contain brief descriptions of specific syndromes of nervous disease, taking into account the general principles previously stressed. Exhaustive descriptions of pathological changes and of differential diagnosis are omitted and the reader will look in vain for lists and tables of diseases and syndromes. Nor will he find detailed analyses of the physiological mechanisms by which symptoms and signs are produced, since this work is based upon clinical methodology, and scientific premises are only mentioned when absolutely necessary for an understanding of clinical principles. The intention has been to make this a book which can be read by the student who wishes to obtain a composite picture of neurological illness, but can also be used for reference if need be. Each chapter is concluded with a list of references to other volumes in which more detailed information can be found and from which the reader can obtain further references to original sources of information, should he wish to consult them.

The book ends with a general review of therapeutic measures which are of value in the field of neurological medicine, but only those appropriate to general practice are considered fully, while more specialised techniques receive mention sufficient only to indicate which patients should be referred to a specialist for these measures to be undertaken.

In preparing this book, I am conscious of the debt I owe to those from whom I learned the principles of neurological diagnosis and management and I wish particularly to thank Professor F. J. Nattrass, Sir Charles Symonds, Dr E. A. Carmichael, Dr Raymond D. Adams and Dr H. G. Miller for the help and encouragement they have given me in the past. No textbook is written without reference to other volumes. I have obtained help particularly from *An Introduction to Clinical Neurology* by Sir Gordon Holmes, Sir Russell Brain's *Diseases of the Nervous System* and the chapters by Dr R. D. Adams in Harrison's *Principles of Internal Medicine*, and wish to express my indebtedness to the authors and publishers concerned. I must also thank the many authors and publishers who have given permission for the reproduction of stated illustrations. I am also grateful to Dr A. E. Clark-Kennedy for his helpful advice and to Dr Peter Nathan, Dr J. B. Foster and Dr David Poskanzer for their valuable criticisms of the manuscript. The work of preparing the typescript was performed by Miss Shirley Whillis and Miss Rosemary Allan, and many of the illustrations were prepared by Miss M. Mustart of the Department of Photography, King's College, Newcastle upon Tyne. I also wish to thank Mr D. K. C. Dickens and the staff of the Pitman Medical Publishing Company Ltd. for their enthusiastic and willing co-operation in the production of this volume.

John N. Walton

Newcastle upon Tyne
July 1959

1 Some General Principles in Neurology

The nervous system of the individual cannot be considered in isolation, for without an adequate supply of oxygen and of nutrients, which depend in turn upon efficient circulatory and respiratory activity, the nervous system cannot survive. The converse is also true, for the activity of the autonomic nervous system exercises a profound and continuing influence upon the behaviour of the heart and circulation, upon respiratory activity, upon the gastrointestinal system, and upon the endocrine glands. These complex and important interrelationships, upon which the normal functioning of the human body depends, are being elucidated increasingly by anatomical and physiological studies; their understanding requires an appreciation of certain homeostatic mechanisms which are already familiar to readers of this volume. But there are still many problems which defy comprehension. Upon what, for instance, does the ability of the brain to control thought processes depend? Disordered activity of the mind is commonly present when modern techniques fail to show any abnormality in the structure or function of the brain; and the influence of the mind upon the behaviour of the viscera can be profound.

Disorders of the mind can sometimes initiate and sometimes accentuate symptoms of physical disease, while conversely some organic diseases are regularly accompanied by psychological manifestations. The mechanisms underlying these relationships are obscure but their importance must be recognised by the physician who deals with sick people. Diseases are not independent entities; it is the patient who suffers from the disease who is real and who shows a personal and individual reaction to it. The pattern of his illness depends upon many factors, for the pathological process is influenced by his genetic constitution, by the condition of other bodily organs apart from that which is primarily affected, and by his state of mind.

Many physical disorders of the nervous system regularly produce a consistent series of symptoms and physical signs independent of the personality and constitution of the individual. The syndrome resulting from division of one median nerve, for instance, is not significantly modified by the patient's mental state. But if the nerve lesion is incomplete, due perhaps to transient compression, the severity of the resultant symptoms and the rate of recovery can be influenced by factors independent of the physical process concerned with the restoration of normal conduction in the damaged nerve fibres. Much may depend, for instance, upon the nature of the lesion; if it was an industrial injury, involving a claim for financial compensation, the patient's disability may be excessive and his recovery delayed.

Many functions of the nervous system, such as those concerned with speech, with seeing and hearing, with the control of movement and with the appreciation of sensation, are subserved by the passage of nervous impulses along pathways which have been clearly delineated. These functions can be disordered if there is a fault in development (a congenital defect). They may also be rendered abnormal by a pathological process, whether it is the result of inherited factors (genetically-determined illness) or whether it is acquired. The lesions so produced will give rise to symptoms and signs depending upon their situation and character and the functions of the pathways which they involve; many subsequent chapters of this book deal with these functions, the means by which abnormalities can be recognised, the lesions responsible localised and their nature determined. The aim of this introduction is to indicate that the clinical effects of these processes are not immutable, and that the resultant disease can be greatly influenced by the personality and constitution of the individual and by his state of mind. Some patients are born physically and mentally less perfect than others and yet show no obvious defect; but constitutionally they are less capable of resistance to stress, and are seriously disturbed by environmental influences which would leave others unaffected. The possible effects of fatigue, of ageing processes, and of other contributory influences which cannot easily be quantified, must also be considered. Are the headaches which the patient describes due to emotional tension or to an intracranial tumour? Are his suspicions that he is suffering from malignant disease well-founded or is he suffering from cancerophobia? Do his insomnia and his anxiety symptoms depend upon constitutional inadequacy and a low resistance to stress, or are they the result of underlying physical disease? These are some common questions which the doctor is called upon to answer, questions which require, for their elucidation, much experience and understanding.

It is also important to consider the use of the term 'functional' as commonly utilised in medicine to identify the nature and cause of a patient's illness, since its use is a common cause of misconception. It would be correct to regard as functional disorders those diseases in which the function of some organ of the body is disordered, but in which there is no recognisable pathological change in the organ concerned, whether structural or biochemical. In neurology, 'idiopathic' epilepsy would be a good example, though it is possible that in this and many other states of altered function, some biochemical or structural abnormality is present which cannot be recognised with techniques at present available. But the term 'functional disorder', as conventionally used, is not generally applied to such diseases, but rather to symptoms and signs which result from a disordered state of mind. Thus when a physician says that a symptom is functional, he usually means that it has no physical cause and, by implication, that its origin is psychological. For instance, headaches due to anxiety or nervous tensions are 'functional', and so too is loss of the voice (hysterical aphonia) in the young singer about to face her first professional engagement. In other words, anxiety reactions, symptoms resulting from mental or emotional fatigue, and those due to a subconscious desire to escape from stress (hysteria) are usually included in this category. It would, be incorrect however to classify as such deterioration of intellectual function (dementia) which results from physical disease of the brain.

Functional disorders, therefore, are those conditions in which symptoms and signs result not from physical disease, but from mental processes, whether conscious or subconscious. These mental processes may in turn influence the physical functioning of the body; the increased heart rate, perspiration and insomnia which commonly accompany anxiety will serve as examples. Hence, the clinical use of the term 'functional', if not strictly correct semantically, is hallowed through common usage and can usefully be employed, provided the doctor appreciates its meaning, and does not regard this as a final diagnosis. For if a disorder is accepted as 'functional' it is then necessary to decide whether it is due to conscious anxiety, whether it is hysterical, or whether it could even be psychotic. In other words, its nature, and if possible its cause, must be determined if treatment is to be effective. Disorders of the mind will be considered in a subsequent chapter, but it is well to appreciate at the outset that the distinction between organic and functional disease is often one of the most difficult differential diagnoses in medicine. And even when there is clear evidence of physical disease it is common for the symptoms and signs to be accentuated or distorted by concurrent psychological factors. The doctor must strive not only to recognise and interpret the symptoms and signs of physical disease which he observes in his patient, but also to understand the workings of his mind and to appreciate the influence which the one may have upon the other.

The Foundations of Neurological Diagnosis

In order to forecast accurately the outcome of a patient's illness and to advise treatment, accurate diagnosis is usually necessary. In diseases of the nervous system, the physical signs often indicate the anatomical localisation of the lesion or process responsible for disordered function, while it is the history of the illness, revealing the evolution of the patient's symptoms, which generally suggests the nature of the pathological process.

Hence the intelligent interpretation of physical signs demands an adequate knowledge, first, of neuroanatomy. This does not imply that the student must be familiar with the finer details of the anatomical organisation of the nervous system, though he should be prepared to consult reference sources in order to find the anatomical information required in a particular case presenting a difficult problem in localisation. He should, however, know which areas of the cerebral cortex control certain major functions, such as those of speech, the control of movement, and the appreciation of visual and somatic sensation. He must also be familiar with the general topography of the cerebral hemispheres, brain stem and spinal cord and with the organisation of the autonomic nervous system, at least in relation to the situation of the more important cranial nerve nuclei and the pathways traversed by the main motor and sensory pathways. Knowledge of anatomy alone, however, is not enough, for one must also understand the normal functions of these structures before being able to decide that these are disturbed. In subsequent chapters we shall deal with disorders of the motor, sensory and other systems and consider how these are recognised, how they are produced, and how the responsible lesion can be localised and identified.

Most symptoms and signs resulting from nervous disease are positive or negative. **Positive symptoms** are those produced by irritation or stimulation of a part of the nervous system, causing it to behave abnormally; focal epilepsy resulting from irritation of or pressure upon the motor area of the cerebral cortex is an example. **Negative symptoms**, by contrast, are those produced by temporary or permanent loss of function, so that an activity or ability, normally present, is lost; paralysis of a limb is one such symptom. Hughlings Jackson's **law of dissolution** said that those functions and skills most recently acquired during the processes of evolution and training are the first to be lost in disease of the brain, while primitive activities and instincts survive longer. A similar principle applies to temporary disturbances of cerebral function produced, say, by anaesthetics or other drugs. Thus a naturalised foreigner may sometimes revert to using his native tongue during recovery from anaesthesia, and only when recovery is more complete can he utilise the language of his adopted country. To take another example, man differs from the higher primates in his ability to move individual fingers and to use opposition of the thumb to the other fingers in order to perform fine and deliberate movements. This can be called the 'precision grip'; the primate possesses only the 'power grip', produced by flexion of all the fingers. In an early lesion of the appropriate area of the motor cortex or of its efferent corticospinal or pyramidal fibres in man the 'precision grip' is impaired as is discrete movement of the individual fingers, at a time when the 'power grip' still seems normal. Similarly, in the leg, movement of the toes is affected early by such a lesion.

Disordered function depends not only upon the situation of pathological change, but upon its severity, its extent and the effects it has upon contiguous nervous tissue and upon interconnected though anatomically remote structures in the nervous system. Thus an acute and extensive lesion may affect more of the brain than its anatomical extent would lead one to expect, for around the edge of the lesion the activity of the surrounding nervous tissue is disturbed by oedema and vascular changes. Furthermore, an acute lesion can produce a state of 'shock' or temporary dissolution of function in related areas of the brain or spinal cord. This is seen in the patient with a hemiplegia which is initially flaccid, later spastic, or in one with an acute spinal lesion; the limbs below the level of the lesion are initially flaccid and totally paralysed but later, as shock wears off, spasticity resulting from bilateral lesions of the corticospinal (pyramidal) tracts develops. By contrast, lesions of equal extent, but of slower development, produce fewer symptoms and physical signs, as it is only those structures which are actively invaded or destroyed whose function is disturbed; the surrounding tissues have more time to adapt to the presence of the lesion. Other forms of adaptation also occur, particularly in the cerebral cortex, for here a function which has been lost through a cortical lesion may be 'adopted', though usually much less efficiently, by another area of the brain. Such adaptation occurs more readily in children than in adults, for the younger the patient the greater the flexibility of cerebral organisation. In the spinal cord, there is less opportunity for this type of reorganisation than in the brain, for the nervous pathways are more stereotyped and less complex. In the peripheral nerves opportunities for adoption of functions in this way are almost non-existent, but these nerves are able to regenerate effectively following injury, while effective regeneration does not occur within the spinal cord or brain.

Pathological Reactions in the Nervous System

A detailed consideration of neuropathology is beyond the scope of this volume, but there are certain fundamental principles which are necessary for an informed approach to neurological diagnosis. Pathological changes in the nervous system can first be classified into three broad groups, namely, **focal lesions**, which cause a localised disturbance of function; **diffuse or generalised disorders**, whether of infective, metabolic, toxic, vascular or other aetiology, which affect nervous and supporting elements throughout the nervous system; and **systemic nervous disease**, in which the pathological process shows a predilection for a particular tissue, structure or group of structures, for example, the anterior horn cells, the cerebellum and its connexions, or the pyramidal tracts. Some focal lesions and diffuse disorders affect nervous tissue by accident and are not primarily neurological diseases. Thus cerebral vascular disease, which can produce a focal cerebral lesion, such as an infarct, is usually a complication of generalised atherosclerosis, while the diffuse pathological changes which occur in the brain in syphilis, for instance, form only one part of the changes resulting from infection of the entire human organism. In the systemic nervous diseases, by contrast, as in motor neurone disease, there is some as yet undefined factor which causes the pathological process to be confined to a particular group of nerve cells or fibre pathways. The tissues of the nervous system vary in their susceptibility to many different noxious influences. Thus ischaemia affects nerve cells more severely than fibres, while plaques of demyelination, as in multiple sclerosis, have a much greater effect upon white matter. There are also differences in the effects of ischaemia, compression and various toxins upon nerve fibres, depending upon whether they conduct motor or sensory impulses.

It is also necessary to subdivide these groups of pathological processes, and particularly the focal lesions, on an aetiological basis. Virtually every pathological lesion of the nervous system will be embraced by one of the following headings—

1 Congenital (developmental disorders)

2 Traumatic (physical or chemical injury)

3 Inflammatory
{ infective
  allergic or postinfective (autoimmune) }
{ acute
  subacute
  chronic }

4 Neoplastic
{ benign
  malignant }
{ primary
  secondary }

5 Degenerative
{ vascular
  other, or of unknown aetiology }

6 Metabolic and endocrine.

For detailed consideration of these pathological processes, the student is referred to textbooks of neuropathology. Most important central nervous lesions of **congenital** origin are clearly apparent as gross disorders of anatomical development and configuration; examples are anencephaly, hydrocephalus due to stenosis of the aqueduct of Sylvius, and meningo-myelocele. Arteriovenous malformations or angiomas, which may develop in the brain or spinal cord, are also of congenital origin. **Trauma** to the nervous system, as elsewhere, produces necrosis, haemorrhage and subsequent scar formation, the scar consisting of proliferated neuroglial cells and fibrils (gliosis) and of mesenchymal fibrous tissue derived from fibroblasts in the supporting tissue of the blood vessels. Among the **acute inflammatory disorders** are the meningitides which produce the typical pathological changes of inflammation and exudation in the meninges.

Meningitis may give rise to superficial degeneration in the underlying nervous tissue or to more extensive ischaemic changes in the nervous parenchyma resulting from an obliterative endarteritis of blood vessels which traverse the subarachnoid space. **Pyogenic infection** of the brain substance or spinal cord begins as a diffuse suppuration, but localisation and abscess formation generally follow with capsule formation, as in a scar following trauma.

Most so-called neurotropic **viruses**, such as those which give rise to virus encephalitis and anterior poliomyelitis, are polioclastic, that is, they show an affinity for nerve cells; inflammatory changes, with perivascular cellular infiltration, and degeneration with phagocytosis (neuronophagia) of nerve cells, are therefore seen in the grey matter of the brain and spinal cord. Sometimes inclusion bodies are found within the nucleus or cytoplasm of infected cells. The herpes zoster virus shows a particular affinity for the cells of the posterior root ganglia. **Syphilis**, despite its decreasing incidence, is still an important chronic infection of the central nervous system. The meningovascular form gives meningeal inflammation and endarteritis of cerebral and spinal arteries; in general paresis there are degeneration of nerve cells, gliosis and minimal inflammatory changes in the cerebral cortex; in tabes dorsalis the most prominent change is gliosis and meningeal fibrosis at the entry zone of the posterior spinal nerve roots with secondary ascending degeneration of the posterior columns of the spinal cord. Gummas of the brain are now very rare. In **allergic or postinfective encephalomyelitis**, in contrast to the virus infections, inflammatory changes are largely confined to the white matter, perivascular collections of inflammatory cells and loss of myelin. The pathological changes in this disease show some resemblance to those observed in the **demyelinating diseases** of unknown aetiology, such as multiple sclerosis, in which there is patchy loss of myelin throughout the white matter of the brain and spinal cord. This primary lesion, in which axons are initially preserved, is eventually replaced by a glial scar.

Most **benign tumours** which affect the central nervous system are extracerebral and extramedullary, lying outside the brain or spinal cord, though within their bony encasements. The two most common are the meningioma, which arises from arachnoidal cells, and the neurofibroma or neurilemmoma, which grows from the sheath of Schwann of the cranial nerves, spinal roots or peripheral nerves. These neoplasms compress and distort but do not invade nervous tissue. The gliomas are the principal **malignant tumours** of the central nervous system; these are invasive tumours whose relative malignancy depends upon whether the principal constituent cell is a relatively mature astrocyte or one of its more rapidly multiplying primitive precursors. Metastatic malignant neoplasms are also common; cancer of the lung, breast and kidney and the malignant melanoma are among those which most often metastasise to the brain. Secondary deposits, often seen at the junction of the white and grey matter, are sometimes single but much more often multiple. Less commonly these deposits, or plaques of reticulosis, involve the meninges; if this occurs in the spinal canal, or if a vertebral body has collapsed following malignant infiltration, spinal cord compression can result.

Vascular disorders of the nervous system are common. Bleeding into the subarachnoid space produces aseptic meningeal inflammation and sometimes a degree of meningeal organisation or arachnoiditis results. Chronic bleeding into the subarachnoid space can produce haemosiderosis of the meninges. Haemorrhage in the nervous parenchyma causes an area of necrosis which is eventually walled off by gliosis and fibrosis; if it is small the necrotic area is absorbed and a scar results, but more often a cavity filled with clear straw-coloured fluid containing bilirubin is left. An infarct, too, shows an area of central ischaemic necrosis. Within 24 hours, activated microglial cells (the histiocytes or scavengers of the nervous system) invade the necrotic area and become distended with the fatty remnants of necrotic myelin. A minute infarct, produced by embolic occlusion of a tiny cortical vessel, may consist of little more than a small cluster of activated microglial cells or a tiny cavity, whereas a large one will show an extensive central area of necrosis surrounded by distended phagocytes ('gitter' cells) and proliferating astrocytes. A large area of infarction may eventually be represented by a contracted glial scar or by a larger cavity, while multifocal infarction sometimes gives many multiple small cavities or lacunes ('status lacunosus').

There remain **degenerative disorders** of the nervous system whose aetiology is at present unknown, but in some of which specific neuropathological changes are seen. In motor neurone disease, for instance, the cells of the motor nuclei of the brain stem, the anterior horn cells of the spinal cord, and the pyramidal tracts show progressive degeneration; in Huntington's chorea there is selective degeneration of the caudate nucleus and of nerve cells in the frontal cortex. But in these and in many other disorders, although the anatomical distribution of pathological change is well-defined, their nature and cause is little understood. We do not know why anoxia affects particularly the cells of the deepest layer of the cerebral cortex, the Ammon's horn area of the hippocampus and the cerebellar Purkinje cells, nor why deficiency of vitamin B_{12}, as in subacute combined degeneration of the spinal cord, damages selectively the posterior columns and pyramidal tracts. Many **metabolic disorders** which seriously disturb nervous function produce relatively little pathological change, although in hypoglycaemia the changes resemble those of anoxia, while in hepatic failure there is astrocytic proliferation, particularly in the basal ganglia. The pathological changes in many forms of **polyneuropathy** are also non-specific, consisting either of segmental loss of myelin, beginning in the region of the nodes of Ranvier (demyelinating neuropathies), or of swelling and fragmentation of axons in the peripheral nerves (axonal neuropathies).

Constitution and Heredity

In considering the aetiological factors which may be responsible for a patient's illness it is easy to overlook important genetic influences. Many neurological disorders, and particularly some of those referred to above as being 'degenerative' in character, are inherited in a strictly Mendelian manner. A disease resulting from a dominant gene situated on one of the autosomes, a so-called autosomal dominant trait, is passed on by an affected individual to half his or her children of either sex if penetrance or expressivity of the gene is complete. Examples of disorders which are often inherited in this way are Huntington's chorea, and facio-scapulo-humeral muscular dystrophy. A recessive gene, carried on an autosome, however, can only produce its effect if it is paired with a similar gene lying on the other chromosome of the pair. Such a trait, autosomal recessive, can only come to light, therefore, when two unaffected heterozygotes marry, and hence there is usually no previous history of the disease in the family, unless there has been intermarriage between relatives (consanguinity). In such families, the likelihood is that the disease will affect one in four of a series of brothers and sisters (a sibship); Friedreich's ataxia, hepatolenticular degeneration and limb-girdle muscular dystrophy are examples.

A recessive gene can produce an effect, however, if it is situated on the unpaired portion of the X-chromosome; such a condition occurs in males and is carried by apparently unaffected females. It is then known as a sex-linked or X-linked recessive character; the disease may have affected maternal uncles and now appears in half the male children of a female carrier. Diseases inherited in this manner include colour-blindness, haemophilia and pseudohypertrophic (the Duchenne and Becker types) muscular dystrophy. Recent evidence indicates that some female carriers may show minor clinical manifestations. Any inherited disease can, of course, appear anew in a family if a previously normal gene has undergone a process of spontaneous change or mutation.

Apart from diseases which are clearly inherited by recognisable genetic mechanisms, there are many other nervous disorders in which genetic influences are important, though less clearly defined. In epilepsy and in multiple sclerosis, for example, more than one member of a family is affected more often than could be accounted for by chance, though no clear pattern of inheritance emerges. From time to time, too, one finds families in which several individuals have died from cerebral tumour or subarachnoid haemorrhage. Furthermore, there is some evidence that an individual's emotional and physical constitution may influence his susceptibility to certain infections or other neurological disorders. Evidence is emerging to indicate that in certain diseases such as multiple sclerosis and myasthenia gravis genetic susceptibility may be related to the histocompatibility (HLA) antigen constitution of the individual. It is therefore of the greatest importance to consider not only the environmental, but also the constitutional influences which may have a bearing upon each patient's disease.

Conclusions

A systematic approach to each patient with symptoms suggesting disease of the nervous system is an essential preliminary to accurate diagnosis. The question should first be asked, where is the lesion or systemic process responsible for these symptoms and signs? Is it extracerebral, in the skull or meninges, in the cerebral cortex, in the white matter, in the brain stem or cerebellum? Or if the clinical picture indicates, say, a disorder of the spinal cord or of the lower motor neurone, is the lesion in the spinal column, the meninges, the spinal cord, the spinal roots, plexuses, peripheral nerves, motor endplates or muscles? And in each of these situations, could it be congenital, traumatic, inflammatory, neoplastic, degenerative or metabolic? What influences are constitutional factors playing in its genesis? Is there disease in the heart, great vessels, lungs or other organs which could be responsible? Are emotional or psychological factors responsible for any part of the patient's disability? While in many cases the answers to some of these questions are self-evident it is well that they should be asked, since it is only through such a comprehensive approach to patients with neurological disease that the student will eventually acquire the skill and experience which will allow him to discard the irrelevant and to concentrate upon those salient facts which lead to accurate diagnosis.

References

Adams, R. D. and Sidman, R. L., *Introduction to Neuropathology* (New York, McGraw-Hill, 1968).

Blackwood, W. and Corsellis, J. A. N., *Greenfield's Neuropathology*, 3rd ed. (London, Arnold, 1976).

Emery, A. E. H., *Elements of Medical Genetics*, 5th ed. (Edinburgh, Churchill Livingstone, 1979).

Holmes, G., *An Introduction to Clinical Neurology*, 3rd ed. revised by W. B. Matthews (Edinburgh, Churchill Livingstone, 1968).

Matthews, W. B., *Practical Neurology*, 3rd ed. (Oxford, Blackwell, 1975).

Pratt, R. T. C., *The Genetics of Neurological Disorders* (London, Oxford University Press, 1967).

2 The Symptoms and Signs of Disease in the Nervous System

In neurology, as in any branch of medicine, prognosis and treatment usually depend upon accurate diagnosis, while diagnosis, in turn, stems from an elucidation of symptoms and signs, combined with information obtained from the appropriate investigations. In some nervous disorders such as epilepsy and migraine, a careful appraisal of the patient's symptoms is all-important if the correct diagnosis is to be reached, and physical examination is essentially negative. Conversely, in many other diseases, the history is singularly uninformative and all will depend upon a meticulous neurological examination. In most cases, however, the history and examination are mutually interdependent, one throwing light upon the significance of the other. In general it is the physical signs which identify the anatomical situation of a lesion responsible for a patient's illness, while the evolutionary pattern of its symptomatology indicates the nature of the pathological process. So many are the individual symptoms and signs which may be the result of a nervous disease that it is essential to have a planned approach to each individual patient, an approach so designed that major manifestations of illness which may at first seem irrelevant are not overlooked, but are fitted into place so that the patient and his disease may be viewed as a whole. In this chapter, bearing in mind the principles previously outlined, an attempt will be made to construct the framework upon which the edifice of neurological diagnosis and management can be erected.

Diagnosis is not, however, an end in itself, not even for the purpose of obtaining medical qualifications, and any examination which takes no account of the candidate's ability to treat patients as people is failing in its object. The doctor is assessed by his patients, who justify his professional existence, not upon his flair for diagnosing rare diseases, but upon his understanding of their needs, of their hopes and fears and of the intensely personal problem which their illness presents. Sometimes fears of cancer or of insanity may play a considerable part in the genesis of the patient's symptoms, and it can be difficult to uncover these or other significant anxieties, which are being consciously suppressed, but are nevertheless of great aetiological importance. Furthermore, the correct management of two identical cases of disabling disease of the nervous system will be totally different if the sufferers differ widely in attitude, emotional constitution and domestic environment. There are many chronic and crippling progressive disorders of the nervous system which continually pose serious problems of management to patient and doctor. These conditions present a challenge which require from the doctor tact, sympathy and understanding, as well as diagnostic expertise and ingenuity in changing circumstances. Acquisition of the skill of communicating clearly, meaningfully and sensitively with the patient and his relatives is also fundamental. These qualities cannot be learned from any textbook but are derived from continuing contact with patients and their relatives, not only in hospital, but in their homes. Diagnosis is only the beginning, and need not necessarily be strictly accurate for management to be correct, provided the broad pattern of the patient's disease is recognised. On the other hand, there are many other conditions, such as meningitis, subdural haematoma and spinal tumour, in which diagnosis must be made early if death or severe disability is to be avoided.

Some Useful Terms in Neurology

Before describing details of the neurological examination it may be useful to quote some terms, largely derived from Greek and Latin, which are in common use in neurological medicine. Thus the prefix 'a-' means absence of, the prefix 'dys-' disturbance of; 'hyper-' means increased and 'hypo-' decreased. If the Greek suffix '-phasis' is taken to denote conceptual skills involved in speech function, then 'aphasia' is used to denote loss of this function, 'dysphasia' when the disorder of function is less severe. Similarly aphonia is loss of the ability to phonate, anarthria means inability to articulate and dysarthria slurring or indistinct articulation. Atrophy of muscles means wasting and hypertrophy enlargement, while hypoaesthesia (often shortened to hypaesthesia) is used to identify reduced sensation, while hyperpathia is taken to indicate an abnormal, unpleasant and increased sensitivity to sensory stimuli.

In much the same way, ataxia means unsteadiness or lack of co-ordination, apraxia loss of motor skills. The suffix '-plegia' means paralysis and '-paresis' weakness. Thus a monoplegia is a paralysis of one limb, a monoparesis weakness of one limb. Similarly a hemiplegia means paralysis of one arm and leg on the same side of the body, tetraplegia or quadriplegia paralysis of all four limbs, and paraplegia paralysis of the lower limbs only. The term diplegia is often used to identify a form of spastic weakness of all four limbs affecting the lower limbs, as a rule, more severely than the upper.

Taking the History

The principles of history-taking in neurological disease do not differ in general from those applicable to any branch of medicine. It is usual to begin by listing the **principal symptoms** of which the patient complains and then to give, in chronological order, a description in his own words of the way in which they developed. Judicious questions may be needed to restrain the garrulous and cut short irrelevancies, as well as to expand and clarify individual points in the history. It is easy to forget that patients have not usually been trained in anatomy and physiology; to them, opinions previously expressed by Dr X, or the fall a few months ago may seem much more important than the transient blurring of vision, say, apparently unconnected with the present complaint, which occurred three years before. Hence, once the patient has given his story, amplified by judicious guidance and prompting, one must ask a number of **leading questions** which have been avoided assiduously at an earlier stage so as not to present the suggestible patient with additional symptoms which he may profess. These should relate to some of the principal symptoms of nervous disease, each of which will be considered individually later. Has there been, for instance, any pain or headache, any loss or impairment of consciousness, either brief or prolonged? Have there been any visual disorders, such as impairment of sight or diplopia, or has the patient noticed any alteration in speech or swallowing? Are memory, behaviour and concentration unimpaired, has he had deafness, tinnitus, giddiness or unsteadiness, or involuntary movements of the head, trunk or limbs? Usually, too, it is wise to enquire specifically about weakness, paralysis or clumsiness of the limbs (though few patients would overlook such striking symptoms) and about numbness, tingling, pins and needles or other unusual sensations. Finally, enquiry should be made as to whether control of the vesical or anal sphincters and/or of sexual function has been impaired and whether there have been other more general symptoms such as breathlessness, weight loss (or gain), anxiety, depression, sleeplessness, anorexia or vomiting.

Having discovered that a particular patient has one or more symptoms, it is usually evident that this knowledge alone is insufficient. If the complaint is of headache, for instance, much more must be known. Where in the head it is situated, and does it spread? What is its character? When does it or did it begin? How long does it last and how often does it occur? Is there any warning of its onset? Does anything precipitate it or make it worse once it has begun, and does anything relieve it? This kind of enquiry may be applied, with minor modifications, to almost any symptom of nervous disease, but should not be learned by rote. It is better to cultivate an inquisitive approach in which each symptom is scrutinised and analysed in detail. Such a spirit of critical enquiry and appraisal is more revealing and profitable to both doctor and patient than a carefully ordered routine learned by heart. On the other hand, the enquiry must be comprehensive. While the experienced physician may reach the heart of the problem with a few well-chosen questions, there are no short cuts for the beginner. This is one of the most important lessons for the student to learn. If history-taking is at first slow and laborious, growing experience, and experience alone, will teach which symptoms may safely be discarded as irrelevant and which are of crucial importance.

In taking the history it should also be recognised that sometimes the patient's own testimony is unreliable. In the unconscious patient it is manifestly necessary to interview relatives or others who may possess the essential information, while it is equally important to have independent evidence about individuals who have experienced lapses of consciousness or mental and behaviour disorders. Few epileptics, for instance, can describe their own seizures, while the history given by demented or psychotic patients, though revealing, is often lacking in essential details.

Having dealt with the history of the patient's present illness one must then enquire as to his **previous health**. Have there been any serious accidents or illnesses in the past, or any unusual sequelae of the common childish ailments? Social and occupational details may also be of considerable importance. What was the patient's educational standard and what occupations has he followed? Is he married, with a family, or does he live alone? Are his domestic circumstances satisfactory or are there financial and/or personal difficulties? And what is known about his physical and emotional constitution? Has he been physically active, athletic and extraverted, or studious, retiring and introspective? Was he excessively nervous or over-protected as a child, did he wet the bed or walk in his sleep, and has he changed his employment frequently? What are his interests and hobbies, and have these changed of late? Questions of this type can be very rewarding, eliciting answers which reveal deterioration in intellect, change in personality, or life-long psychopathy and failure of adjustment to the demands of society. Such information about the patient as an individual may throw important light upon the nature and significance of his symptoms. Clearly, too, the consumption of alcohol, of tobacco and of drugs should be recorded.

Finally, the **family history** can be very important, as some neurological disorders are clearly inherited, while in other conditions an inherited predisposition plays a part. Hence enquiry should be made as to the existence of nervous or mental disease in the sibs, parents and more distant relatives; if further cases of disease come to light, then a pedigree should be drawn. Important diseases of other systems should also be noted in other members of the family; for instance, a strong family history of coronary artery disease may suggest that atherosclerosis of the cerebral, rather than of the coronary arteries, accounts for the patient's symptoms.

Clearly this guide to history-taking in nervous diseases is incomplete, but if these general principles are followed, few mistakes will be made and the amplified descriptions of symptoms and symptom-complexes which appear in subsequent chapters will help to stress those interrelationships between individual symptoms which must always be borne in mind.

The Neurological Examination

Whereas in taking the history, an inspired virtuosity born of experience may yield results superior to those achieved by a didactic and methodical approach, a comprehensive neurological examination depends much more upon a carefully itemised routine. Many schemes for examining the nervous system have been recommended and most are satisfactory, provided they are complete. The outline given below is of a method for examining the nervous system which the author has found satisfactory in practice. A full examination performed in this way is admittedly time-consuming, but once it has been learned and practised assiduously, experience will teach which parts of it may be discarded or abridged in any individual case. However, when experience is limited, attempts to abbreviate the process will lead to inevitable and important oversights.

The Mental State

Disease of the brain may have a profound effect upon the patient's behaviour and awareness, so that accurate assessment of the mental state is of great importance. Individual symptoms and signs will be considered in later chapters; it is therefore unnecessary at this stage to define terms but brief outlines will be given of certain common abnormalities.

First, the patient's state of awareness must be assessed. Is he comatose or semicomatose, confused or disorientated, or is he alert and well orientated in time and in place? Secondly, is his mood normal, or is he euphoric, elated, depressed, anxious or agitated? Thirdly, are his behaviour and social adjustments normal or is he anti-social and amoral, dirty in his habits and blandly unconcerned? Does he show disordered thought processes with ideas of persecution (paranoia) or other delusions, or are there visual or auditory hallucinations? While questions of this type can be answered through careful observation and by questioning the patient, simple tests of a more formal nature may be required in order to assess memory and intellect and the powers of abstract thought. To assess attention and concentration it is usual to ask the patient to repeat a series of numbers forwards and then backwards; the normal individual can easily remember seven figures forwards and five backwards. Similarly, the patient is asked to subtract serial sevens from 100 and the number of mistakes made as well as the time taken are recorded. It is generally possible to tell whether memory for the remote past is intact when the history is being taken. In assessing recent memory and the ability to record and retain new impressions it may be necessary to ask the patient for details of his last meal or to give him a name, address and the name of a flower to remember; he should be asked to repeat these several minutes later. It may be useful to ask him to repeat the Babcock sentence, viz. 'One thing a nation must have to be rich and great is a large secure supply of wood'. Most normal individuals can repeat this correctly by the third attempt. In testing the patient's ability to think in an abstract manner, one may ask for an interpretation of common proverbs or of a fable. A defect of abstract thought will be apparent, for instance, in the individual who suggests that people who live in glass houses should not throw stones as they would break the glass. Finally, in assessing the patient's intellectual state, it is usual to ask for the names of recent monarchs, Prime Ministers and US Presidents, the names of six large cities in Britain, or of European capitals. For accurate assessment of minor changes, detailed psychometric testing by a psychologist will be required, but these simple tests will often reveal important defects of cerebral function.

Praxis and Gnosis and the Body Image

Praxis is the ability to perform purposive skilled movements; if this function is impaired, those skills most recently acquired may be the first to be lost. In testing this function it is usual to ask the patient to perform movements of moderate complexity, such as those involved in dressing, in shaving, in opening a box of matches and striking one or in constructing a model with toy bricks. Inability to perform these movements in a patient without obvious motor weakness or sensory impairment may indicate a disorder of praxis, known as apraxia.

Gnosis is the ability, based upon the reception of sensory stimuli, either visual or tactile, to recognise the nature and significance of objects. This may relate to articles in the patient's environment, but may also be concerned with the parts of his own body. In testing this function the patient may be asked to interpret humorous drawings or pictures which tell a story, or to identify objects, such as coins placed in the hands. He is also asked to identify parts of his or the examiner's body, for example, one ear, a knee or individual fingers. The patient's awareness of his own body and of its relationship to extrapersonal space is known as the body image and a loss of awareness of a part of that image is a form of agnosia or impairment of gnosis. This may also involve an inability to distinguish right from left; this faculty should also be tested.

Speech

The function of speech may be subdivided into first, the higher or cortical control of speech, and secondly the lower or peripheral mechanism responsible for phonation and articulation. Reading (understanding of the written word) and writing (expression by means of the written, rather than the spoken word) are closely related to speech function, as is the ability to calculate. An inability to express one's thoughts in words when the peripheral mechanisms of articulation are intact, and understanding of the spoken word is preserved, is known as motor, expressive or Broca's aphasia; while a failure to understand the spoken word is called sensory, receptive or Wernicke's aphasia. These and related functions are most easily tested by asking the patient to name a series of common objects of progressive difficulty (hand, mouth, pen, radiator, spectacles, stethoscope, etc.) and by giving simple commands, or by asking simple questions. A patient with slight motor aphasia may be accurate in his speech but yet hesitant and at a loss for simple words, while one with sensory aphasia may fail to obey commands or name simple objects or may use totally inappropriate words in his reply to questions, since words to him, as symbols, have lost their meaning and significance. When the exact answers to these questions have been recorded the patient should then be asked to read, interpret and perhaps paraphrase a short passage from a book, to write from dictation and to write down his name and address and some of his outstanding symptoms. The ability to do a number of simple sums should also be tested.

A patient with complete paralysis of the muscles of articulation is generally well able to understand and interpret the spoken and written word and to express himself fluently in writing. If he cannot make a sound (phonation) this is called aphonia, but if the sound is uttered and cannot be moulded into words, this sign is entitled anarthria. Complete anarthria is rare, but slurring or indistinctness of speech is much more common and is called dysarthria. The patient should be asked to repeat a number of set phrases if dysarthria is suspected; 'British constitution' and 'Methodist episcopal' are good examples in common use.

The Skull and Skeleton

Inspection and palpation of the skull is an essential part of the neurological examination. The size and shape of the skull and any asymmetry should be noted, as should the presence of any abnormal bony protuberances or points of tenderness. Auscultation in the temporal fossae and over the globes of both eyes should also be carried out while the patient holds his breath, so that the presence or absence of a **cranial bruit** or murmur may be recorded. Auscultation for such a bruit over the carotid, vertebral and subclavian arteries in the neck is also necessary; very rarely a bruit is heard over the vertebral column (a spinal bruit). Cranial bruits are often heard in normal children but if a bruit is unilateral this is more likely to be significant. In adults one must be sure that a bruit heard in the neck is not being conducted from the heart (as in aortic stenosis). In the remainder of the skeleton, any bony deformities (abnormal spinal curvature, pes cavus, etc.) should be noted as should limitation of movement in the spine (cervical, dorsal or lumbar) or in limb joints. Restricted straight leg raising with pain down the back of the thigh may be due to meningeal irritation (Kernig's sign) or to compression of one of the nerve roots which form the sciatic nerve, as by a prolapsed intervertebral disk (Lasègue's sign).

The Special Senses

The sense of **smell** (the olfactory nerves) should be tested in each nostril independently with the other occluded. Camphor, coffee, peppermint and oil of cloves are convenient test substances.

Taste should be tested on either side of the tongue. Testing on the anterior two-thirds is feasible in clinical practice, on the posterior third almost impossible, though often attempted. The four modalities of taste which can be recognised are sweet (sugar), salt (salt), bitter (quinine) and sour or acid (vinegar). The tongue should be protruded and dried and held with gauze while a fine brush dipped in a solution of one of the test agents is applied to its surface. The patient is then asked to point to one of four cards on which these four modalities are given. Taste sensation from the anterior two-thirds of the tongue is carried in the chorda tympani (facial nerve) and from the posterior one-third in the glossopharyngeal nerve.

Vision (The Optic Nerves)
In testing vision it is customary first to test the **visual acuity** in each eye independently, the other being covered. Usually, Snellen's test types are used, and the patient is asked to read, at a distance of 6 m, the letters on the card. Each line of type is numbered and the acuity is recorded as 6 over the number of the lowest line of type which can be read accurately; for instance, 6/6 is normal. If the patient normally wears spectacles it is then reasonable to record the acuity when they are worn, the so-called corrected acuity. The test is appropriate to distance vision, while near vision may be tested with Jaeger's reading card, in which case acuity is expressed as from J1 to J6, J1 being normal, J6 severely impaired acuity. The cards approved by the London Faculty of Ophthalmologists use N6 for normal reading acuity (to correspond to 6/6 for normal distance acuity) and N12, N24, N36, etc., when acuity for reading is progressively impaired. There are, of course, cases in which vision in one or both eyes is so severely impaired that none of the test types can be seen. Here one records that sight is limited to 'counting fingers', 'hand movements' or 'light perception only', whichever is the case. In patients who claim to be blind and in whom hysteria is suspected, it may be of value to see whether blinking occurs at the threat of a blow.

Colour vision is rarely impaired as a result of disease, but colour-blindness is present from birth in about 8 per cent of males and in occasional females, being inherited as an X-linked recessive character.

This function is tested most satisfactorily with the Ishihara charts with which full instructions are supplied.

The **visual fields** must also be tested, and it is usual to begin by testing on confrontation. The patient and the examiner sit face to face and the patient is instructed to gaze steadily at the bridge of the examiner's nose. One eye is covered and a test object (such as a hat-pin with a white head) is brought into the patient's field of vision from all angles, the patient being instructed to say 'now' whenever it first comes into view. The procedure is then repeated with the other eye. In this way, gross defects in the peripheral visual fields may be detected and must then be confirmed by accurate charting on a perimeter. Even the perimeter, however, is insufficiently accurate to plot in full the important area of central vision, the area around the fixation point, which is subserved by the macular area of the retina. To examine this area, especially if small scotomas (small areas of visual loss) are to be detected, central vision should be charted on the Bjerrum screen. Patients with central scotomas, due to disease of the macula or of the nerve fibres from this area, may have greatly reduced visual acuity and may be quite unable to read, even though the peripheral fields as charted with a perimeter are full. The visual field for large objects is larger than that for small, and for white objects it is more extensive than for red; a scotoma for red is sometimes detected before one for white can be found.

The **optic disks and fundi** are next inspected, after dilatation of the pupils with homatropine if necessary. The optic disk is normally faintly pink in colour, but the temporal half is paler than the nasal. A deep physiological cup into which the vessels enter can give a mistaken impression of pallor of the central and temporal areas of the disk until a pink rim of normal-appearing disk is seen to its temporal side. Some blurring of the nasal margin of the disk is common in normal individuals and sometimes only the extreme temporal margin is clear-cut. In papilloedema, or swelling of the optic nerve head, not only are the disk margins blurred and sometimes impossible to define, but the vessels are seen to be 'heaped up' in the centre of the disk, no physiological cup is present, the veins are distended, and there may even be haemorrhages and exudates in the surrounding retina. In optic atrophy, by contrast, the disk is flat and dead-white in colour with clearly-defined and often irregular margins. In the type of optic atrophy often seen in multiple sclerosis, the temporal half of the disk is strikingly pale. In examining the fundus, abnormal pigmentation, patches of retinal degeneration, haemorrhage, exudates and vascular changes (arterial narrowing, 'nipping' of veins at arteriovenous crossings, micro-aneurysms) and any other abnormality should all be noted and described if present.

Any abnormal position of the globe of one or other eye, such as proptosis (asymmetrical protrusion), exophthalmos (uniform protrusion), or enophthalmos (sunken eye) must also be recorded, as must the state of the **eyelids and pupils.** Drooping of the eyelids, or ptosis, may be observed, or alternatively lid-lag, revealing white sclera above the cornea on downward ocular movement. The size, equality or otherwise, and regularity of the pupils should now be examined, along with the changes which occur on shining a bright light into the eye; the effect upon the other pupil (the consensual reaction) as well as the direct reaction should be observed. Changes occurring on accommodation-convergence, when transferring the gaze rapidly from a distant to a near object, such as a finger placed a few inches from the eyes, should also be tested. The afferent pathway for the pupillary reflex to light is in the optic nerve, the efferent pathways are in the parasympathetic constrictor fibres of the oculomotor nerve and in the dilator fibres of the ocular sympathetic.

Ocular movements (controlled by the oculomotor, trochlear and abducent nerves) must now be examined. The patient is asked to follow with both eyes an object, such as a finger or hat-pin, which is moved quickly from right to left and then up and down in front of the eyes. If diplopia (double vision) occurs in any direction of gaze, this is noted, as well as the position of the two images in relation to one another. When diplopia is present, noting which image disappears when each eye is covered in turn is helpful in identifying the particular external ocular muscle which is weak or paralysed, as the false image is projected in the direction in which the paretic muscle would normally move the eye. Any deviation of the ocular axes during movement should be recorded as well as the occurrence of nystagmus, an oscillatory or rotatory movement which can be a very important physical sign. If it occurs, its character and direction should be carefully observed, as well as the ocular movements which produce it. In some cases, it is not the movement of one or other eye which is defective, but movement of the two together, either laterally, upwards or downwards, is impaired. These are movements which are necessary for the maintenance of binocular vision. Such defects of conjugate ocular movement have considerable localising value and should, if present, be carefully defined. Similarly, the ability to converge the ocular axes when watching an object approach the bridge of the nose, may be lost in disease and should be examined.

Hearing and Labyrinthine Function (The Auditory and Vestibular Nerves)
A crude clinical assessment of a patient's **hearing** can be obtained by recording the distance at which a whispered voice or the ticking of a watch can be heard by each ear, with the other temporarily occluded. If comparison with a normal subject suggests that one or both ears is deaf, then it is necessary to decide whether this is due to middle ear disease (conduction deafness) or to disease of the cochlear or auditory nerve (nerve, perceptive or sensorineural deafness). This may be done with a 256-frequency tuning fork. Normally air conduction is better than bone conduction and in nerve deafness this principle is still true though hearing by either means may be greatly diminished; in middle-ear deafness, by

contrast, bone conduction is better. In **Rinne's test,** a vibrating tuning fork is applied to the mastoid process and when the sound is no longer heard the fork is held at the external auditory meatus; the normal and those with nerve deafness will still hear it, while those with middle-ear deafness will not. While performing this test the contralateral ear must be occluded. Even if this is done, the results of the test are easily misinterpreted as the sound produced when the fork is applied to one mastoid process is often heard in the contralateral ear even when the ipsilateral one is totally deaf. In **Weber's test** the vibrating fork is applied to the vertex; normal individuals hear the sound equally in the two ears, while patients with nerve deafness hear it louder in the normal ear, in contrast to those with conductive deafness to whom it seems louder in the affected ear. Accurate measurement must, of course, depend upon audiometry.

Clinical assessment of **labyrinthine** function may be difficult, but in patients with vertigo it is reasonable to alter suddenly the position of the head to see whether this produces nystagmus or vertigo. For instance, a patient may be asked to lie down suddenly and the head is then turned sharply to one or other side. This test is particularly useful in patients who complain of giddiness brought on by change in posture. Caloric tests, mentioned in Chapter 3, constitute an important means of testing the function of the labyrinths and of central vestibular connexions.

The Motor System

Foremost in examining the motor system in the patient who is able to walk, is observation of the **gait**. Some neurological diseases produce striking abnormalities, many of which are distinctive. The hemiplegic patient drags or circumducts his weak and spastic leg, while the arm is commonly flexed at the elbow and lies across the abdomen when he walks; the patient with a spastic paraparesis, by contrast, shows a stiff and clumsy mode of progression, in which both feet seem to drag along the ground. The festinant gait of Parkinsonism is even more striking; the patient shuffles along with short hurried steps, the head bowed and the back bent, as if he were having continually to press forwards to prevent himself from falling on his face. By contrast, the individual with cerebellar ataxia walks on a wide base, the feet unusually far apart; he staggers occasionally from side to side and if asked to stop suddenly or to turn round he may be very unsteady and may even fall. He finds heel-toe walking ('tandem' walking in the USA) difficult if not impossible. Equally characteristic is the 'clopping' or slapping gait of the individual with unilateral or bilateral foot-drop resulting from weakness of the dorsiflexors of the feet, while the waddle, protuberant abdomen and accentuated lumbar lordosis of the patient with pelvic girdle weakness due to muscular dystrophy (or to other forms of myopathy or spinal muscular atrophy) is also virtually diagnostic. Another important abnormality is the high-stepping unsteady gait of the patient with sensory ataxia, as in tabes dorsalis, who slaps his feet down hard as if he is not sure where they are in space.

Having observed the gait it is also necessary to note any **abnormalities of posture** or **involuntary movements**. These are abnormalities which cannot be corrected, and movements which cannot be prevented, by willed effort on the part of the patient. If involuntary movements are present, their situation, nature, amplitude, rhythmicity and frequency should be assessed and it is also important to observe whether changes in posture are permanent or temporary and whether they are influenced by volitional activity.

One must next turn to detailed examination of the **neuromuscular system**. It is customary first to inspect the muscles of the cranium, trunk and limbs, for the presence or absence of **atrophy** (wasting or reduction in muscular bulk), **hypertrophy** (muscular enlargement) or **fasciculation** (involuntary twitching or isolated bundles of muscle fibres). Next, contractures or irreversible shortening of muscles and tendons, possibly resulting in skeletal atrophy or deformity, should be looked for before going on to an examination of muscular **power**.

Beginning with the **motor cranial nerves**, the muscles of mastication (temporals, masseters and pterygoids), supplied by the motor division of the fifth or trigeminal nerve, are tested by asking the patient to clench the teeth or to move the jaw from side to side against resistance while the bulk and firmness of the muscles on the two sides are compared. The function of the seventh or facial nerve is first assessed by inspection of the face and then by asking the patient to close the eyes tightly and to show the teeth. Inability to bury the eyelashes adequately on one side may be significant, while differences in power between the upper and lower facial muscles should be noted. If emotional movement of the face, as in smiling, is normal, while volitional movement on command is impaired, this is important. Movement of the palate on saying 'ah' may reveal a disorder of one or other vagus nerve; thus if the uvula moves to one side this implies weakness of the opposite side of the palate, possibly resulting from a lesion of the nerve. Similarly, atrophy and weakness of one trapezius and sternomastoid can imply disease of the homolateral spinal accessory nerve, while atrophy and fasciculation of the tongue and deviation to one side when it is protruded indicate a lesion of the twelfth or hypoglossal nerve on the side to which the tongue protrudes.

In testing the **power of the trunk and limb muscles**, most can be tested individually if necessary. Rational application of simple anatomical knowledge will indicate how this can be done, but unless there is striking atrophy of single muscles or muscle groups, so detailed an examination is rarely necessary. In a routine examination it is usual to test representative groups, which are contracted against resistance from the examiner; such muscles are those concerned in abduction of the shoulder, flexion and extension of the elbow, extension and flexion of the fingers (the grip) in the upper limbs. The upper and lower abdominal muscles may be compared in the recumbent patient by noting whether the umbilicus deviates upwards or downwards on lifting the head. In the lower limbs it is usual to test hip flexion, flexion and extension at the knee, and dorsi- and plantar-flexion at the ankle.

No single method of assessing the power of individual muscles is perfect in view of subjective variations from one examiner to the next, but that given in the Medical Research Council's pamphlet *Aids to the Examination of the Peripheral Nervous System* (HMSO 1976) is most widely used and gives numerical gradings from 5 to 0 to identify degrees of power as given below:

5 = Normal power.
4 = The muscle, though able to make its full normal movement, is overcome by resistance.
3 = The muscle is able to make its normal movement against gravity but not against additional resistance.
2 = The muscle can only make its full normal movement when the opposing force of gravity is eliminated by appropriate positioning.
1 = There is a visible or palpable flicker of contraction, but no resultant movement of a limb or joint.
0 = Total paralysis.

Grades 4−, 4 and 4+ are used to indicate movement against slight, moderate and strong resistance respectively.

If examination reveals weakness of one or more major muscle groups it may then be necessary to examine in detail the power of individual muscles in order to determine whether the pattern of weakness indicates, for instance, disordered function of a single peripheral nerve or nerve root. Details of methods of examination of all of the limb and trunk muscles are outside the scope of this volume. However, methods of testing a number of representative muscles are illustrated in Plate I.

In certain circumstances it is also necessary to test for muscular **fatigability**. Thus, in patients with myasthenia gravis an initial contraction (say of deltoid in abducting the shoulder) can be quite powerful, but if the movement is repeated several times it becomes progressively weaker. By contrast, in **myotonia** muscular contraction may be powerful, but on relaxing (say after making a fist) the fingers 'uncurl' abnormally slowly. Direct percussion of a myotonic muscle gives a 'dimple' which slowly disappears; this phenomenon must be distinguished from myoidema, a localised ridge which forms after a direct blow upon a muscle belly and which is usually seen in malnourished, cachetic, or hypothyroid patients.

The **tone** of the limb muscles is next tested by noting and comparing the resistance which the muscles show to passive movement at the shoulder, elbow, knee and ankle joints. This may be a most difficult examination as some patients find it almost impossible to relax the limb being tested and try to help by carrying out the movements themselves. If tone is reduced (hypotonia) the limbs are limp, 'floppy' and excessively mobile with little resistance, while if it is increased (hypertonia) they may be spastic, in which case there is a severe initial resistance which suddenly 'gives' (clasp-knife rigidity); alternatively the tone may be increased throughout the entire range of movement (plastic or lead-pipe rigidity) or intermittently normal and increased (cog-wheel rigidity). In spastic limbs, a muscle which is being stretched may show the phenomenon of **clonus** (rapid intermittent involuntary contraction and relaxation); this may be seen best at the ankle on sudden dorsiflexion of the foot, at the knee on pushing sharply against the upper border of the patella, and occasionally on sudden extension of the fingers.

Tests for **co-ordination** are next carried out in order to elicit signs of cerebellar disease. The patient is asked to touch his nose and the examiner's finger alternately, with the tip of his index finger, and any tremor or past-pointing should be noted. In the lower limbs, the heel–knee test, in which the heel of one foot is placed on the opposite knee and then moved smoothly down the shin, is used. Other valuable tests for the clumsy inco-ordinate movements of cerebellar disease include rapid tapping with the fingers or toes on the opposite limb or a convenient surface, 'playing the piano' on a table top, or rapid alternating pronation and supination of the hands and forearms; clumsiness in performance of the latter test, one of the least useful, is called dysdiadochokinesis.

There are a number of **primitive reflexes**, which, present in the newborn, disappear with maturation but may persist in infants with cerebral palsy; some may reappear in adults suffering from diffuse degenerative brain disease. The tonic neck reflex is elicited by turning the head and neck to one side; extension of the limbs occurs on the side towards which the head is turned. In the normal infant this reflex is no longer obtainable after the sixth month; it is typically present in adults with severe cerebral or brain stem lesions giving a 'decerebrate state'. The sucking reflex of the normal neonate and the closely-related snout reflex (a pout or snout evoked by a sharp tap on the closed lips) may reappear in adults with diffuse brain disease or with bilateral corticospinal tract lesions in the upper brain stem or above. In normal adults the contraction of both orbicularis oculi muscles (blinking) induced by a tap on the centre of the forehead above the nose (the glabellar tap sign) quickly habituates if the tap is repeated, but in patients with Parkinsonism the blinking continues to occur rhythmically in time with the taps. For the interpretation of infantile automatisms (including the Moro, 'placing', and parachute reactions) the reader is referred to more detailed texts.

Of particular value in assessing the integrity of the brain stem in comatose patients are the **oculocephalic** and **oculovestibular reflexes**. When the eyelids are held open and the head is rotated from side to side or if it is flexed, the eyes show conjugate deviation away from the direction to which the head is moved. They return rapidly to the midline even if the head remains rotated or flexed. This oculocephalic reflex (the doll's head phenomenon) may be lost in severe pontine lesions, as is the oculovestibular reflex (nystagmus elicited by irrigation of the external auditory meatus with cold or warm water).

Finally, the **deep and superficial reflexes** should be tested. First the jaw jerk is elicited by placing a finger across the patient's chin, with the mouth slightly open and then tapping sharply downwards on the finger. A brisk contraction of the masseters is a positive jaw jerk, which is present in about 10 per cent of normal individuals but is exaggerated when there is bilateral corticospinal tract disease in the upper brain stem. In the upper limbs, the biceps jerk is elicited by a blow on a finger which is placed across the biceps tendon with the elbow flexed; the radial jerk by a brisk stimulus to the tendon of the brachioradialis as it traverses the lateral aspect of the lower end of the radius; and the triceps jerk by tapping the tendon of the triceps just above its insertion into the olecranon, again with the elbow flexed. To produce a finger jerk the examiner's fingers are tapped as they lie in contact with the palmar aspect of the tips of the patient's fingers; these should be partially flexed. Like the jaw jerk, the finger jerk is present in some normal individuals and in those who are tense; if it is present only on one side, however, this may be significant. Concomitant flexion of the terminal phalanx of the thumb when the finger jerk is elicited, usually indicates that this reflex is exaggerated. Similar flexion of the terminal phalanx of the thumb occurring when the terminal phalanx of the middle finger is flicked sharply downwards between the examiner's finger and thumb (Hoffmann's sign) may also indicate corticospinal tract dysfunction, particularly if present on one side only. In the lower limbs, the knee jerk is elicited by a blow on the patellar tendon with the knee in a semiflexed position, while the ankle jerk is obtained by tapping the tendo Achilles while the foot is dorsiflexed passively. Sometimes reinforcement (Jendrassik's manoeuvre) is necessary to bring out these reflexes; the patient is asked to grip an object or to clasp the hands firmly when any tendon is about to be tapped.

Turning to the superficial reflexes, the first to be tested are usually the abdominals; to elicit these, brisk strokes are made downwards and inwards in each quadrant of the abdomen with a sharp instrument such as the point of a pin when the umbilicus should move towards the stimulus. The cremasteric reflex is less valuable clinically; it consists in an upward movement of the ipsilateral testis on stroking the inside of the thigh. The superficial anal reflex consists of contraction of the external sphincter when the skin around the anus is stroked. Finally, a most important reflex is the plantar response. A firm stroke is made along the sole from the heel to the base of the fifth toe, along the outer side of the foot. Plantar-flexion of all the toes is a flexor or normal response, while dorsiflexion of the great toe with plantar-flexion and 'fanning' of the other toes is the extensor or Babinski response.

When it is necessary to assess the integrity of the parasympathetic outflow from the second and third sacral segments of the spinal cord, it may be necessary to elicit the anal sphincter reflex (contraction of the internal sphincter around an examining finger) or the bulbocavernosus reflex (contraction of bulbocavernosus elicited by pinching the glans penis).

When examining the deep tendon and abdominal reflexes the patient should be resting comfortably and the muscles being tested should be relaxed. Furthermore it is best to compare each reflex on one side of the body with the corresponding one on the opposite side, observing any asymmetry of response. Conventionally, each reflex is recorded as −, +, + + or + + + depending upon its activity, while the plantar responses are recorded as ↓ (flexor), ⇡ (equivocal) or ↑ (extensor).

The Sensory System

It is usual to test the different modalities of sensation independently, as they follow different pathways in the spinal cord and brain. The perception of pain may conveniently be tested by pinprick and that of touch with a fine wisp of cotton wool. Each of these forms of sensation can be tested quantitatively by applying painful stimuli of graduated weight (algesiometers) or hairs which are calibrated so that a particular force is required to bend them (von Frey hairs). Such refinements are, however, unnecessary in clinical practice. Abnormalities of sensory perception should be sought on the face, trunk and limbs, by exploring representative areas with the two types of stimuli mentioned; the corneal reflexes, evoked by touching each cornea with a fine wisp of cotton wool, should also be compared. If an area of diminished pain sensation (hypalgesia) or touch sensation (hypaesthesia) is discovered, or even one of apparent hypersensitivity (hyperpathia), this should be outlined by applying repetitive stimuli from within to without the area and *vice versa,* asking the patient to say when any change occurs. The area of sensory change should then be charted on a drawing of the human body, each modality being recorded separately. If pain loss is found, then temperature perception should be tested within the same area, using test-tubes filled with hot and cold water.

The finer and more discriminative aspects of sensibility should also be tested. Thus the patient may be asked to identify objects placed in the hands when his eyes are closed, or figures drawn on the skin. He is also asked to state the direction of movement each time the terminal phalanx of a finger or the great toe is moved passively upwards or downwards and any defects in position and joint sense, so elicited, must be recorded. In the normal individual, movements of 1 mm are easily appreciated. The appreciation of vibration should also be tested with a 128-frequency tuning fork over bony prominences such as the sternum, elbow, knuckle, anterior superior iliac spine, patella and external malleolus. The ability to perceive

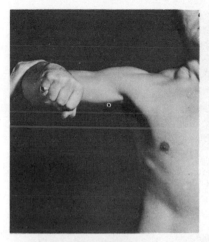

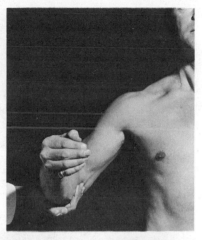

A. Deltoid (axillary nerve; **C5**, C6). The patient is abducting the upper arm at the shoulder joint against resistance.

B. Pectoralis major; sternocostal head (lateral and medial pectoral nerves; **C7**, C8). The patient is adducting the upper arm at the shoulder joint against resistance.

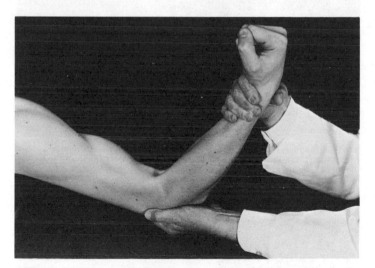

C. Biceps brachii (musculocutaneous nerve; C5, C6). The patient is flexing the supinated forearm at the elbow joint against resistance.

Plate I. Methods of examining the power of some representative skeletal muscles (Reproduced from *Aids to the Examination of the Peripheral Nervous System*, 1975, revised from War Memorandum No. 7, 1943, by permission of the Medical Research Council and Her Majesty's Stationery Office. Plates A, B, D and E were prepared in the Department of Medical Illustration, the National Hospital, Queen Square, Plates C and F to L inclusive in the Department of Medical Illustration and Photography, Guy's Hospital Medical School).

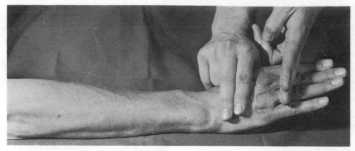

D. Extensor digitorum (radial nerve; **C7,** C8). The patient's hand is firmly supported by the examiner's right hand. Extension of the fingers at the metacarpophalangeal joints is maintained against the resistance of the fingers of the examiner's left hand.

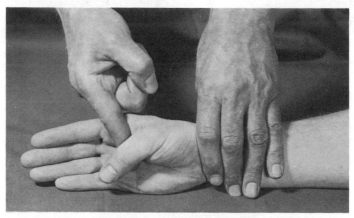

E. Opponens pollicis (median nerve; C8, **T1**). The patient is attempting against resistance to touch the base of the little finger with the tip of the thumb while the thumb nail remains in a plane parallel to the palm.

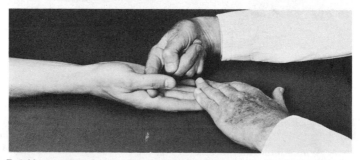

F. Adductor pollicis (ulnar nerve; C8, **T1**). The patient is adducting the thumb at the metacarpophalangeal joint against the resistance of the examiner's finger.

Plate I (contd.)

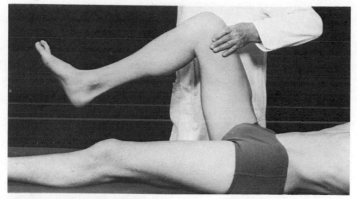

G. Iliopsoas (femoral nerve and branches from L1, 2 and 3 spinal nerves; **L1, L2, L3**). The patient is flexing the limb at the hip joint against resistance with the leg flexed at the knee.

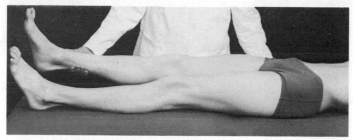

H. Gluteus maximus (inferior gluteal nerve; **L5, S1, S2**). The patient is lying on his back with the limb extended at the knee joint and is extending the limb at the hip against resistance while the examiner's left hand palpates the belly of the muscle.

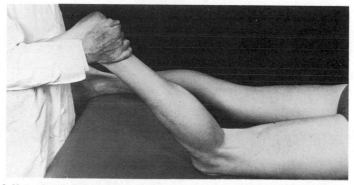

I. Hamstrings (sciatic nerve; semitendinosus and semimembranosus L4, L5, **S1, S2**; biceps femoris L5, **S1, S2**). The patient is flexing the leg at the knee joint against resistance.

Plate I (contd.)

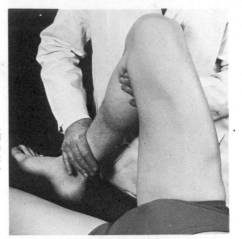

J. Quadriceps femoris (femoral nerve; L2, **L3,** L4). With the limb flexed at the hip and knee, the patient is extending the leg at the knee joint against resistance. To detect slight weakness the leg muscle is fully flexed initially.

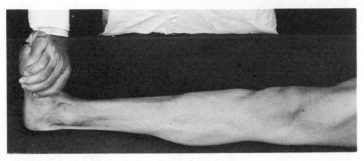

K. Tibialis anterior (peroneal nerve; L4, L5). The patient is dorsiflexing the foot at the ankle joint against resistance.

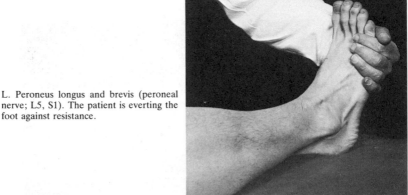

L. Peroneus longus and brevis (peroneal nerve; L5, S1). The patient is everting the foot against resistance.

Plate I (contd.)

whether the tips of the fingers or the soles of the feet are being touched with one or two points may also be noted. The normal threshold for two-point discrimination on the tips of the fingers is 2–3 mm, while on the sole of the foot it is 2–3 cm. Another useful test for eliciting very minor defects of sensation is to touch similar points on opposite limbs, sometimes independently and sometimes together, while asking the patient to say which has been touched. A patient who can feel perfectly stimuli applied independently may only feel the stimulus on one side when both are touched at the same time. This phenomenon is known as tactile inattention.

Testing of sensory function carries many pitfalls for the unwary and needs much practice and experience before it can be accurately performed. One reason for this is that many suggestible individuals may easily produce spurious areas of cutaneous sensory loss, and hypalgesia is one of the commonest neurological signs of hysterical origin. Furthermore, many less intelligent patients find it difficult to understand what is required of them, while the more intelligent may find sensory changes which are more dependent upon unintentional variation in intensity of stimulus than upon organic disease. A circumspect approach free from suggestion and combined with dispassionate objectivity is therefore required.

Signs of Disease in Other Systems

The human body cannot function as an isolated nervous system and neurological manifestations may result from dysfunction in other systems. Cerebral infarction, for instance, can follow cardiac infarction, a brain abscess may be the result of bronchiectasis, otitis, or paranasal sinusitis, or a confusional state can result from uraemia due to renal disease, from pernicious anaemia or from liver failure. Hence even though the patient's symptoms and signs indicate disease of the nervous system, examination of the patient as a whole must be no less assiduous, for the essential clue to the nature of the patient's illness may lie elsewhere.

Discussion and Differential Diagnosis

A detailed clinical history and a physical examination recorded in meticulous detail will be of no value unless it can be interpreted and it is upon this interpretation that treatment may depend. It is at this stage particularly that experience plays the greatest part, but experience can only be acquired if the student or young doctor learns to sift the accumulated data, discarding the irrelevant and tabulating the significant. He must therefore at this stage apply his powers of inductive and deductive reasoning in order to decide first the situation and secondly the nature of the pathological changes responsible for the patient's disease. He must be expected to tabulate in order of likelihood the possible diagnoses which he is considering, and must then decide which ancillary investigations, if any, are required in order to establish whichever is correct. For the history and examination are but a means to an end, the end being diagnosis, upon which management of the patient must depend.

References

Adams, R. D. and Victor, M., *Principles of Neurology*, 2nd ed. (New York, McGraw-Hill, 1981).

Bickerstaff, E. R., *Neurological Examination in Clinical Practice,* 4th ed. (Oxford, Blackwell, 1980).

Gordon, N. *Paediatric Neurology for the Clinician,* (Spastics International Medical Publications, London, Heinemann, 1976).

Holmes, G., *An Introduction to Clinical Neurology*, 3rd ed. revised by W. B. Matthews (Edinburgh, Livingstone, 1968).

de Jong, R., *The Neurologic Examination*, 5th ed. (New York, Hoeber, 1979).

Klein, R. and Mayer-Gross, W., *The Clinical Examination of Patients with Organic Cerebral Disease* (London, Cassell, 1957).

Mayo Clinic, Section of Neurology, *Clinical Examinations in Neurology*, 5th ed. (Philadelphia, Saunders, 1981).

Medical Research Council, *Aids to the Examination of the Peripheral Nervous System* (London, HMSO, 1976).

Paine, R. S. and Oppé, T. E., *Neurological Examination of Children,* Clinics in Developmental Medicine, 20/21 (London, The Spastics Society and Heinemann, 1966).

Spillane, J. D., *An Atlas of Clinical Neurology*, 2nd ed. (London, Oxford University Press, 1975).

3 Investigation of the Patient with Neurological Disease

In considering the ancillary investigations which are used as aids to diagnosis in a patient whose symptoms and signs suggest a disorder of the nervous system it is important to appreciate that symptoms of neurological dysfunction may result from disease in another part of the body. The patient must therefore be viewed as a whole if he is not to be subjected to a series of unpleasant tests designed to demonstrate a primary nervous disease, when the lesion responsible may be in some other organ far removed from the brain and spinal cord. A second principle too often forgotten is that investigations should be planned to give the maximum required information about the patient's illness with the least possible discomfort and risk. There is an unfortunate tendency in some centres to submit all patients to a routine series of disturbing, irrelevant and often expensive laboratory or radiological studies. Such a rigid and mechanistic approach, as observed in certain 'diagnostic' hospitals and clinics, is mentioned only to be deplored. A system of this type takes little account of the patient as an individual and of his comforts and discomforts. Whereas a thousand routine barium enema studies may perhaps reveal one unsuspected early carcinoma of the large bowel, one must ask whether the other nine hundred and ninety-nine could be justified on this score, taking into account the time spent by skilled radiologists, the patient's discomfort and the cost to him or to the community.

In many patients with neurological disorders there is no need for investigations either for diagnosis or for guidance on management. Migraine, for instance, is a condition in which the diagnosis is usually made on the history alone and in which ancillary tests are rarely needed. In other cases, investigations should be designed to establish or exclude the diagnoses which are suggested by the patient's symptoms and signs. It is reasonable to begin by carrying out the simpler tests which the doctor can do himself, before proceeding, if still in doubt, to the more difficult investigations which need specialised apparatus and skilled technical help. Ethical considerations must always be considered in assessing potential risks on the one hand against the information which may be derived from investigation on the other.

General Medical Investigations

The central and autonomic nervous systems play an important role in regulating the body **temperature.** Hence in a febrile patient with neurological symptoms and signs it is important to determine whether the pyrexia is due to inflammatory changes in the nervous system or elsewhere, or whether it is due to a lesion of the neuraxis giving a disorder of temperature regulation. Pyrexia and fever are of course seen in patients with meningitis and encephalitis, whether infective or postinfective, and a remittent fever characteristic of suppuration may occur in those with an intracranial or spinal abscess. An aseptic or chemical meningitis, resulting from bleeding in the subarachnoid space, also gives fever. Lesions of the pons and hypothalamic region, however, may give hyperpyrexia, with temperatures of 40°C (105°F) or more; this typically results from pontine haemorrhage, brain-stem injury or massive haemorrhage into the third ventricle with consequent compression of hypothalamic centres in its floor. But drowsiness, headache and neck stiffness (meningism) sometimes occur in patients with pneumonia, especially in childhood, while a stuporose or delirious febrile patient at first thought to have a primarily neurological illness could alternatively be suffering from enteric or some other specific fever.

Examination of the **pulse** is of considerable value in neurology. A slow pulse in a patient with neurological symptoms and signs may indicate increased intracranial pressure, giving rise to compression of medullary centres, but when this is so, there is usually some impairment of consciousness. Bradycardia in the alert and conscious patient is more probably constitutional, or rarely due to heart block. A rapid pulse, on the other hand, is a terminal feature in some fatal brain diseases (e.g. cerebral haemorrhage or tumour), but in the conscious patient, tachycardia will often be the result of anxiety (when there is usually other evidence of nervousness), or of systemic disease such as infection or thyrotoxicosis. Irregularity of the pulse is also important; sinus arrhythmia and extrasystoles have little pathological significance, but auricular fibrillation occurring in a patient with a hemiplegia may indicate that the hemiplegia was the result of cerebral embolism from a thrombus in the left auricle. Similarly a full, bounding pulse may suggest hypertension and its neurological complications, while a collapsing pulse, resulting from aortic valve incompetence, could suggest that the patient's neurological symptoms are due to neurosyphilis. Recording of the **blood pressure** is also essential in any physical examination. If the sphygmomanometer reading, combined with the presence of haemorrhage, exudates and vascular changes in the retina, indicate a diagnosis of malignant hypertension, this may explain neurological signs and symptoms such as headaches, drowsiness, convulsions or even coma. Hypertension is usually severe, too, in patients with cerebral haemorrhage, but in cases of so-called cerebral thrombosis it is atheroma rather than hypertension which is the primary offender and the blood pressure is sometimes normal. However, atheromatous changes can be seen in the retinal arteries of such cases on **ophthalmoscopy**, and **electro-cardiography** (ECG) may show that there is also atherosclerosis of the coronary arteries, with cardiac ischaemia; irregularities of the pulse, and abnormalities of the serum potassium which can cause neurological symptoms, will also be defined by this investigation. Occasionally intra-cranial disease and subarachnoid haemorrhage in particular can produce transient abnormalities in the ECG.

Examination of the **urine** is also of value. The presence of *glycosuria* may suggest that the patient has diabetes mellitus and will therefore explain why he has signs of peripheral neuropathy. *Polyuria* is occasionally a functional or psychiatric symptom, but if much urine of low specific gravity is passed, it may indicate diabetes insipidus due to a disorder of the hypothalamus–pituitary axis. *Albuminuria* and the *abnormal cells* and *casts* in the urine may indicate primary renal disease causing uraemia and drowsiness, or hypertension and consequent cerebral symptoms. Alterna-tively, minimal albuminuria with some red cells may be due to embolism (as in subacute bacterial endocarditis) or diffuse arterial disease (as in polyarteritis nodosa) and these conditions also give neurological manifesta-tions. A number of biochemical tests also give useful information. Thus *bilirubin* in the urine may be an expression of liver disease, in which episodes of confusion and disturbed behaviour may occur, while a dark port-wine coloured urine which goes darker on standing is indicative of *porphyria*, a condition in which confusion, abdominal pain and peripheral neuropathy occur. Furthermore, there may be a diminished urinary output of *17-oxogenic steroids* in patients with hypopituitarism resulting from a chromophobe adenoma destroying the pituitary gland. Alternatively, in Cushing's syndrome, which is usually of adrenal origin but occasionally results from a basophil adenoma of the pituitary, the oxosteroid output is raised. Assay of urinary *growth hormone* output is sometimes necessary to confirm the diagnosis of acromegaly. Estimation of *sodium and potassium output* can also be of value in patients suffering from intermittent attacks of flaccid muscular paralysis, for some have a nephritis causing excessive salt loss and consequent hypokalaemia, while others, in whom there is a diminished output of sodium, may have attacks of paralysis caused perhaps by excessive adrenal aldosterone secretion. Estimation of *heavy metals* in the urine is also useful; thus in a painter or battery-maker with unilateral wrist drop, or in a child with convulsions due to lead encephalopathy, there is an excessive lead output, while in Wilson's disease (hepatolenticular degeneration) the urinary copper content is increased. In some chronic degenerative neurological diseases the urinary excretion of *amino acids*, determined by paper chromatography, is abnormal.

Examination of the **blood** often gives useful clues as to the significance of neurological symptoms and signs. One valuable test is estimation of the *erythrocyte sedimentation rate* (ESR). Primary disorders of the nervous system, save for the suppurative infections, rarely influence this reading, though it is occasionally slightly raised in patients with intracranial haemorrhage or primary intracranial neoplasms. A moderate rise in the ESR, however, to above 10 mm/hr (Westergren) in men, or above 15 mm/hr in women, may indicate an infective or inflammatory disorder or malignant disease, while an excessively high reading in the region of 50–100 mm/hr is often indicative of one of the 'connective tissue' group of disorders such as rheumatism, polyarteritis nodosa, lupus erythematosus, cranial arteritis, or dermatomyositis, or of multiple myeloma.

Haematological studies also shed important light on certain manifestations of nervous disease. Thus dysphagia, at first suggesting a paresis of swallowing, may be associated with hypochromic anaemia. In addition to microcytosis and a low colour index, the *serum iron* is then low. More frequent are the neurological complications (subacute combined degeneration of the spinal cord and brain, or rarely optic atrophy) of pernicious anaemia. Most such cases have a macrocytic anaemia with an increased mean cell volume, while megaloblasts are found in profusion in the bone marrow. Occasionally, however, typical neurological signs appear before any of these haematological findings develop, and the diagnosis must then rest upon the finding of histamine-fast achlorhydria in the **gastric juice**, an abnormally low value of *serum B_{12}* (less than 160 ng/l) and an abnormal Schilling test.

Some cases of macrocytic anaemia are due to folate deficiency resulting either from malabsorption, anticonvulsant therapy or dietary deficiency, while dementia and/or polyneuropathy have been attributed in certain cases to folate lack; a low serum folate (less than 2 μg/ml) may assist in diagnosis. And several systemic diseases which may have neurological manifestations (malignant disease and 'connective tissue' disease are examples) can produce a normocytic and orthochromic anaemia. By contrast there are often neurological symptoms (headache, giddiness and minor 'strokes') in patients with polycythaemia vera, in whom the *red and white cell components of the blood* (as well as the platelets) are greatly increased.

A *differential white cell count* is also a valuable aid in neurological diagnosis. A polymorphonuclear leucocytosis is found in many infective disorders, while leucopenia or eosinophilia may occur in 'connective tissue' diseases, such as lupus erythematosus or polyarteritis nodosa. Some disorders of the reticuloendothelial system also produce neurological complications; thus meningoencephalitis and/or poly- or mononeuropathy are occasional complications of infective mononucleosis (glandular fever). Furthermore, leukaemic deposits in the central nervous system can give focal neurological symptoms and signs of which facial palsy is one of the commoner; leukaemia is usually identified by blood and marrow examinations. Neurological signs, particularly those of cord compression, can also result from reticulosis, such as Hodgkin's disease, but here blood examination is usually uninformative and diagnosis often rests upon the result of **lymph node biopsy**. Similarly, multiple myeloma can compress the brain, optic nerves or spinal cord, and in this condition diagnosis depends upon the identification of myeloma protein in the serum and/or upon marrow biopsy and radiological changes in the bones. Haemorrhagic disorders, such as haemophilia or thrombocytopenic purpura, can also give rise to neurological complications of which subdural, intracerebral and subarachnoid haemorrhage are the most frequent and these conditions will usually be identified by estimation of the *bleeding* and *clotting time*, or other tests of blood coagulation and the *platelet count*.

Many more neurological diagnoses can be established by the determination of the absolute values of various **biochemical substances** in the serum. Thus in some individuals with long-standing respiratory insufficiency a syndrome of chronic cerebral anoxia and carbon dioxide narcosis gives rise to a severe confusional state, and this is identified first by the clinical evidence of chronic lung disease (usually emphysema and chronic bronchitis) and by estimation of the *arterial oxygen* and *carbon dioxide tension*. The coma or drowsiness of uraemia will be recognised by the clinical evidence of acidosis and by the finding of a high blood urea, while diabetic ketosis is confirmed by *blood-sugar estimation* and by finding acetone in the breath and urine. Another important cause of coma, sometimes with focal neurological signs, is hypoglycaemia, which is identified by a blood-sugar estimation carried out during an attack. A five-hour *glucose tolerance curve*, repeated blood-sugar estimation during prolonged fasting (for up to 48 hours), and insulin or tolbutamide tolerance tests may be needed in patients with frequent fainting spells or epileptic seizures in whom there is reason to suspect either reactive or organic hyperinsulinism. Examination of the *serum electrolytes* is also of value, as muscular asthenia and drowsiness are common features of Addison's disease, in which condition the serum sodium is usually low, while hypokalaemia or hyperkalaemia are important causes of periodic attacks of generalised flaccid muscular paralysis. Estimation of the *serum cortisol* (low in Addison's disease and high in Cushing's syndrome) or prolactin and many other specialised studies may be necessary to identify neurological complications of various endocrine disorders; thus measurement of serum osmolarity may be necessary to identify the syndrome caused by inappropriate secretion of anti-diuretic hormone which may occur in some cases of intracranial tumour (usually in the area of the hypothalamus). In mentally retarded patients with epilepsy it is important to estimate the *serum calcium* and *phosphorus* as some such patients have idiopathic hypoparathyroidism and may be helped by calciferol or similar therapy which raises their abnormally low serum calcium. Furthermore, fainting attacks and muscular weakness may occur in patients with hypercalcaemia whether due to hyperparathyroidism or to renal disease.

Neurological complications of liver disease often take the form of intermittent confusion and abnormal behaviour, associated with a curious flapping, or wing-beating, tremor of the hands (asterixis). Some adults with cirrhosis develop movements suggestive of combined chorea and athetosis (*see* p. 412). In any patient presenting with such symptoms, it is necessary to carry out a battery of *liver function tests*, including the serum bilirubin and alkaline phosphatase; one of the most valuable estimations is that of the blood ammonia, which is usually greatly raised in cases of 'hepatic encephalopathy'. In such individuals, there is often an abnormal pattern of serum proteins, and this may be confirmed by electrophoresis. Identification in this way of a rise in *serum γ-globulin* is also a valuable aid in the diagnosis of 'collagen' disease. Measurement of the fractions of *γ-globulin* (IgA, IgG, IgM) by means of immunoelectrophoresis has proved of increasing value in the diagnosis of a variety of primary and acquired dysglobulinaemias, some of which are occasionally accompanied by neurological manifestations.

A rise in the *serum cholesterol* may help in the diagnosis of myxoedema, a condition which occasionally presents with mental symptoms or with stiffness, aching and sluggishness of the skeletal muscles. Confirmation of the diagnosis is obtained from the *serum thyroxin, protein-bound iodine* and *radio-iodine uptake* studies, and by the detection of anti-thyroid antibodies in the serum. Estimation of the *serum copper*, copper oxidase and caeruloplasmin content are valuable in children with extra-pyramidal disorders, as these values are low in patients with Wilson's disease. Estimation of the *serum alphafetoprotein* in maternal blood has proved to be valuable in identifying fetal abnormalities such as anencephaly and spina bifida: confirmation by means of a similar estimation carried out on amniotic fluid obtained by amniocentesis (*see below*) may be needed before therapeutic abortion can safely be recommended.

A number of **microbiological** studies are also applicable in neurological diagnosis. In addition to the *culture of organisms* from the cerebrospinal fluid or from abscesses in or near nervous tissue, blood culture is indicated if there is any clinical evidence to suggest a bacteraemia. *Agglutination reactions* are also important, not only in the diagnosis of enteric, abortus and glandular fever, but also in suspected cases of leptospirosis (Weil's disease and canicola fever) in which the nervous system is often involved. *Virological studies* are of increasing importance, not only in the diagnosis of recognised viral infections such as poliomyelitis, but also in the investigation of cases of lymphocytic meningitis and encephalomyelitis of unknown aetiology. Thus herpes simplex virus, for example, which may cause an acute necrotising encephalitis, can be identified sometimes by a fluorescent antibody technique and may quickly be recognised in brain biopsy material under the electron microscope. Other viruses can sometimes be cultured from blood, faeces or cerebrospinal fluid and viral antibody tests performed on serum are also sometimes of considerable diagnostic value. In addition to the well-known *Wassermann, Kahn* and *VDRL reactions* utilised in the diagnosis of syphilis as well as the more specific *treponema-immobilisation* and *fluorescent treponemal antibody absorption (FTA–ABS) tests*, there are also available a number of other complement-fixation and agglutination reactions which aid in the recognition of less common infective and parasitic disorders of the nervous system, such as toxoplasmosis and cryptococcosis.

Biopsy techniques, other than lymph-node biopsy which was previously mentioned, are of great value in the investigation of suspected nervous disease; in certain cases, skin, liver or renal biopsy and other methods commonly used in general medicine may be applicable. *Muscle biopsy* has, however, a more immediate relevance to neurological medicine as this method can be very useful in deciding whether muscular weakness and wasting is due to a disease of the motor nerves (neuropathy) or of the muscles (myopathy), and in identifying the nature of the myopathic affliction. It may also be of help in the diagnosis of 'connective tissue' disease and particularly of polyarteritis nodosa. Sural *nerve biopsy* is occasionally of use in investigating cases of peripheral neuropathy, while *brain biopsy* is utilised in the diagnosis of cerebral tumour or of diffuse degenerative or metabolic disease; these techniques have relatively restricted clinical applications.

In some rare inherited disorders of the nervous system in which specific enzymatic abnormalities have been detected, these can be identified in skin fibroblasts or white blood cells in culture; similar techniques applied to amniotic cells obtained by *amniocentesis* can be used for antenatal diagnosis with a view to therapeutic abortion on eugenic grounds.

The Cerebrospinal Fluid (CSF)

Formation and Composition

From experimental work carried out in the early part of this century it was found that the choroid plexuses of the cerebral ventricles play an important part in forming the cerebrospinal fluid. Blockage of the aqueduct of Sylvius was found to cause a striking dilatation of the lateral and third ventricles, due to the continued production of cerebrospinal fluid for which there was no longer an outlet. From these observations and from the fact that hydrocephalus could follow blockage of the sagittal sinus and was then presumed to result from impaired re-absorption of the fluid, the classical view of CSF formation and circulation evolved. According to this view, the fluid is formed in the choroid plexuses, not by simple diffusion or dialysis but by a process of active secretion; that secreted in the lateral ventricles then passes through the foramina of Monro, the third ventricle, the aqueduct and fourth ventricle, to enter the basal cisterns of the subarachnoid space through the foramina of Magendie and Luschka. It then flows upwards over the surface of the cerebral hemispheres, while some flows down into the spinal subarachnoid space; reabsorption into the blood stream then occurs through the arachnoidal villi which protrude into the sagittal and other venous sinuses. Work on the passage of radioactive substances into the CSF has confirmed that this mechanism of secretion and reabsorption operates and the mean rate of formation is about 0.35 ml/min. In addition there is a constant process of dialysis, with

Table 1 Normally Accepted Values Relating to CSF Obtained at Lumbar Puncture*

Pressure (at lumbar puncture)	50–200 mmH$_2$O
Volume	100–130 ml
Specific gravity	1.003–1.008
Cells adults	0–4 mononuclears
infants	0–20 mononuclears
Total proteins (mostly albumin)	0.15–0.45 g/l
Globulin	0–0.06 g/l
Colloidal gold (Lange)	000110000
Urea nitrogen	0.05–0.10 g/l
Creatinine	0.004–0.022 g/l
Non-protein nitrogen	0.12–0.30 g/l
Uric acid	0.003–0.015 g/l
Glucose	0.50–0.85 g/l
Sodium	144 mEq/l
Chloride	120–130 mEq/l
Calcium	0.04–0.07 g/l
Phosphate	0.012–0.020 g/l
Magnesium	0.01–0.03 g/l
Potassium	2.06–3.86 mEq/l
Cholesterol	0.0006–0.005 g/l

*Modified from Johnson (1972) by kind permission of the author, editors and publisher.

exchange of chemical constituents between the CSF and blood, occurring across the arachnoid membrane at all levels. Large molecules cannot enter the fluid as they are unable to pass the vascular endothelium which effectively constitutes the blood-brain barrier, but there is a rapid exchange of substances of small molecular weight between the CSF and the extracellular fluid of the central nervous system. Thus in some ways the CSF acts as a 'sink' in preventing the extracellular fluid from achieving true equilibrium with the blood plasma. The composition of the ventricular fluid is very different from that in the lumbar subarachnoid space and many constituents of the lumbar fluid are added to it by diffusion across the spinal arachnoid membrane.

The CSF acts as a cushion protecting the brain and cord against external pressure waves. It has no nutritional function but removes metabolites from the nervous system, and through its hydrogen ion concentration (its pH is in equilibrium with that of the extracellular fluid of the brain) it influences the respiratory volume and rate, cerebral blood flow and other aspects of cerebral metabolism.

The total volume of cerebrospinal fluid in the normal adult is between 100 and 130 ml. The fluid is clear and colourless; it contains less than four white blood cells per mm^3 and all of these are lymphocytes. The protein content of the lumbar fluid is 0.15–0.45 g/l, the respective values for

Table 2 The Composition of CSF (Average Values) Compared with Plasma*

Constituent	Ratio CSF: plasma	CSF	Plasma	Units
pCO_2	1.28	50.2	39.5	mm Hg
Chloride	1.21	125	103	
Sodium	1.03	144	140	
Bicarbonate	1.01	25.1	24.8	mEq/l
Magnesium	0.8	2.4	3	
Urea	0.8	0.12	0.15	
Glucose	0.64	0.64	1.0	g/l
Potassium	0.52	2.1	4	
Calcium	0.33	1.7	5	mEq/l
Protein	0.0033	0.20	6.0	
Cholesterol	0.0002	0.0014	1.75	g/l

*Modified from Johnson (1972) by kind permission of the author, editors and publisher.

ventricular and cisternal fluid being 0.05–0.15 g/l and 0.15–0.25 g/l; most of the protein present is albumin. Normally, too, the fluid contains 0.50–0.80 g glucose and 120–130 mEq chloride (expressed as NaCl) per 1. The concentrations of these and other substances in the CSF are given in Table 1 and comparative concentrations in CSF and plasma are listed in Table 2. Thus the protein content of the fluid is low when compared with that of the blood serum, the sugar level is also lower than in the serum, while the chloride is higher. Sodium, potassium, urea and some drugs such as sulphonamides, pass freely into the fluid and are there found in concentrations equal to that in the serum, whereas other substances such as antibodies, salicylates, penicillin and streptomycin pass into it in relatively minute quantities even if the serum concentration is high. Bromide, too, is found in the lumbar CSF in only about one-third the concentration in which it is present in the blood. Clearly, therefore, the entry of many chemicals into the CSF is a selective matter and does not depend upon a simple process of diffusion across a semipermeable membrane. Disease, and particularly inflammation of the arachnoid, may influence this process and in some cases of meningitis, penicillin, say, and bromide enter the fluid more easily.

Lumbar Puncture

Cytological and chemical examination of the CSF is of great value in neurological diagnosis and specimens of fluid are most easily obtained by lumbar puncture, which is usually a comparatively simple and safe procedure though never to be undertaken lightly. The exploring needle is inserted into the lumbar subarachnoid space below the termination of the spinal cord, and as the roots of the cauda equina are pushed aside by the needle, the risks of damage to nervous tissue are negligible. The investigation is, however, dangerous if the intracranial pressure is high, and particularly if an intracranial tumour is present, since reduction in the fluid pressure in the lumbar subarachnoid space can result in impaction of the cerebellar tonsils in the foramen magnum or of the medial aspects of one or both temporal lobes between the brain stem and the edge of the tentorium cerebelli, with fatal results. Hence papilloedema is usually a contra-indication and lumbar puncture should be avoided if the patient's symptoms suggest that the intracranial pressure is raised; should manometry reveal that the pressure is unexpectedly high, it is wise to remove only a few drops of fluid. Even this precaution, however, will not always avoid cerebellar or tentorial herniation, as persistent leakage of fluid can occur through the hole in the spinal dura mater left by the exploring needle. This mechanism, with consequent reduction of the intracranial pressure below normal, is probably the cause of the common post-lumbar-puncture headache.

In carrying out lumbar puncture, the patient should lie horizontally on the left side with his neck firmly flexed, the knees drawn up to the chin and the trunk flexed. The skin of the back is cleaned with a suitable antiseptic; a line is then drawn down the spinous processes of the vertebrae and another joining the highest points of the iliac crests. This line usually crosses the spine of the fourth lumbar vertebra and the needle may be inserted either in the intervertebral space above or in the one below this line. Full aseptic precautions are essential; the operator should wear a mask and sterile gloves, and the lumbar puncture outfit, including needles, stylets and manometer, should have been autoclaved. Harris's or similar needles are satisfactory. After infiltration of the skin and subcutaneous tissue with local anaesthetic (e.g. 1 per cent procaine hydrochloride solution) the needle is then inserted with its stylet in position and is passed horizontally inwards in a slightly cephalad direction. It passes through the interspinous ligaments and then encounters the resistant ligamentum flavum. After penetrating this ligament resistance suddenly lessens as the needle enters the subarachnoid space. The stylet is now removed from the needle and the fluid drips out slowly. Care must be taken not to insert the needle too far, as a vertebral vein may then be punctured or an intervertebral disk can be damaged.

It is usual to measure the pressure of the fluid by attaching a manometer to the needle and the height of the fluid column in mm of CSF is measured when it ceases to rise in the upright tube. The normal pressure in the recumbent adult is 50–200 mm of fluid; when he is sitting upright the pressure in the lumbar subarachnoid space is about 200–250 mm. It is important that the patient is lying comfortably relaxed during this procedure. Coughing or straining causes an increased pressure in abdominal veins and consequently in the vertebral veins; this displaces CSF from the spinal canal and its pressure therefore rises. Similarly, if there is a free communication between the cerebral and lumbar subarachnoid spaces, a temporary increase in the intracranial pressure is reflected in the manometer. Such an increase may be produced by compressing one or both internal jugular veins in the neck, thus reducing venous outflow from the cranium. In carrying out this procedure, known as Queckenstedt's test, there is usually a sharp rise in pressure to 300 mm or more, with an equally rapid fall when the pressure is released. If there is a block to the free passage of fluid in the subarachnoid space, then no rise in pressure occurs during the manoeuvre, while if the block is partial the rise and fall are both abnormally slow. This test has been used to diagnose thrombosis in one lateral sinus when digital compression of one jugular vein produces a rise in pressure but no rise occurs on the affected side; it has also been used in various positions of the head to diagnose cervical spondylosis utilising precise techniques of electromanometry. But the increasing sophistication of radiological techniques such as myelography and angiography and the relative imprecision of Queckenstedt's test, which gives too many false negative results to be reliable, has meant that it has been largely discarded in clinical practice except where neuroradiological facilities are not immediately available. Even in such circumstances, if transfer to a neurological unit is possible, when a spinal tumour is suspected, lumbar puncture is better avoided as withdrawal of CSF distal to a spinal block can render subsequent myelography difficult or impossible.

After pressure readings have been taken it is then usual to collect fluid in two separate sterile and chemically clean test-tubes or other appropriate containers. One specimen is used for bacteriological, the other for cytological and chemical studies. When the examination is complete, the stylet is reinserted into the needle, it is withdrawn and the track is sealed by a simple dry dressing. Failure to obtain fluid (a 'dry tap') may mean that the puncture has been performed incorrectly or vertebral disease may have narrowed the interspace; if the first puncture is unsuccessful, another attempt should be made in the interspace above or below. A genuine 'dry tap', when the needle is in the subarachnoid space but no fluid can be withdrawn, even on suction, means either that the space is blocked at a higher level or that the lumbar sac is filled by a neoplasm or developmental lesion such as a lipoma.

Cisternal Puncture

Cisternal puncture is a more difficult and dangerous procedure than lumbar puncture, since if the needle is inserted too far into the cisterna magna, the lower part of the medulla oblongata is pierced. Hence this method is only used if lumbar puncture is impossible owing to spinal deformity, if contrast medium is to be injected to define the upper level of a spinal lesion causing a block, if it is necessary to compare the chemical constitution of the lumbar and cisternal fluids, or if intrathecal injections of therapeutic agents are to be given and there is a block in the spinal subarachnoid space.

In preparation, the neck is shaved to the level of the external occipital protuberance and the head is flexed. After skin preparation and local anaesthesia, the needle is inserted about 1 cm above the highest palpable spinous process and is passed upwards and inwards until it strikes the posterior atlanto-occipital ligament. It is then passed through the ligament and advanced cautiously for another 0.5 cm; the stylet is now withdrawn, as the tip should be lying in the cisterna magna. Sometimes the fluid fails to flow from the cistern, as the pressure here is considerably lower than in the lumbar subarachnoid space, and gentle suction with a syringe is often needed to obtain a specimen of fluid. This technique is one which, unlike lumbar puncture, should only be performed by a skilled operator working in a specialised unit.

Ventricular Puncture

Direct needle puncture of a lateral cerebral ventricle is sometimes necessary in order to relieve symptoms of increased intracranial pressure prior to an operation for intracranial tumour, or in order to inject air for ventriculography. Rarely, when there is inflammatory exudate in the subarachnoid space and lumbar or cisternal puncture do not produce a free flow of CSF, this route is used to administer antibiotics. In infants the ventricles can be entered directly by a needle inserted in the lateral angle of the fontanelle which is then passed through the cerebral substance. In older children and in adults, cranial burr-holes must first be made. In view of its potential hazards, this technique is one for the specialist.

Examination of the Cerebrospinal Fluid and Some Common Abnormalities

Pressure

An increase in the CSF pressure above 200 mm in a relaxed, recumbent patient usually implies raised pressure inside the cranium. This is usually due to an increased brain volume produced by oedema or by a lesion such as a tumour, abscess or haematoma. A moderate rise occurs in patients with severe arterial hypertension. An unusually low pressure is much less significant if there is no other evidence of spinal block, and is generally of no diagnostic value, although some patients in whom the pressure is low initially seem more liable to develop headache as a sequel of lumbar puncture. A syndrome of intracranial hypotension has been postulated as an explanation of this finding, but the evidence that such a condition exists is inconclusive, although dehydration, as in a 'hangover', may temporarily reduce CSF pressure.

Naked-eye Appearance

Turbidity of the fluid usually indicates a polymorphonuclear pleocytosis; excessive lymphocytes, even in large number, rarely give visible changes. Some specimens of fluid which contain an excessive quantity of protein may clot on standing; a fine cobweb-like **fibrin deposit** appearing after a few hours also implies an increased protein content; it is seen in tuberculous meningitis and less commonly in poliomyelitis and meningovascular syphilis. Frank **blood** in the CSF may be present owing to puncture of a vertebral vein by the exploring needle, in which case the contamination of the fluid becomes less as it flows; if two test-tubes are filled, the second is less stained than the first, and if the specimen is centrifuged the supernatant fluid is clear. Uniform blood-staining is, however, seen in subarachnoid haemorrhage or if a primary cerebral haemorrhage has extended to the subarachnoid space; in such a case, the supernatant fluid, after centrifuging, generally shows a yellow coloration or **xanthochromia**. A faint colour, generally orange, appears within four hours of a subarachnoid bleed and is then due to the presence of oxyhaemoglobin; within 48 hours the deep yellow colour of bilirubin appears. This colour may persist for six weeks after a haemorrhage but usually disappears in from two to three weeks. Xanthochromia is also seen in CSF with a very high protein content (as in spinal tumour), in some patients with subdural bleeding, and in others who are deeply jaundiced. Spectrophotometric analysis of samples of fluid has shown that methaemalbumin is another pigment occasionally found in the CSF but this only appears as a rule as a result of extensive brain damage (as in severe head injury or cerebral haemorrhage).

Cytology

Many techniques of counting the white cells in the CSF are in common use. That most commonly used is to draw up 0.1 ml of methyl green diluting fluid in a white-cell-counting pipette and to fill the pipette with CSF. After mixing, the number of cells seen in the entire lined area of a Neubauer counting chamber is counted; this gives the number per mm^3 of fluid. Staining is usually good enough for red cells, lymphocytes and polymorphonuclear leucocytes to be identified. Tumour cells, yeasts and other abnormal cells are occasionally found but require specialised cytological techniques and skilled scrutiny for their recognition and interpretation.

A small number of **red cells** may be present due to the trauma of the puncture but if they persist in several specimens this can indicate a cerebral infarct, a haemorrhage approaching the surface of the brain, or bleeding into the subdural, as distinct from the subarachnoid space; the possibility of minor leakage from an intracranial aneurysm must also be considered. An increase in **white cells** generally implies inflammation in the meninges and this can be primary, as in meningitis, or secondary to diffuse cerebral disease, as in encephalitis. In general, polymorphonuclear leucocytes predominate in pyogenic infections such as coccal or influenzal meningitis and many thousands of cells may be present per mm^3 of fluid. As the condition resolves, so the polymorphs are gradually replaced by lymphocytes in decreasing numbers. In a case of cerebral abscess, without obvious meningitis, it is usual to find between 20 and 200 cells/mm^3 of which most are polymorphs. In tuberculous meningitis there is a polymorphonuclear reaction at the beginning of the illness but within a few days the pleocytosis is generally entirely mononuclear (lymphocytes and histiocytes) and usually of from 200 to 1,000 cells/mm^3. Meningovascular syphilis generally gives a mononuclear pleocytosis of up to 200 cells/mm^3, but some polymorphonuclears are present in the more acute cases; patients with tabes dorsalis rarely show an excess of cells in the fluid, but in patients with general paresis counts of from five to 50 lymphocytes/mm^3 are usual.

In viral infections such as encephalitis, lymphocytic meningitis and poliomyelitis, a moderate lymphocytic reaction, up to 1,000 cells/mm^3 is general, but in poliomyelitis a number of polymorphs, and even a predominance, may be seen in the first few days of the illness.

A slight pleocytosis, nearly always of lymphocytes, can also be found in many miscellaneous conditions, including cerebral tumour (primary or secondary), cerebral infarction, venous sinus thrombosis and multiple sclerosis. Only rarely in these conditions does the count exceed 40 to 50 cells/mm^3. In subarachnoid haemorrhage, too, the aseptic meningitis produced by blood in the CSF excites a moderate lymphocytic pleocytosis, and the number of white cells present is proportionately greater than would be expected from the number of red cells present. In occasional cases of intracranial tumour, particularly medulloblastomas in childhood, neoplastic cells, which look very like lymphocytes, are present in the fluid in comparative profusion. Specialised cytological techniques are sometimes helpful in identifying other varieties of tumour cells and are particularly valuable in diagnosing carcinomatosis of the meninges. Even with precise modern cytological techniques, malignant cells are detected in the fluid in only 10 per cent of cases of glioma and 20 per cent of patients with intracranial metastases. Immunofluorescent techniques of examining fresh or cultured cells obtained from CSF are being increasingly used in the rapid diagnosis of viral encephalitis.

Chemical Abnormalities

Protein

An increase in the protein content of the CSF is one of the commonest abnormalities discovered in neurological practice and also one of the most difficult to interpret. A rise to 0.5–5.0 g/l is usual in inflammatory disorders of the meninges such as meningitis and a lesser increase persists after the pleocytosis is no longer present; this is also true of poliomyelitis, in which disease a rise in protein without an increase in cells is sometimes seen only four or five days after the onset. A moderate increase, usually to about 1.0 g/l or less may be found in encephalitis, cerebral abscess, cerebral infarction, neurosyphilis (excluding tabes dorsalis), intracranial venous sinus thrombosis and multiple sclerosis. A similar moderate rise is common in patients with intracranial gliomas and metastases but extra-cerebral neoplasms such as meningiomas often give a higher value and the protein content of the fluid is usually well over 1.0 g/l in a patient with an acoustic neuroma. Particularly high values for CSF protein, often to as much as 10 g/l, are found in patients with postinfective polyneuropathy (the Guillain–Barré syndrome), and in these cases there is usually no pleocytosis ('*dissociation albuminocytologique*'). Virtually the only other circumstance in which similarly high readings are found in the lumbar CSF is in cases of spinal block, usually due to a spinal neoplasm, but occasionally resulting from vertebral collapse and angulation, extra-dural tumour or abscess, or arachnoiditis, which may be of undetermined aetiology, but sometimes follows chronic (especially tuberculous) meningitis. Often this fluid with a high-protein content is xanthochromic, and these signs, combined with a Queckenstedt test indicating a block, constitute Froin's syndrome. Minor degrees of spinal cord compression without complete block, as in cervical spondylosis, show less striking rises in the protein content of the fluid, rarely to above 1.0 g/l. A moderate rise usually below that value is also found sometimes in patients suffering from a recent prolapse of an intervertebral disk, either lumbar or cervical.

Albumin–globulin ratio. In the normal CSF the albumin–globulin ratio is approximately 8:1 but in many of the inflammatory conditions referred to above there is a selective rise in globulin. Pandy's test for the presence of excess globulin is now outmoded. Various techniques of electrophoresis, immunoprecipitation and electroimmunophoresis are now being used not only to estimate γ-globulin as a fraction of total CSF protein but also to fractionate IgG, IgA, IgM and IgD. These methods have shown that the total γ-globulin content of the fluid is usually raised in such diseases as multiple sclerosis, neurosyphilis and subacute sclerosing panencephalitis. If a relatively crude zinc sulphate precipitation method is used to measure total γ-globulin, this constitutes more than 25 per cent of the total protein in more than 40 per cent of cases of multiple sclerosis. However, with more precise modern techniques, over 14 per cent is now considered abnormal and in multiple sclerosis most of this is IgG; in this disease and in neurosyphilis the excess IgG present in CSF (when compared with the serum) appears to be produced in the central nervous system. Isoelectric focusing of CSF proteins seems likely to be of further diagnostic value.

Gold colloidal (Lange) curve. Selective changes in the protein content of the CSF account for variations in this curve, charted by noting the numbered colour reactions produced when various dilutions of fluid are added to Lange's colloidal gold solution. The test is outdated but is still used when estimation of CSF γ-globulin is not possible.

The normal Lange curve is 0000000000, but slight rises to 1 or even 2 in any of the tubes are not significant. The *paretic* or 'first-zone' curve (e.g. 5544322110) is characteristic of general paresis but also occurs occasionally in meningovascular syphilis, tabes dorsalis, multiple sclerosis (about 30 per cent of cases) and after subarachnoid haemorrhage. The *luetic* or tabetic curve (e.g. 0123322100) is usually found in tabes dorsalis or meningovascular syphilis, while the *meningitic* curve (e.g. 0001223210) is seen in meningitis of various types.

Sugar
Sugar disappears completely from the CSF in pyogenic meningitis, but in tuberculous meningitis, in meningeal carcinomatosis and sometimes in cerebral sarcoidosis, unlike lymphocytic meningitis, a moderate fall in glucose to about 0.20–0.45 g/l is often found.

Chlorides
The chlorides in the CSF run parallel to those in the blood and are therefore reduced in patients who have vomited frequently. For this reason they are usually low in tuberculous meningitis, but this has no diagnostic value.

Bromide
The CSF bromide level in the normal human is negligible, but if a patient is given a dose of bromide by mouth or injection, the drug soon appears in the CSF in one-third the concentration of that in the blood. In tuberculous meningitis, more than in any other condition, this serum–CSF bromide ratio after a dose of the drug is reduced from 3 to about unity and this has been used as a diagnostic test. A similar finding may be obtained in carcinomatosis of the meninges.

Hydrogen Ion Concentration
The hydrogen ion concentration of the blood is normally maintained within narrow limits at a pH of about 7.31. While the most important factor in controlling pulmonary ventilation is the CO_2 tension (pCO_2) of the arterial blood and its effect upon chemoreceptors in the medulla, the pH of the

CSF also has some influence through its effect upon the pH of the cerebral extracellular fluid with which it is in equilibrium. In chronic hypercapnia the brain produces increased amounts of ammonia which are reflected in the CSF by an increase in glutamine. The CSF pH and hence that of the cerebral extracellular fluid also influence cerebral vascular resistance; hypercapnia produces vasodilatation, hypocapnia vasoconstriction.

Enzymes
Much work has been done in recent years upon the concentration of various enzymes (such as the aminotransfcrascs, lactate dehydrogenase, creatine kinase, non-specific esterases and various proteinases) in the CSF, and while abnormalities have been found in various disease states, these have not been shown to be of diagnostic value.

Sterols
Desmosterol appears in the CSF after the administration of triparanol and the CSF cholesterol is raised in patients with glioma, but the specificity of this finding remains uncertain.

Amines
5-hydroxyindoleacetic acid (5-HIAA), a metabolitc of scrotonin, and homovanillic acid (HVA), a metabolite of dopamine, are both present in the CSF. They are each reduced in concentration in Parkinson's disease and may rise after treatment with levodopa. Changes in these amines in patients with migraine and various mental diseases have also been reported.

Microbiological Examination
If turbid CSF is removed, a smear should be stained with Gram's stain and examined for micro-organisms and another specimen cultured. In pneumococcal, staphylococcal, streptococcal and influenzal meningitis the causal organisms are usually profuse in a direct smear, but meningococci may be difficult to find and culture. Tubercle bacilli should also be looked for in preparations stained by the Ziehl – Neelsen or auramine techniques and are usually found in cases of tuberculous meningitis after an assiduous search, particularly if a fibrin 'web' can be examined. If no bacilli are found, confirmation of the diagnosis depends upon finding the organisms on culture on Lowenstein-Jensen slopes or guinea-pig inoculation, but these measures take about six weeks. In some cases of chronic meningitis, special culture media (e.g. Sabouraud's medium for cryptococcosis and Korthof's for leptospirosis) are required for the identification of some rare infections. Virological studies carried out on CSF tend to give results only when the illness is over but are useful even at this stage in establishing the nature of the organism responsible for some obscure infections of the nervous system. However, newer techniques of immunofluorescent staining for

viral antibodies have added precision to early diagnosis. Serological tests for syphilis, such as the Wassermann, Kahn, VDRL, treponema immobilisation, and the even more specific fluorescent treponema antibody absorption (FTA–ABS) reactions are sometimes positive in the CSF but negative in the blood of cases of neurosyphilis.

Electroencephalography (EEG)

Electroencephalography is a technique of recording the electrical activity of the brain through the intact skull. Electrodes are applied to the scalp and the potential changes so recorded are amplified and presented for interpretation as an inked tracing on moving paper. Machines in common use have eight, sixteen or more channels so that the activity from many different areas of the head can be recorded simultaneously. The technique is simple and harmless and may give valuable diagnostic information.

In the normal adult the dominant electrical activity in the EEG from the post-central areas is usually a sinusoidal wave form with a frequency of 8–13 Hz. This is the alpha rhythm; it commonly disappears on attention, as when the eyes open. Normally there is often some faster or so-called beta activity (14–22 Hz) in the frontal regions; this is accentuated by barbiturates and sometimes by anxiety. In young infants the EEG is dominated by generalised slow activity of delta frequency (up to 3.5 Hz); gradually during maturation this is replaced by theta activity (4–7 Hz) and subsequently by the alpha rhythm. Theta activity disappears last from the posterior temporal regions, particularly on the right side, and the record is usually fully mature, showing no theta activity, by the age of from 12 to 14 years. During drowsiness and sleep in the normal adult, theta activity and later delta activity reappear. Some common EEG appearances are illustrated in Fig. 1.

The EEG is of particular value in the diagnosis of **epilepsy**. In **petit mal** it often shows regular, rhythmical, generalised outbursts of repetitive complexes, each consisting of a spike and a delta wave (spike-and-wave), and recurring at a frequency of about 3 Hz. In idiopathic or 'centrencephalic' **major epilepsy**, the inter-seizure record may show brief generalised outbursts of spikes or sharp waves, or of mixed spikes and slow activity (an irregular spike-and-wave discharge). In patients suffering from **focal epilepsy**, including **temporal lobe or 'psychomotor' attacks**, there are often spikes, sharp waves or rhythmical outbursts of slow (delta or theta) activity arising in the epileptogenic area of cortex. Unfortunately, a single record taken in an epileptic patient is often normal; positive findings are commoner in children and less common the older the patient. Many other patients show non-specific abnormalities, such as excessive temporal theta activity, a finding often attributed to immaturity in the broadest sense. Hence, it may be necessary to take repeated recordings or to use various

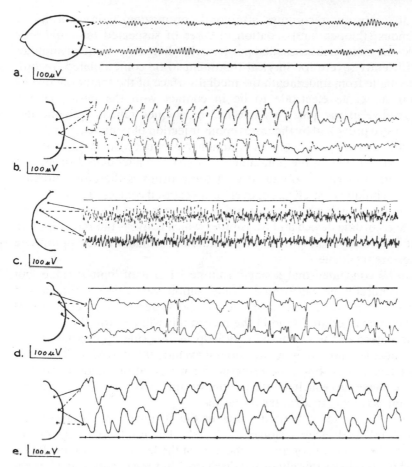

Fig. 1. Some common appearances in electroencephalographic (EEG) recordings.
a. A normal alpha rhythm recorded from both occipital regions and disappearing (in the centre of the recording) when the eyes are open.
b. A 3Hz spike-and-wave discharge of petit mal epilepsy, recorded in this illustration from the right temporal region.
c. High-frequency discharges (mainly muscle artefact) recorded from the left fronto-temporal region during a major epileptic seizure.
d. A right anterior-temporal focus of spike discharge in a patient suffering from temporal lobe epilepsy.
e. A focus of high-amplitude delta activity seen in the right mid-temporal region in a patient suffering from a cerebral abscess in this situation.

activation techniques in order to uncover epileptic discharges. Overbreathing for from two to three minutes is particularly effective in evoking the discharges of petit mal, while photic stimulation (repetitive light flashes of variable frequency) can also bring out epileptic discharges. Since temporal spikes or sharp waves often appear in early sleep it has become conventional to carry out recordings after oral (promazine hydrochloride) or intravenous (thiopentone) sedation in cases of suspected temporal lobe epilepsy. In some such cases, and particularly when the patient's symptoms are sufficiently severe for surgical treatment to be contemplated, recordings are made from underneath the medial surface of the temporal lobe by inserting a needle electrode to lie in contact with the basi-sphenoid. Occasionally, in the past, when other techniques failed, epileptic discharges were provoked by the intravenous injection of pentylenetetrazol or bemigride, but these substances commonly produce clinical convulsions and may do so even in the non-epileptic if given in adequate dosage. The interpretation of results obtained with these drugs is therefore difficult, and this technique is rarely used, even in specialised centres. Telemetering, a technique through which prolonged recording is possible using a simple portable recording device and transmitter which conveys the recording to a distant laboratory, has proved of considerable value where appropriate facilities are available.

It can be concluded that a single routine EEG is of limited value, but should generally be performed, using simple activation techniques if necessary, in most patients suspected to be suffering from epilepsy. If epileptic discharges are found in the record this will confirm the diagnosis and the nature of the discharge may help in choosing appropriate treatment. Negative findings, however, do not exclude this diagnosis. The more difficult techniques should be reserved for use in intractable or problem cases or those in which confirmation of the diagnosis is particularly important, say, for, medico-legal reasons.

The EEG is also of limited value in the diagnosis of **focal cerebral lesions**. A relatively acute lesion of one cerebral hemisphere usually gives a focus of delta activity in or around the area of the lesion. It is not the lesion itself which produces this abnormal discharge, but the changes which it has produced in the surrounding brain. A **cerebral abscess** usually produces a very slow discharge of high amplitude, and similar though less striking abnormalities result from **tumour, haemorrhage, local injury** or **infarction**. Thus the EEG can give some clue to localisation, but is of little help in pathological diagnosis, which must depend upon clinical and other information, or upon progressive changes occurring in a series of records. An abnormality due to a tumour usually becomes worse, while that due to an infarct tends to improve. In the case of lesions which are more chronic or more deeply situated in the cerebral hemisphere, focal theta activity of low amplitude, or even absence of the alpha rhythm or of beta activity which is present on the other side, may be the only abnormality. Indeed in some patients with chronic, slowly growing tumours, such as meningiomas, the record is normal. However, some localised abnormality is found in upwards of 70 per cent of patients with cerebral neoplasms. A **subdural haematoma** is another condition which may be revealed by the EEG, as such cases often show a unilateral suppression of the alpha rhythm and some irregular slow activity on the affected side. While the EEG was regularly used in the past as an aid to diagnosis of such intracranial space-occupying lesions, if only because the more precise radiological methods were more risky and uncomfortable for the patient, the advent of the CAT scan (*see below*) has meant that the EEG is now rarely used for this purpose.

Certain rare conditions such as **subacute sclerosing panencephalitis (SSPE)** also show characteristic findings, but in many chronic neurological disorders such as **Parkinsonism** and **multiple sclerosis** the EEG is usually normal. In SSPE isolated bizarre slow-wave complexes occur simultaneously in all channels against a background of comparative electrical silence, while in some children with cerebral lipidosis or in adults with certain rapidly progressive degenerative disorders of the brain (e.g. **Creutzfeldt–Jakob disease**) generalised and almost continuous irregular spike-and-wave discharge may be seen. A similar severe abnormality, often called hypsarrhythmia, may be found in records from infants suffering from so-called **infantile spasms** (*see* p. 127). Tumours in the posterior fossa or deeply situated lesions near the midline often give paroxysmal outbursts of theta or delta activity at the surface, but these changes are by no means specific as they occur in patients with many diffuse cerebral disorders including **meningitis, subarachnoid haemorrhage** and **encephalitis** or conditions causing **disorders of cerebral metabolism** such as anoxia, uraemia, hyperglycaemia, hepatic coma or pernicious anaemia. Similar non-specific abnormalities are found in patients who are confused or comatose from any cause.

The EEG is of little value in **psychiatric diagnosis** although anxious and obsessional patients often show excessive frontal fast activity, while **psychopaths** and children with **behaviour disorders** have typically immature records with excessive temporal slow activity, particularly on the right side posteriorly. Patients with **organic dementia** often show a dominant rhythm of theta rather than alpha frequency; this is in a sense a reversion to the childhood pattern and may even occur in ageing without dementia; it is certainly not specific.

Hence the EEG has considerable value in the diagnosis of epilepsy and of certain uncommon brain diseases in which relatively specific abnormalities are found; it is now less useful in the investigation of patients with suspected intracranial tumour or haemorrhage. Repeated studies often help in assessing the response to treatment of certain diffuse metabolic disturbances. The method also has considerable research applications.

Evoked Potential Recording

The increased sophistication of electrophysiological techniques and of equipment for stimulating and recording, as well as the introduction of small computers and microprocessors, has resulted in the increasing utilisation of techniques of evoked potential recoding in neurological diagnosis. These generally require a variety of methods of summation and averaging of the potentials which are to be recorded and are still available only in a limited number of centres. However, methods of visual evoked potential recording, using light flashes or more often patterned visual stimuli, and recording electrodes placed over the occipital lobes, have been successful in identifying delays in the transmission of the stimuli indicating, for example, unsuspected lesions of one or both optic nerves in patients with known or suspected multiple sclerosis. Similarly it is possible to measure auditory evoked potentials which give information about the integrity of the cochlea, the auditory nerve and the auditory cortex, and methods of evoked potential audiometry are now in common use. Information about the integrity of ascending sensory pathways in the spinal cord and brain can also be obtained from stimulating an extremity and then recording the arrival of the stimulus over the spinal column (the spinal evoked potential) or over the sensory cortex (the somatosensory cortical evoked potential).

Echo-encephalography

Ultrasound has been used in neurological diagnosis for over 25 years. A number of simple and relatively inexpensive machines are available commercially which pass an ultrasonic beam horizontally through the intact skull and an 'echo' is recorded from mid-line structures (the 'A' scan). A 'shift' of the mid-line can readily be demonstrated and this method, which carries no risk to the patient, is of value in confirming rapidly the presence of a space-occupying lesion in or overlying one cerebral hemisphere. Thus, the method can be used for rapid screening of patients in whom, for instance, a subdural or extradural haematoma or a cerebral tumour is suspected. More complicated and refined techniques have been introduced in order to define the 'echoes' arising from intra-cranial structures other than those in the mid-line (the 'B'-scan) but these have been largely supplanted by the more accurate technique of computerised transaxial tomography (the CAT scan).

Gamma-encephalography

Scanning of the radioactivity recorded over the skull surface following the intravenous injection of a suitable isotope (^{99}Technetium is commonly used) has been widely employed in neurological and neurosurgical units as an aid to the diagnosis of intracranial lesions. The blood vessels, and probably the cells of certain tumours, show a selective affinity for such

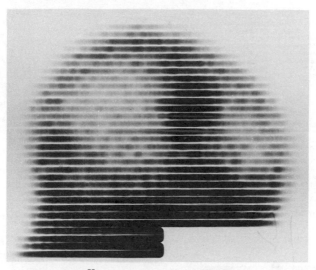

A. Right lateral ^{99}Technetium scan from a female patient aged 42 years, showing increased radioactivity in the posterior frontal region resulting from a large arteriovenous malformation.

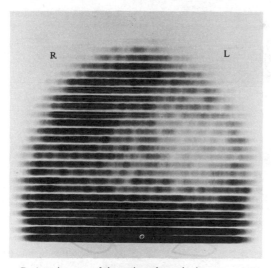

B. Anterior scan of the patient shown in A.

Plate II. Some representative gamma-encephalograms.

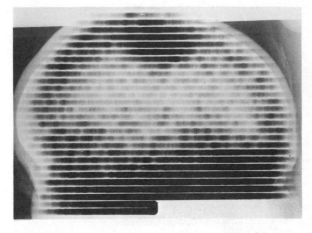

C. Right lateral ^{99}Technetium scan from a female patient aged 54 years. There is increased uptake of the isotope in the right fronto-parietal region caused by a parasagittal meningioma.

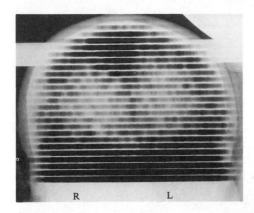

D. Anterior scan of the patient shown in C.

R   L

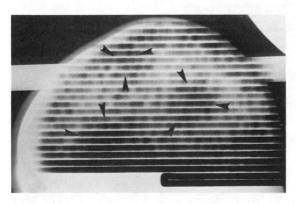

E. Left lateral ^{99}Technetium scan from a male patient aged 55 years. There are multiple areas (arrowed) of increased radioactivity due to cerebral metastases from a primary bronchogenic carcinoma.

Plate II (contd.)

isotopes so that the tumour is shown as an area of increased radioactivity. With lateral and anteroposterior 'scans', localisation may be very accurate. However, uptake may also be increased in an infarct, This technique is particularly valuable in demonstrating multiple intracranial lesions (e.g. metastases)—see Plate II.

Isotope Ventriculography

If a small amount of radio-iodinated serum albumin (RISA) is injected by lumbar puncture in a normal individual and the skull is then 'scanned', a few hours later radioactivity is seen in the subarachnoid space over the brain surface and not, as a rule, in the cerebral ventricles. If, however, the lateral ventricles soon show radioactivity and if little or no isotope flows over the surface towards the sagittal sinus, then communicating hydrocephalus is likely to be present. This technique is also useful in detecting fistulous communications between the subarachnoid space and the middle ear or paranasal sinuses such as may occur after head injury, otitis media, or sinusitis.

Studies of Peripheral Nerve and Muscle Function

Many methods of electrodiagnosis are in common use to study peripheral nerve function. It has long been known that motor nerves respond to an applied electrical current of brief duration (faradism) and that muscle, even when it has lost its motor nerve supply, will contract, though sluggishly, in response to a long-duration current (galvanism). In Erb's **reaction of degeneration** (R.D.) there is loss of the response to faradism and retention of that to galvanism, a finding which implies denervation. However this classical method did not indicate whether this was partial or complete; to overcome this difficulty, the method was replaced by the charting of **strength-duration** (S.D.) curves which are more quantitative.

To chart an S.D. curve, a square-wave electrical stimulator is used, so designed as to give a current (or voltage) which remains constant independently of varying resistance in the patient's tissues. An electrode is applied to the motor point (where the motor nerve enters) of the muscle under test, and an earth electrode is placed on the skin elsewhere. A square wave of long duration is then applied repetitively and the current (or voltage) is gradually increased until a muscular contraction is just produced. The procedure is then repeated with square waves of increasingly brief duration and the current (or voltage) required on each occasion is charted. Typical curves are obtained for normally innervated, totally denervated and partially denervated muscle. Since many muscles can be tested it is therefore possible to determine which have lost their nerve supply, and approximately to what extent.

This technique is of some value in studying patients with **peripheral nerve lesions** and in some with **neuromuscular disease**. It also has a prognostic value, as characteristic changes occur during re-innervation. It may also suggest a diagnosis of **myasthenia gravis** since, in some such cases, muscular contractions become progressively more feeble during repeated nerve stimulation. In **myotonia**, by contrast, there is a prolonged after-contraction with delayed relaxation. While this method is still used in some departments of physical medicine and rehabilitation, it has gradually been discarded in favour of newer methods of electromyography and nerve conduction velocity measurement.

Electromyography (EMG)

Electromyography is a technique of recording the electrical activity produced by muscle at rest and during contraction. Surface electrodes can be used but are only useful for physiological studies, in determining, for instance, which muscles contribute to a particular movement, or for recording the frequency of involuntary movements (e.g. tremor). For most diagnostic work, bipolar concentric needle electrodes are inserted into the muscle being tested; the electrical activity is then passed through a high-gain amplifier and is presented for interpretation both on an oscilloscope screen and in a loudspeaker. Sometimes the visual trace is more valuable, sometimes the auditory pattern, but the combination is more valuable than either alone. **Normal voluntary muscle** is electrically silent at rest, but on contraction motor-unit potentials are seen and appear in increasing number and frequency as contraction increases, to give a continuous trace across the screen and a low-pitched rumble in the loudspeaker. These potentials are smooth, monophasic, diphasic or triphasic waves, each about 5–8 msec in duration and about 1 mV in amplitude. They are generally known as motor unit action potentials, as it was once thought that each resulted from the contraction of all of the muscle fibres innervated by one anterior horn cell and its axon (a motor unit). It now seems more probable that these potentials are due to the contraction of only a few component fibres of the motor unit which happen to be close to the recording electrode (a 'sub-unit').

When a muscle **loses its nerve supply,** spontaneous **fibrillation** or contraction of individual muscle fibres begins within 14 to 21 days and can be recorded from the relaxed and resting muscle; it takes the form of a series of repetitive small spikes on the screen and a ticking noise in the loudspeaker. If the muscle has lost only a part of its nerve supply, some motor unit potentials will still appear on attempted contraction, but the pattern of voluntary effort will be much reduced. During re-innervation after nerve regeneration complex polyphasic potentials of long duration appear, so-called **recovery potentials**; their long duration is due to the fact that regenerating nerve sprouts, which re-innervate previously denervated muscle fibres, conduct at different rates. Hence in patients with disease of the motor neurone at any point from the anterior horn cell to the motor end-plate the EMG will show spontaneous fibrillation and a **reduced pattern** of motor units on voluntary effort. When the lesion is in the anterior horn cells some of the surviving motor unit action potentials (**'giant' units**) may be unusually large (up to 5 mV in amplitude and 10 msec in duration); this is because collateral axonal sprouts from surviving neurones may 'adopt' and re-innervate some denervated muscle fibres. Sometimes in disorders of the anterior horn cell there are also spontaneous **fasciculation potentials** which look like normal motor unit potentials but are recorded from the resting muscle, while if there is nerve or nerve root irritation, groups of two or three motor unit potentials may be recorded, again from a muscle which is apparently at rest.

In **primary diseases of muscle**, such as muscular dystrophy, the pattern is different. Spontaneous activity such as fibrillation is scanty or absent, and on volition the motor unit potentials are seen to be broken-up, **polyphasic** and of **short duration**. Hence the pattern is complex and spiky and the noise in the loudspeaker is a crackling sound, like hail on a tin roof. The phenomenon of **myotonia** also gives a characteristic EMG; chains of oscillations of high frequency are seen which give a typical 'snarling' or 'dive-bomber' sound in the loudspeaker.

The technique of **single fibre electromyography**, introduced recently, involves the use of a needle multielectrode which has many tiny openings in its 'shell', so that the different exposed parts of the core each function as electrodes recording from the surface of the individual muscle fibres with which they come into contact. If one supposes that the axon derived from one anterior horn cell divides within the muscle so that each terminal branch innervates a single muscle fibre, this type of electrode can be used to record contraction of the individual fibres. If for some reason the nerve impulse in one nerve twig arrives after that in another branch has reached the adjacent muscle fibre, then there will be an interval between the potentials derived from each of the muscle fibres; this interval is known as **jitter**. And if, during repeated muscular contraction, whether voluntary or electrically induced, one such potential disappears, this is known as **blocking** and may indicate either a failure of conduction in the nerve branch concerned, or more probably a failure of neuromuscular transmission at its motor end-plate, as in myasthenia gravis. The measurement of these phenomena has proved to be of considerable diagnostic value.

The electromyogram is thus of considerable value in neurological diagnosis. It is of particular use in investigating peripheral nerve injuries and in studying cases of muscular wasting and weakness in which it is especially helpful in distinguishing disease of the muscle from that of the motor nerves.

Nerve Conduction Velocity

By stimulating a motor nerve at two separate points along its course and by recording the motor unit potentials so produced from an appropriate muscle, it is possible to measure the stimulus–contraction delay interval in each case and hence to calculate the rate of conduction of the impulse along the nerve. For accurate recording the temperature of the limb must be carefully controlled. Nerve conduction is slowed in some forms of polyneuropathy and the technique can also be utilised to localise focal lesions in nerves, such as compression of the median nerve in the carpal tunnel, of the ulnar nerve at the elbow or of the common peroneal nerve at the neck of the fibula. Thus, if one applies a supramaximal stimulus to the median nerve in the cubital fossa and records the muscle action potential evoked in the opponens pollicis, a similar action potential can then be obtained by stimulating the nerve at the wrist. By measuring the stimulus–contraction latency in each case and the distance between the stimulating electrodes, the conduction velocity in the forearm segment of the nerve can be calculated. If the nerve is compressed in the carpal tunnel then 'terminal latency' (normally 5 msec or less) is increased.

The normal conduction velocity in the adult is 50–60 m/sec in the median, ulnar and radial nerves and 45–50 m/sec in the common peroneal. In demyelinating peripheral neuropathies conduction is markedly slowed, while in those accompanied by axonal degeneration the surviving axons conduct at a normal rate but the amplitude of the evoked muscle action potential is reduced. Measurement of the conduction velocity in sensory fibres, stimulated by ring electrodes on a digit and picking up the sensory volley by an electrode over the nerve trunk, is also widely used for diagnosis. These techniques involve the measurement of sensory nerve action potential (SNAP) amplitude and latency in such nerves as the median and ulnar in the upper limbs and the common peroneal and sural in the lower.

If one refers to the action potential recorded from, say, the calf muscles on stimulation of the sciatic nerve as the M-response, there is a second wave form of longer latency which follows it and is called the H-reflex. This results from the fact that the stimulus applied to the trunk of the nerve also produces an afferent volley in the sensory fibres of the nerve and this volley reflexly excites anterior horn cells in the same segment of the cord to send a further action potential down their axons to produce this second muscle action potential. A somewhat similar wave form can be seen in the small muscles of the hands after stimulation say of the ulnar nerve and is called the F-wave. Measurement of these wave forms and of their latencies can give information about conduction velocity in proximal segments of the respective nerves.

Studies of Sensory Nerve Function

If a nerve is made ischaemic, by inflating a sphygmomanometer cuff around a limb to above the systolic arterial blood pressure, ischaemic paraesthesiae develop in the skin areas supplied by the nerve concerned within 5 to 10 minutes. On release of the cuff post-ischaemic paraesthesiae are experienced. If the blood supply of the nerve concerned is already reduced due to pressure, ischaemic paraesthesiae appear earlier, perhaps within one or two minutes and post-ischaemic paraesthesiae are more severe. This technique is of some value in diagnosing pressure lesions of peripheral nerves, such as median nerve compression in the carpal tunnel.

Motor End-plate Dysfunction

If repetitive supramaximal shocks are applied to the ulnar nerve at the elbow at 3–5/sec and the evoked motor action potential is recorded from the hypothenar muscles, then in a patient with myasthenia gravis in whom these muscles are affected by the disease it is usual to find a progressive decrement in the amplitude of the evoked response. This abnormality may be corrected temporarily by an intravenous injection of edrophonium hydrochloride (*'Tensilon'*); a similar decrement usually occurs at fast rates (50/sec) of stimulation which produce a muscle tetanus. By contrast, in the myasthenic-myopathic (Eaton–Lambert) syndrome which may complicate bronchial carcinoma, the evoked potential is initially of low amplitude and a striking increment in amplitude is obtained at fast stimulation frequencies. Weakness in this condition is little influenced by edrophonium but may be corrected by guanidine hydrochloride.

As mentioned above, increased jitter and blocking in single fibre electromyography are also of considerable help in the diagnosis of myasthenia.

Radiology

Radiological methods are among the most helpful and widely-used of all the ancillary techniques used in neurological diagnosis. While final diagnosis often depends upon highly specialised methods involving computerised tomography or the use of air or other contrast media, each of these techniques, which will be considered below, is time-consuming, expensive and some are disturbing to the patient. It must therefore be remembered that valuable and even conclusive information can sometimes be obtained from plain radiographs of the skull and/or spine and even of other parts of the body. Thus in patients with a clinical picture suggestive of intracranial tumour, or in others with a subacute meningitic illness, it is important to X-ray the chest, as in one case a bronchogenic carcinoma may be revealed suggesting a metastatic intracranial lesion, while in another the appearances of pulmonary tuberculosis may be discovered. In other cases changes in the skeleton will cast light upon the significance of neurological symptoms and signs as, for instance, in cases of prostatic carcinoma or multiple myelomatosis.

Straight Radiography of the Skull

It is usual to take routine anteroposterior and lateral views of the skull, while in most specialised centres an anteroposterior view is also taken with the brow depressed some 35° so that the petrous temporal bones become visible (Towne's view), and another of the skull base. Stenver's view is also utilised to examine the petrous temporal bone. Usually the **skull vault** is first examined to see if there is reasonable uniformity of bony thickness or whether there is any **erosion** or **bony overgrowth** (as may result from a meningioma) or **abnormal vascular markings** due to dilatation of the middle meningeal artery which is supplying a meningeal tumour or vascular malformation. Sometimes, as in carcinomatosis or myelomatosis, there are multiple areas of **bony rarefaction** in the skull vault or there is a general thickening or 'woolliness' of the bone as in Paget's disease. In young children, hydrocephalus due to any cause gives **separation of the cranial sutures** and a characteristic **'beaten copper' mottling** of the bone. However, the latter appearance is so often seen in normal individuals, even in adult life, that in itself it is not diagnostic. Fractures of the vault are, of course, noted if present, and it is also wise to examine the frontal, maxillary and sphenoidal paranasal sinuses for opacities which would suggest infection or neoplasia. **Hyperostosis** of the inner table of the frontal bone is not uncommon but has no definite pathological significance.

The **base of the skull** is next examined, first in the lateral projection. Here the relationship of the upper **cervical spine** to the **foramen magnum** is observed and it is noted whether there is any protrusion of the odontoid process of the axis above Chamberlain's line which joins the posterior margin of the hard palate to the posterior lip of the foramen magnum. If the odontoid does show above this line, or if there is an abnormal tilt of the body of the atlas implying invagination of the basi-occiput, then **basilar impression,** which may give important neurological symptoms and signs, is present. However, the most important structure in the skull base which is visible on the lateral projection is the **sella turcica**. Its size and shape and the integrity and density of the anterior and posterior clinoid processes which form its lips are noted. In patients with primary pituitary neoplasms the sella is expanded or ballooned and partially decalcified. In those with suprasellar lesions the sella is also expanded, but is shallower and flattened and there is often erosion of the clinoid processes. Moderate flattening and expansion of the sella with decalcification of the posterior clinoid processes may occur in any patient with increased intracranial pressure whether there is a lesion near the sella or not.

Also to be noted on the lateral projection is the presence or absence of **intracranial calcification**. If present, such calcification is then more accurately localised in anteroposterior views, or sometimes by stereoscopic lateral projections. In about 50 per cent of adults, and even in some normal children, the **pineal gland,** which lies above and behind the sella, is calcified and may even measure up to 0.5 cm in diameter. If the gland is calcified it is important to measure its distance from the inner table of the skull at either side on anteroposterior radiographs, as lateral displacement may indicate the presence of a space-occupying lesion in one cerebral hemisphere. Other intracranial structures which occasionally calcify in the normal individual are the choroid plexuses, the falx cerebri and the petro-clinoid ligaments. **Pathological intracranial calcification**, if mottled in type and suprasellar in situation, usually indicates a craniopharyngioma, but many other intracranial tumours, including meningiomas, gliomas and oligodendrogliomas, occasionally show a fine spidery pattern of calcification. Fine curvilinear lines of calcification are rarely seen in the wall of a large aneurysm, while calcific stippling or even dense calcification may occur within a haematoma or in an arteriovenous angioma. Rare causes of intracranial calcification include cysticercosis (calcified cysts), toxoplasmosis (mottling in the basal ganglia) and hypoparathyroidism (also in the basal ganglia). A form of calcification outlining clearly the gyri of one occipital and/or parietal lobe is seen in diffuse cortical angiomatosis associated with a port-wine naevus of the face (the Sturge–Weber syndrome).

In anteroposterior, Towne's, Stenver's and the basal views, the most important feature to look for is **enlargement or erosion of cranial exit foramina. Sclerosis and overgrowth of bone** may also occur, particularly in the wings of the sphenoid, in patients who have a meningioma in this region. Otherwise it is usual to examine the optic foramina, superior orbital fissures, and internal auditory meati particularly. A funnel-shaped erosion of the internal auditory meati, revealed by Towne's and Stenver's views, is characteristic of acoustic neuroma. The basal view may reveal bony erosion due to malignant infiltration of the base of the skull or enlargement of one foramen spinosum due to a meningioma producing dilatation of one middle meningeal artery.

Radiology of the Spinal Column

In examining radiographs of the spine we are concerned first with changes in the **vertebrae** themselves, secondly with the **intervertebral disks** and thirdly with the **intervertebral foramina**. It is usual to carry out anteroposterior and lateral views to study the vertebrae and disks, but to examine the intervertebral foramina, oblique views are needed. In the vertebrae themselves one may observe **congenital abnormalities** such as **fusion** of several vertebral bodies (if in the cervical region this is called the Klippel–Feil syndrome) or **spina bifida**, either of which may be responsible for, or associated with, neurological signs. Fracture, fracture-dislocation, Paget's disease, osteomyelitis, neoplasia, either benign or malignant, of vertebral bodies, any one of which can give vertebral collapse and spinal cord compression, are generally revealed by routine X-rays. **Bony erosion** and, in particular, enlargement of the relevant intervertebral foramen is typically seen, often with the extraspinal soft tissue shadow of a dumb-bell tumour, in cases of spinal neurofibroma. Less striking but of equal diagnostic importance is a **variation in interpedicular distance**. The distance between the vertebral pedicles is large in the cervical region, diminishes to a minimum in the mid-dorsal region, and then expands again in the lumbar region, corresponding to the cervical and lumbar enlargements of the spinal cord. If successive interpedicular distances are measured and one or more measurement falls outside the expected arithmetical progression, this indicates an expanding lesion within the spinal cord or spinal canal in this region. Dorsal meningiomas may produce no more radiological change than this, whereas neurofibromas commonly give bony erosion as well. Measurement of the **anteroposterior diameter** of the spinal canal is also of value, particularly in the cervical region; an unduly wide canal is seen, for instance, in some cases of syringomyelia. A narrow canal may contribute to the early development of symptoms of myelopathy in patients with spondylosis.

In a patient with an acute **intervertebral disk prolapse**, radiographs of the spine are often normal or reveal simply narrowing of the disk space concerned. The prolapsed disk is not itself radio-opaque. If one or more disk protrusions have been present for months or years, the margins of the prolapsed tissue gradually become calcified, giving posterior (and often anterior) **osteophyte formation** at the upper and lower borders of the contiguous vertebrae. As the prolapsed tissue often projects laterally as well, osteophytes also tend to encroach upon the intervertebral foramina and this change is shown on oblique views. A combination of changes of this type, which are most often found in the cervical and lumbar regions, is referred to as **spondylosis**.

Computerised Transaxial Tomography (the CAT, CTT or CT scan)

The introduction of this technique, largely in the last decade, has transformed the practice of clinical neurology, especially in relation to the diagnosis of intracranial lesions, just as it seems likely that the more widespread use of the whole-body scanner will facilitate the more accurate diagnosis, for example, of lesions within the thoracic and abdominal cavities (and in the spinal column and canal) in the next decade.

The first apparatus commercially available, developed by Dr Godfrey Hounsfield of Bristol, was manufactured by the British Company, EMI Ltd, and hence the earliest records were often called Emiscans. The technique depends upon the movement of an X-ray generator along a tangent in relation to the skull and the simultaneous movement on the opposite side of the head of a crystal which detects the photon beam transmission. The method gives scans of the head in a series of horizontal slices each 8 mm in depth. In one traverse 160 readings of photon transmission are obtained. As the instrument is rotated 180° around the head to give new readings after each degree of movement, the entire skull, the orbits and the intracranial and orbital cavities are scanned, giving a total of 28,800 readings of photon transmission. These readings are analysed by computer so that on a cathode ray tube images corresponding to the relative densities of the tissues scanned are recorded and can be photographed and stored on magnetic tape or disks. The entire procedure takes about 20 minutes; it gives rise to no discomfort and is harmless, the total exposure to X-rays simply corresponding to that involved in taking a series of routine skull X-rays. Confused or restless patients and children may require sedation as the head must be held still during the recording.

Using this technique the brain parenchyma, ventricular system, the CSF cisterns, the pineal, falx cerebri, brain stem, cerebellar hemispheres, orbital contents and even individual intracranial arteries can be visualized. In general, most neoplasms can be seen as areas of increased density unless their centre is necrotic or cystic when a rim of dense tumour around a translucent area is seen, an appearance which may resemble that of an abscess. Areas of haemorrhage, too, usually show typical increased density, whether in the extra-dural, subdural, subarachnoid or ventricular spaces or within the brain substance. Infarcts are generally apparent as areas of reduced density, as are plaques of demyelination, while cerebral atrophy can be diagnosed when the cortical sulci are widened and the ventricles enlarged. The use of contrast enhancement, following the intravenous injection of meglamine iothalamate (*Conray*) increases the absorption coefficient of some normal and many abnormal intracranial tissues so that vascular malformations, many tumours and even areas of haemorrhage may show greatly increased density afterwards, for several hours. Several representative CAT scans are illustrated in Plate III.

The CAT scan at present is rather less successful in identifying lesions in the posterior fossa than in the cerebral hemispheres. For a lesion to be visualised it must have a density different from that of the surrounding brain and must be 5 mm or more in diameter. Nevertheless the diagnostic yield of this technique is far greater than that of any of the contrast methods (to be described below) upon which neurologists and neurosurgeons were compelled to rely before its introduction. Whether the newer technique of positron emission computerised tomography, now being introduced, will add even greater precision to diagnosis will become apparent within the next decade.

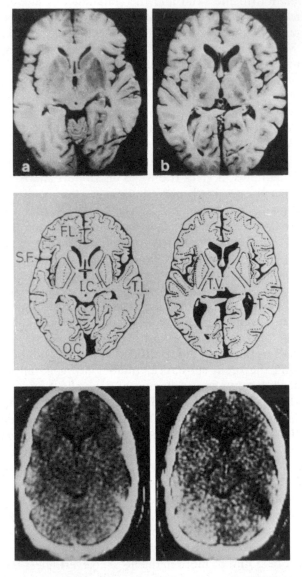

A. A normal computerised transaxial tomogram (a CAT scan) above, showing the cerebral ventricular outlines at different sagittal planes, as seen in the brain slices below and the diagram in between.

Plate III. Some representative CAT scans

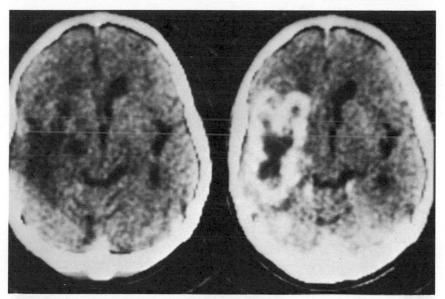

B. A CAT scan showing an encapsulated cerebral abscess in the L. temporal region. This is seen as an area of reduced density in the left-hand scan. The scan on the right, after contrast enhancement, shows the capsule of the abscess clearly.

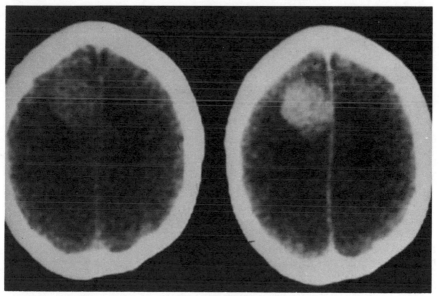

C. A CAT scan showing a left frontal haematoma due to head injury, without (on the left) and with (on the right) contrast enhancement.

Plate III (contd.)

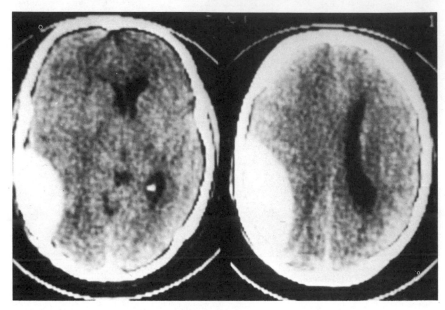

D. A CAT scan of a large left temporo-parietal extracerebral haematoma.

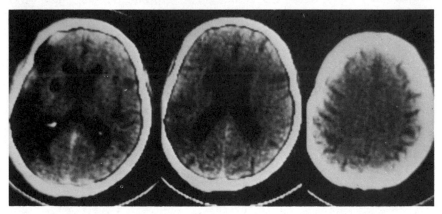

E. A CAT scan showing ventricular dilatation and widened sulci due to cortical atrophy in a patient with presenile dementia.

Plate III (contd.)

Contrast Methods

Before the advent of the CAT scan, the methods most often used in the diagnosis of intracranial lesions were first the outlining of the cerebral ventricular system with air or oxygen either by injection through a lumbar puncture needle (**air encephalography or pneumoencephalography**) or by **ventriculography**, which involved inserting a needle into one lateral ventricle via a burr-hole in the skull vault. Sometimes for greater diagnostic accuracy air ventriculography was followed by the injection of an oily or a water-soluble contrast medium into the ventricular system. Air encephalography was usually performed in patients in whom intracranial tumour, communicating ('low-pressure') hydrocephalus or cortical atrophy were suspected but in whom there were no symptoms or signs of increased intracranial pressure which contraindicated lumbar puncture, while ventriculography was felt to be needed in patients with suspected posterior fossa tumours or in those with suspected neoplasia in one or other cerebral hemisphere in whom angiography and the gamma scan had given inadequate or conflicting information. Now, in centres where the CAT scan is available, these investigations are virtually never performed.

Cerebral angiography, however, whether by injection or catheterisation of the carotid or vertebral arteries or of the aortic arch, continues to be a useful investigation providing some information which the CAT scan cannot reveal. Thus in cases of intracranial haemorrhage or infarction it may reveal an aneurysm or angioma as a cause of the haemorrhage and occlusion or stenosis of an intracranial or extracranial artery or vein. And in some patients with intracranial neoplasia the pattern of the vascular supply of the tumour can give a useful indication of pathology.

In the investigation of suspected spinal cord compression, **myelography** using either oily or water-soluble contrast media, or, less commonly, air or oxygen, injected by lumbar puncture, remains the method of choice, but may with time become less necessary as the use of the whole-body CAT scan increases. When oily contrast medium is used and this is allowed to run into the posterior cranial fossa along the clivus, the technique has been found useful in identifying neoplasms lying in relation to the brain stem and especially early acoustic neuromas as the internal auditory meati can readily be visualised in this way in normal subjects. **Spinal cord angiography**, achieved by injecting contrast medium into the aorta, is also useful in demonstrating arteriovenous angiomas of the cord.

Now that the CAT scan gives so much information without risk or discomfort, the need for invasive investigations has diminished greatly. Thus now, even more than in the past, it should be stressed that these uncomfortable and sometimes potentially hazardous investigations should only be performed if the information which they yield cannot be obtained in any other way. Since the CAT scan is not yet available in all neurological centres throughout the world, even those methods which are now becoming obsolescent will be described and are illustrated in Plate IV.

Air Encephalography

Air encephalography, like lumbar puncture, is generally contra-indicated in patients with papilloedema or other evidence of increased intracranial pressure, in view of the dangers of cerebellar or tentorial herniation. It should only be performed if skilled neurosurgical aid is immediately at hand, in patients suspected of having an intracranial neoplasm.

To perform an air encephalogram a lumbar puncture is done with the patient sitting upright. After a few drops of CSF have been allowed to flow, sufficient only to determine that the needle is in position, 5 ml of air is injected slowly and radiographs are taken as the bubble of air passes through the basal cisterns and fourth ventricle. Then 5 ml of CSF is removed, 10 ml of air is injected and subsequently 10 ml of fluid is withdrawn. The procedure is continued until 25–30 ml of air has been injected and adequate filling of the ventricular system has been obtained. Usually this amount of air can be manipulated in order to give a complete demonstration of the entire ventricular system and of the basal cisterns. The procedure usually produces a severe headache and sometimes even prostration and vomiting; the severity of these symptoms is usually in direct proportion to the amount of air injected. It is usual to give pethidine or a similar analgesic both as a premedication and subsequently, and haloperidol or chlorpromazine may be required in order to prevent or relieve vomiting. General anaesthesia is usually required when this investigation is to be carried out in children or in restless or confused adults.

Using this procedure the upper limits of a **pituitary neoplasm** can be defined by distortion of the basal cisterns or a **posterior fossa neoplasm** by displacement of or encroachment upon the fourth ventricle. Similarly, **neoplasms of the cerebral hemispheres** are localised by signs of distortion and displacement of the lateral and third ventricles (Plate IVA). A localised dilatation of some part of the ventricular system may indicate a localised area of **cerebral atrophy** in this situation, while enlargement of the cerebral ventricles and/or pooling of air in widened cortical sulci results from diffuse cortical atrophy, as in presenile dementia (Plate IVB). If air enters the ventricles but none appears over the cortex, this may indicate communicating hydrocephalus which can then be confirmed by isotope ventriculography; clinical deterioration following the procedure is said to be characteristic of cases of so-called 'low-pressure' communicating hydrocephalus. By contrast, while a failure to fill the cerebral ventricles may be indicative of obstruction to the exit foramina of the fourth ventricle, this is much more often due to technical failure.

Ventriculography

To perform ventriculography, air is injected into one lateral ventricle through a needle which has been inserted through a burr-hole in the skull and then passed through brain tissue. The procedure is not without risk as the needle may pierce a vessel during its passage through brain tissue,

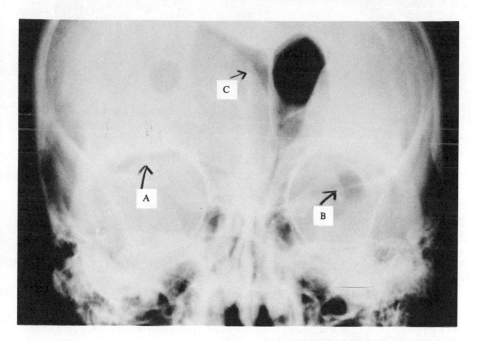

A. A ventriculogram demonstrating the presence of a right temporal glioma which is causing elevation of the right temporal horn and is also infiltrating the basal ganglia to give distortion and displacement of the lateral ventricles. A = right temporal horn, B = left temporal horn, C = displaced and distorted right lateral ventricle.

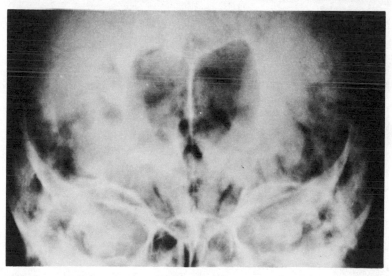

B. A lumbar air encephalogram demonstrating diffuse ventricular dilatation with pooling of air in the sulci in a case of presenile dementia.

Plate IV. Some important radiological abnormalities seen in patients with neurological disease.

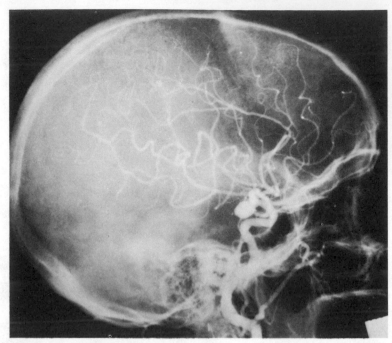

C. Right carotid arteriogram demonstrating a supraclinoid aneurysm of the internal carotid artery arising at the origin of the posterior communicating artery.

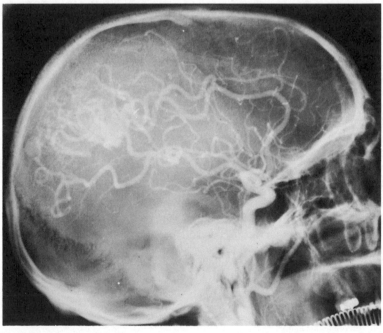

D. Left carotid arteriogram demonstrating an arteriovenous malformation in the posterior occipital region in a man of 29 years.

Plate IV (contd.)

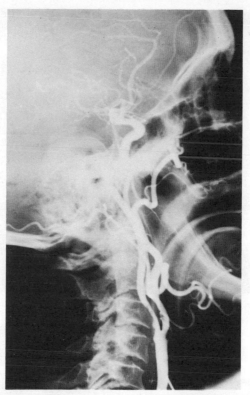

E. Left carotid arteriogram demonstrating stenosis at the origin of the internal carotid artery.

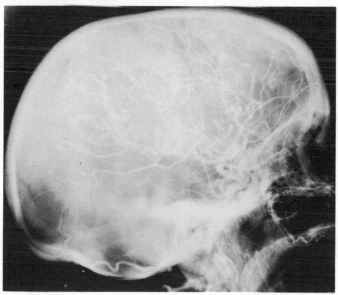

F. Right carotid arteriogram (late arterial phase) demonstrating the sinusoidal pathological circulation of a highly malignant glioma in the parietal region.

Plate IV (contd.)

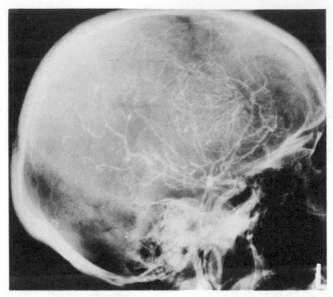

G. Left carotid arteriogram demonstrating a frontal meningioma (aterial phase).

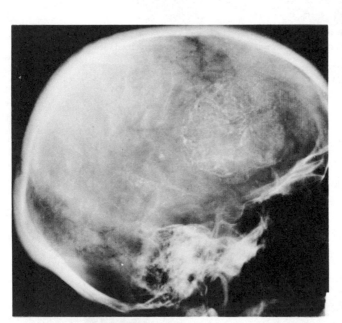

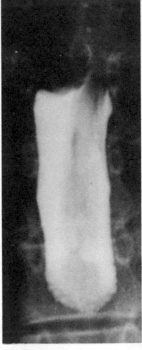

H. Left carotid arteriogram demonstrating a frontal meningioma (the same as that seen in G—venous phase showing a 'blush').

J. A myelogram (antero-posterior view) demonstrating a smoothly rounded extramedullary but intrathecal space-occupying lesion in the dorsal region which is displacing and compressing the spinal cord. The spinal cord is seen outlined as an area of decreased density running down the centre of the myodil column.

Plate IV (contd.)

while a sudden release of pressure in one lateral ventricle sometimes results in herniation of the contralateral cerebral hemisphere across the midline beneath the falx cerebri. Immediate puncture of the other lateral ventricle or even operative decompression is then necessary. Hence this investigation should only be carried out when it is possible to proceed with the appropriate neurosurgical operation without delay.

The information obtainable by this method is comparable to that derived from air encephalography and hence before the advent of the CAT scan it was usually performed in patients with suspected **cerebral tumour** in whom the intracranial pressure was high. A **stenosis of the aqueduct of Sylvius,** giving internal hydrocephalus, is also demonstrated by this method, as the air fails to pass through the aqueduct into the fourth ventricle. Sometimes, when despite manipulation it is impossible to demonstrate the fourth ventricle adequately, it is necessary to inject 1–2 ml of oily contrast medium such as myodil into the lateral ventricle and to observe its flow downwards through the third and fourth ventricles. This technique must only be used in carefully selected cases as the myodil acts as a cerebral irritant unless it can flow down into the spinal theca after the examination.

Cerebral Angiography

Three techniques of cerebral angiography are in common use. In the first, **carotid arteriography**, the common carotid artery is injected with an iodine-containing contrast medium such as Urografin (60 per cent) or Conray 80 (46 per cent). With this technique, which is carried out by percutaneous injection under either local or general anaesthesia, the internal carotid artery and its branches (middle and anterior cerebral and their radicals) are demonstrated. The second technique, **vertebral arteriography**, can also be performed by percutaneous injection of the vertebral artery in the neck, and the vertebral, basilar and posterior cerebral arteries are then filled; this method is, however, difficult and is much less often used than carotid injection. In skilled hands, complications are few, but undue trauma to the wall of the injected artery may cause it to go into spasm, and in the elderly, hypertensive or atherosclerotic individual this can lead to cerebral or brain stem ischaemia or infarction with transient or even occasionally permanent residual paresis. Many radiologists now prefer to inject contrast medium into the vertebral arteries through a catheter inserted into a limb artery such as the femoral or radial; a similar technique can be utilised when it is necessary to demonstrate the **aortic arch** and its main branches in cases of cerebral vascular disease.

Normally at least three lateral, anteroposterior and oblique views are taken at one- or two-second intervals to give early and late arterial and venous filling, but much more frequent pictures can be taken, giving a more comprehensive demonstration of the vascular tree (rapid serial angiography).

Angiography is particularly valuable in the diagnosis of **vascular lesions** and the techniques of magnification and subtraction greatly increase the diagnostic yield. Thus **intracranial aneurysms** and **arteriovenous angiomas** (Plates IVc and D) are readily demonstrated and localised; the technique must be used with some caution in cases of presumed cerebral ischaemia or infarction because of the danger of complications, but in many such cases obstruction or **stenosis of the internal carotid artery** (Plate IVE), or of other major vessels in the neck or cranium are clearly demonstrated. **Subdural haematoma**, too, can be diagnosed with confidence, by finding an avascular area beneath the vault of the skull in the anteroposterior view.

Carotid arteriography also assists in the diagnosis and localisation of **space-occupying lesions** of the cerebral hemispheres. An unusually wide 'sweep' of the pericallosal branches of the anterior cerebral arteries is usually indicative of dilatation of the lateral ventricles. Distortion and displacement of vessels may also localise the lesion whether it be tumour, abscess or haemorrhage, while many tumours show a typical pattern of vascularisation. **Astrocytomas** are relatively avascular, while **glioblastomas** commonly show a tangle of small abnormal blood vessels (Plate IVF); **meningiomas** often give a characteristic 'blush' in the venous phase of the angiogram (Plates IVG and H), owing to retention of contrast medium in the tiny vessels of the tumour. Vertebral arteriography may help in the diagnosis of tumours in the posterior fossa and is of great value in patients suspected of having vascular anomalies of the hind-brain circulation.

Myelography
Myelography is a valuable means of localising lesions which compress or distort the spinal cord. It is usual to inject contrast medium into the lumbar subarachnoid space and then to observe its flow up and down the spinal canal under the screen (fluoroscope) on tilting the patient. Anteroposterior and lateral radiographs are also taken at intervals. It is only necessary to use cisternal injection when there is a block beyond which contrast medium injected in the lumbar region will not pass and information is required concerning the upper limit of the lesion. The investigation has few complications, though some pain and paraesthesiae in the lower back and legs, along with mild fever, may persist for a few days afterwards. Very rarely a transient 'cauda equina syndrome' occurs, or else lumbar or sacral root pain, presumably due to irritation or mild arachnoiditis, persists for some weeks or months. Traditionally oily contrast medium (Myodil or Pantopaque) has been used, and in the United States this was always removed afterwards for medicolegal reasons. Now water-soluble and absorbable media (such as metrizamide) are being used increasingly so that this is no longer necessary.

An **extramedullary neoplasm** will almost always be localised accurately on myelography, either by the presence of a block or by a characteristic filling defect in the column of contrast medium (Plate IVj). Expansion of the spinal cord, indicative of an **intramedullary neoplasm**, or of **syringomy-**

elia can also be demonstrated, while an outline of abnormal vessels in patients with **spinal vascular malformations** may also be seen. It is of particular importance to carry out myelography with the patient in the supine as well as in the prone position, especially when the foramen magnum area is being examined, as supine views may demonstrate descent of the cerebellar tonsils (a Chiari anomaly) or, less commonly, arachnoiditis around the foramen magnum, disorders with which the syndrome of syringomyelia is generally associated. **Prolapsed intervertebral disks** and spondylotic changes are demonstrated best in lateral views, when indentations in the contrast column are seen opposite the disk space or spaces concerned; lateral protrusions may result in a failure of certain root sleeves to fill, and this is seen best in the anteroposterior view. Until supplanted by whole body CAT scans, myelography will be an essential preliminary to any operation performed for the relief of spinal cord compression, as clinical signs in themselves are never sufficiently accurate for exact localisation of the lesion.

The Special Senses

Visual and Oculomotor Functions

Methods of examining the visual apparatus which are part of the routine neurological examination have been described in Chapter 1. These include testing of the visual acuity, charting of the peripheral and central visual fields, examination of the pupils, of the ocular movements and ophthalmoscopy. The principles of visual evoked potential recording have also been mentioned (p. 54).

Slit-lamp examination is occasionally helpful in neurological diagnosis, either for detecting early cataract, or in looking for the peripheral corneal pigmentation which occurs in Wilson's disease (the Kayser–Fleischer ring).

Recording of ocular muscle imbalance on a **Hess's chart** is also valuable in the investigation of cases of diplopia, since repeated recordings may give an objective assessment of the patient's progress.

Ophthalmodynamometry, a technique of measuring the pressure in the retinal arteries by applying a simple instrument to the globe of the eye, is occasionally helpful in the diagnosis of occlusion of the internal carotid artery, as the ophthalmic artery is a branch of the internal carotid and retinal artery pressure on the affected side is reduced.

Fluorescein retinal angiography is helpful in confirming the presence of early papilloedema and in elucidating other ocular fundal lesions. It may also be useful to elicit **optokinetic nystagmus** by rotating a striped drum or unrolling a piece of vertically-striped cloth in front of the patient's eyes, first in one direction and then in the other, as this reflex response gives valuable information about the integrity of the visual pathways.

Auditory and Vestibular Function

Simple tuning-fork tests for assessing auditory function are described in Chapter 2. For a more accurate assessment of degrees of deafness **audiometry** is necessary. Each ear is tested independently and sounds of different frequencies are used, produced by an electronic instrument which gives pure tones. At each frequency, the intensity of sound (measured in decibels) is increased until the patient can just hear it. Thus the degree of deafness, if any, which is present in each ear can be measured and it can also be determined whether it affects all frequencies. Evoked response audiometry is especially useful in children.

In disease of the cochlear end organ (as in Ménière's syndrome), the phenomenon of **recruitment** may occur. This means that impaired hearing in the affected ear decreases progressively as the intensity of the stimulus is increased so that eventually it is heard equally loudly in the unaffected and diseased ears. Recruitment does not occur in patients with lesions of the auditory nerve (e.g. acoustic neuroma).

Vestibular function can be tested by **caloric tests.** The head is tilted backwards 60° so that the lateral semicircular canal is vertical and the ear is then irrigated with cold water (at 30°C). This produces nystagmus with the quick phase to the right if the left ear is irrigated or *vice versa.* The test is then repeated using warm water (44°C), when the quick phase of the nystagmus occurs in the opposite direction, that is to the side of the ear being tested. The two ears are stimulated independently and the total duration of the nystagmus obtained in each of the four tests is recorded. The accuracy of recording may be improved by **electronystagmography**. In lesions of the peripheral vestibular system (Ménière's disease) or of the vestibular nerve, stimulation of the affected labyrinth by caloric tests either produces no nystagmus at all or else its duration is greatly reduced (**canal paresis**). This finding is often of diagnostic value. In some patients with lesions of the brain stem or of the temporal or parietal lobes of the contralateral cerebral hemisphere, the duration of the nystagmus occurring to the side opposite to the cerebral lesion is reduced, whether it is produced by warm water in one ear or cold in the other. This finding, known as **directional preponderance**, is not due to a labyrinthine lesion but to a lesion of the central pathways which are responsible for conducting and recording labyrinthine stimuli. In stuporose or comatose patients a modified caloric test, involving only the injection of cold water into the internal auditory meati, to see whether nystagmus is evoked, often gives valuable evidence as to the integrity of the vestibular nuclei and is thus invaluable in the diagnosis of brain stem dysfunction and of 'brain death'.

Psychological Testing

Simple tests of intellectual function have been described in Chapter 1. Many methods for assessing intelligence and personality are available.

Detailed consideration of these psychometric tests is beyond the scope of this volume, but they are widely used to assess objectively the mental changes which occur in organic neurological disease. The Wechsler–Bellevue series are particularly valuable in confirming the presence of early dementia and in assessing degrees of deterioration. A comparison of verbal and performance tests will sometimes reveal specific defects in the utilisation of language or in the execution of skilled motor activity which may not be immediately apparent on routine clinical examination. In neurological medicine these tests are most helpful in confirming objectively subjective impressions of early intellectual deterioration. Other tests designed for the assessment of personality rather than intellect, such as the Rorschach ink-blot test, have more application to psychiatry than to neurology.

References

Davson, H., *The Physiology of the Cerebrospinal Fluid* (London, Churchill, 1967).

Dubowitz, V. and Brooke, M. H., *Muscle Biopsy: A Modern Approach,* Major Problems in Neurology, No. 2 (London, Philadelphia, Toronto, Saunders, 1973).

Fishman, R. A., *Cerebrospinal Fluid in Diseases of the Nervous System* (Philadelphia, Saunders, 1980).

Johnson, R. H., 'Cerebrospinal fluid', in *Scientific Foundations of Neurology*, Ed. Critchley, M., O'Leary, J. L. and Jennett, B., p. 281 (London, Heinemann, 1972).

Kiloh, L. G., McComas, A. J. and Osselton, J. W., *Clinical Electroencephalography*, 4th ed. (London, Butterworth, 1981).

Krayenbuhl, H. A. and Yasargil, M. G., *Cerebral Angiography*, 3rd ed. (London, Butterworth, 1972).

Lenman, J. A. R. and Ritchie, A. E., *Clinical Electromyography*, 2nd ed. (London, Pitman Books, 1976.)

Mayo Clinic, *Clinical Examinations in Neurology*, 5th ed. (Philadelphia, Saunders, 1981).

Newton, T. H. and Potts, D. G., *Radiology of the Skull and Brain* (St. Louis, Mosby, 1974).

Oldendorf, W. H., *The Quest for an Image of Brain* (New York, Raven Press, 1980).

Ramsey, R. G., 'Computed tomography of the brain', Vol. 9 in *Advanced Exercises in Diagnostic Radiology* (Philadelphia, Saunders, 1977).

Robertson, E. G., *Pneumoencephalography*, 2nd ed. (Springfield, Ill., Thomas, 1967).

Shapiro, R., *Myelography*, 3rd ed. (Chicago, Year Book Medical Publishers, 1975).

Sutton, D., 'Recent advances in neuroradiology', in *Recent Advances in Neurology and Neuropsychiatry,* Eds. Brain, the late Lord, and Wilkinson, M., Chapter 10, 8th ed. (London, Churchill, 1969).

Toole, J. F. (Ed.), *Special Techniques for Neurologic Diagnosis,* Contemporary Neurology Series, Vol. 3 (Philadelphia, F. A. Davis, 1969).

Walton, J. N. (Ed.), *Disorders of Voluntary Muscle*, 4th ed., Chapters 26–30 (Edinburgh, Churchill Livingstone, 1981).

Weisberg, L. A., Nice, C. and Katz, M., *Cerebral Computed Tomography* (Philadelphia, London, Toronto, Saunders, 1978).

Wood, J. H. (Ed.), *Neurobiology of the Cerebrospinal Fluid* (New York, Plenum Press, 1980).

4 Pain

Pain is one of the most common and disturbing of human experiences. While it may have many causes, the appreciation of painful sensations depends upon the stimulation of pain-sensitive nerve endings in the skin, muscles, skeleton, blood vessels, viscera and membranes, and upon the conduction of nerve impulses into the central nervous system where the sensation finally enters consciousness. The central pathways along which impulses conveying painful sensations travel and the effects of disease of the central nervous system upon its appreciation will be considered in Chapter 10, while methods used to relieve pain are discussed in Chapter 20. In this chapter some common neurological syndromes in which pain is a prominent symptom will be mentioned, with particular reference to its pathophysiology.

It should first be noted that individuals vary widely in their response to painful experiences, some remaining relatively impassive when experiencing sensations which produce in others an intense reaction. This individuality in emotional responses to painful stimuli means that although the threshold stimulus intensity required to produce pain (the pain threshold) is relatively constant, the reaction to painful stimuli which exceed this threshold intensity may be specific to the individual and can even vary in the same patient, depending upon circumstances.

There are no specific sensory receptors in the skin concerned with pain perception; painful cutaneous stimuli are recorded by multiple fine cutaneous nerve endings. In general nerve-fibre networks of this type are most luxuriant in those areas of skin which are most sensitive. There is also good evidence that pain sensation can be conveyed in peripheral nerves both by large heavily-myelinated A fibres and/or by small unmyelinated C fibres. In their so-called 'gate theory', Melzack and Wall proposed that cells in the substantia gelatinosa of the spinal cord act as a gate which is normally kept open by tonic activity in small nerve fibres and that this allows the central transmission of painful stimuli via the first central transmission (T) cells in the dorsal horn of the cord which stimulate central mechanisms controlling response and perception. Forms of peripheral sensory stimulation causing increased discharge along large fibres may, however, close the gate, thus inhibiting or modifying the onward transmission centrally of painful sensation.

Analysis of the pain which follows cutaneous stimulation has shown that it has two components, the first immediate and the second delayed; probably these two forms of the sensation are conveyed by nerve fibres which conduct at different rates. A sensation of deep pain is also felt after stimulation of deeper structures such as tendons, blood vessels and the periosteum. Painful lesions of muscles or viscera sometimes give pain in the overlying skin, or else it is experienced in a cutaneous area which is comparatively remote (referred pain). The mechanism of reference of painful sensations can be explained by the 'gate theory', in that it is suggested that there are central summation effects produced by a widespread, diffuse monosynaptic input to the T cells, often from relatively distant afferents.

Many types of pathological change can give rise to pain, through stimulation of pain-sensitive nerve endings in the diseased organ or organs. Thus, trauma and inflammation are two important causes of cutaneous and skeletal pain; malignant disease, including metastases in bone, can also be very painful. Visceral pain, particularly that arising in the abdominal organs, most often results from excessive contraction of plain muscle, producing pain-carrying impulses which travel along afferent fibres accompanying sympathetic nerves, though distension of hollow organs or inflammation of their enveloping membranes (such as the peritoneum) may also be painful; in the latter case the impulses are carried by somatic afferents. Pain arising in skeletal muscle is commonly due to prolonged over-activity, cramp, fatigue or postural abnormality, though repeated activity of a muscle with an inadequate blood supply (ischaemic work) can also be responsible; this principle applies also to cardiac muscle (angina of effort).

Since the sensory nerve fibres and central structures concerned in the reception and appreciation of painful stimuli are themselves sensitive to inflammation or irritation, and since there are other pain-sensitive structures within the cranium and spinal canal, pain is a relatively common symptom of disease of the nervous system. We must therefore consider in turn headache, facial pain and pain in the back, trunk or limbs which may result from such disease. It should also be noted that a reduction in the ability to perceive painful stimuli is known as **hypalgesia**; an excessively painful response has been called **hyperalgesia**, but it is more correct to call such an unpleasant or abnormal sensation **hyperpathia**.

The 'gate' theory explains hyperpathia either by excessive continuing stimulation of C fibres, thus keeping the gate open, or by a selective loss of A fibres which reduces inhibition as in post-herpetic neuralgia.

While central pathways conducting painful sensation are described in Chapter 10, it should be noted that there are few cortical neurones which show any selective response to painful stimuli. Electrical stimulation of the sensory cortex does not produce painful sensations, but such stimulation of cells in the posterior thalamus and intralaminar reticular substance may do so. However, the receptive fields of these cells are huge and they appear incapable of recording spatial information; it therefore seems likely that our ability to localise painful sensations depends upon the fact that painful stimuli invariably activate simultaneously nearby receptors concerned with touch.

Recent neuropharmacological evidence indicates that many neurones concerned with pain perception, and especially those in the periaqueductal grey matter of the midbrain, possess opiate receptors with which morphine and its analogues combine to produce their analgesic effects. When morphine or other opiates combine with receptors on neurones in this area, they appear to activate a descending serotoninergic system which inhibits the transmission of pain in the spinal cord. There is also evidence that the pituitary gland, and very probably other parts of the brain, produce β-endorphin which in turn contains a pentapeptide called enkephalin which is a powerful natural analgesic. The part which it plays when it combines with cerebral lipoproteins to form endogenous ligands in those disorders of the brain associated with disorders of pain perception is still uncertain.

Headache

Headache is produced by the stimulation of pain-sensitive structures within the cranium or in the extracranial tissues of the head and neck. Sensitive extracranial structures include the occipital, temporal and frontal muscles, the skin of the scalp, the arteries which traverse the subcutaneous tissue, and the periosteum. The cranial bones themselves are insensitive. Within the skull the sensitive areas are the meninges, particularly the basal dura mater and that forming the walls of the venous sinuses, as well as the large arteries at the base of the brain, forming the circle of Willis and its branches. Most of the cerebral substance itself is insensitive to stimuli which are painful if applied to appropriate receptors.

One of the commonest causes of **headache of extracranial origin** is emotional tension. **Tension headaches** are typically occipital, but sometimes frontal, in situation, and result from continuous partial contraction of muscles attached to the scalp. Usually these headaches come on towards evening when the patient is tired; the posterior neck muscles are often tender and this symptom may be relieved by rest if the patient can be taught to relax properly. The headaches of so-called **eye-strain** are probably similar in aetiology; if an uncorrected visual refractive error is present, then the continuous effort required to compensate for this defect also causes muscular tension, giving rise to headaches which are relieved by appropriate spectacles. Headache of purely **psychogenic origin**, of the type which occurs in neurotic, hypochondriacal or hysterical individuals, is often vertical in situation and is typically described in over-elaborate terms, perhaps in order to impress; a common example is to say that the top of the head feels as if it were being lifted off. Often such patients also experience true tension headaches towards the end of the day. Headaches described as being like 'a sense of pressure' or like 'a tight constricting band' are usually of this type and depressed patients may complain of headaches occurring in the mornings when depression is often at its worst.

Disorders of the **extracranial arteries** can also give rise to headache and indeed the symptoms of migraine, which will be discussed below, may be attributed in part to alterations in calibre occurring in the branches of the external carotid artery. Other 'vascular' headaches, such as that of a 'hangover', or of hypertension, can probably be attributed at least partly to dilatation of extracranial rather than intracranial arteries. The pain of temporal arteritis is also extracranial in origin, being due to inflammatory changes in the temporal arteries. Other causes of extracranial headache are **paranasal sinusitis** and **middle-ear disease** in which the pain results either from the increasing tension of pus in a confined space or from spread of inflammation to the bone and its coverings.

Headache of intracranial origin is due to inflammation, compression, and distortion of or traction upon the pain-sensitive meninges and blood vessels within the skull. Such headaches are usually felt in the frontal or occipital regions or both, though a unilateral lesion sometimes produces a unilateral headache, say, in one or other temple. When this is the case it can be assumed with reasonable confidence that the lesion concerned lies upon the same side of the head as the headache.

The headache of **diffuse meningeal inflammation**, as in meningitis, subarachnoid haemorrhage and following air encephalography, is generally severe, continuous and unvarying and associated with neck stiffness. Like that of **increased intracranial pressure**, whether resulting from a single space-occupying lesion or from diffuse brain swelling or hydrocephalus, it is characteristically made worse by sudden movements of the head, by stooping, or by coughing and straining. Each of these mechanisms increases the distortion of pain-sensitive structures already present, either through movement, or through a sudden brief increase in intracranial pressure produced by delaying the outflow of venous blood from the cranium. Typically this type of headache is throbbing in nature, perhaps due to the transmission of arterial pulsation to tissues already under increased tension. It is often present on waking but tends to improve as the day wears on. If a cerebral abscess or tumour is the cause, then vomiting and papilloedema may also occur.

A headache similar in character to that described above is due to a similar mechanism in cases of **reduced intracranial pressure**, in which there is again traction upon pain-sensitive arteries and meninges. This is the basis of the **post-lumbar puncture headache** which is presumed to be due to continued leakage of CSF through the hole in the spinal dura left by the exploring needle. The headache of dehydration has a similar cause and some believe that a clinical syndrome of **intracranial hypotension**, characterised by this type of headache, occurs spontaneously; this seems unlikely, as the pressure in the spinal theca on lumbar puncture may be low in healthy patients who make no complaint of headache. Dehydration caused by the diuretic effect of alcohol probably contributes to the 'hangover' headache. A benign syndrome of '**cough headache**' does, however, occur in which severe headache, typically of 'intracranial' type, accompanies coughing. While some such patients have emphysema and are presumed to have an unusually large increase in intracranial pressure during coughing owing to delayed venous return to the heart, others have no evidence of severe chest disease and in them the aetiology of the syndrome is obscure. While the possibility of intracranial tumour should always be considered in such patients, many cases of this type carry an excellent prognosis, though little can be done to relieve this symptom except to advise avoidance of the circumstances which induce coughing.

Migraine

Migraine is one of the commonest neurological disorders and may also be one of the most disabling. It occurs in both sexes, but is more common in women, and generally begins in adolescence or early adult life, often in patients who have had bilious attacks in childhood. Rarely migrainous headaches begin first at the time of the menopause, usually in hypertensive women, and attacks are particularly liable to occur during or just before the menstrual periods. Often there is a strong family history of the condition, while it has been thought, probably erroneously, to occur most often in the more intelligent and industrious, though intense and obsessional, members of the community. Attacks of migraine tend to be more frequent during or after episodes of emotional stress.

Migraine has been defined as a paroxysmal unilateral headache, preceded by visual and sensory phenomena and accompanied or followed by nausea and vomiting. While this description fits a 'typical' case, there are many patients with undoubted migraine in whom no visual or sensory aura is ever experienced and in whom the headache is never one-sided. Its paroxysmal occurrence is its most important feature. Some patients experience an aura alone, without subsequent headache but with vague malaise only, in some attacks.

The pathophysiology of the migrainous headache is now quite well understood. The initial disturbance is one of vasospasm in the extra- and intra-cranial arteries and their branches, often on one side of the head, and this is followed some 10 to 30 minutes later by a dilatation of the same vessels. The arterial constriction is responsible for the symptoms of the aura, the dilatation for the headache. The aetiology of these alterations in vascular tone, however, remains obscure. There is evidence of excessive fluid retention in the body before each attack, followed by a subsequent diuresis, a finding which has suggested a metabolic or endocrine cause.

Certainly there is no definite evidence that allergy or a disorder of the autonomic nervous system is responsible. Recent biochemical studies have revealed an increased urinary excretion of 5-hydroxindolacetic acid (5-HIAA) during attacks, suggesting an intermittent release of 5-hydroxytryptamine (serotonin) into the circulation. Paroxysmal headaches of migrainous type may be prominent in patients harbouring intracranial arteriovenous angiomas or even aneurysms, but in these individuals the headache is usually strictly unilateral, occurring on the same side of the head as the vascular anomaly; the reason for this association is not known.

Usually the migrainous attack begins soon after waking. A visual aura is the most common, resulting from spasm of the retinal arteries or of branches of the posterior cerebral artery supplying one or both occipital lobes. The patient then experiences either a hemianopic field defect, a less well-defined scotoma or rarely transient blindness, jagged lines ('fortification spectra'), or bright dancing or shimmering lights (teichopsia) in one half-field. Alternatively a sensory aura, with paraesthesiae (tingling, numbness and pins and needles) in the corner of the mouth and in the arm, or less commonly in the leg on the same side, may occur, presumably due to spasm of those branches of the middle cerebral artery which supply the sensory cortex. In a few patients the aura (vertigo, diplopia, bilateral paraesthesiae) suggests that the hind-brain rather than the fore-brain circulation is involved (basilar artery migraine) and sometimes fainting occurs either during the aura or at the height of the headache. Attacks of epilepsy occur in sufferers from migraine slightly more often than can be accounted for by chance. Rarely there is actual transient weakness of one arm and leg (hemiplegic migraine) or paresis of one oculomotor nerve (ophthalmoplegic migraine); however, some patients with the latter condition have an aneurysm of the internal carotid artery compressing the nerve trunk within the cranium.

As the aura passes off the headache usually begins and mounts in intensity; why some patients experience an aura after the headache has developed is difficult to explain. The headache can be unilateral and frontal (above one or other eye), bifrontal, bioccipital, or generalised. Sometimes it is comparatively mild, though accompanied by lassitude and depression, but more often it is prostrating, and there is photophobia, so that the patient must lie down in a darkened room. Typically the headache lasts all day, passing off after a night's sleep, but sometimes it wanes in an hour or two. Alternatively, it may persist, though with diminishing intensity, for a few days or even for as long as a week. Characteristically it is accompanied by nausea, sometimes by vomiting and occasionally by retching. There are some individuals who never have an aura, and others who occasionally have it without headache; indeed numerous variants occur. 'Bilious attacks' in childhood are almost certainly migrainous, while some believe that the same is true of recurrent abdominal pain or cyclical vomiting in children and adolescents.

Attacks of migraine can be mild and infrequent, occurring once every few months and having only a nuisance value, but in other cases they are severe and prostrating, occurring every few days, and causing serious disability. The condition tends to improve as middle age approaches and to disappear at the menopause, but the form which first develops in post-menopausal women may be particularly intractable. A temporary exacerbation with frequent attacks often accompanies a paramenopausal depressive illness. Treatment is considered in Chapter 20 (*see* p. 443).

Migrainous Neuralgia

There are some patients who experience episodes of severe and continuous pain, often burning in character, in, around or behind one eye or in the cheek, forehead and temple. These attacks occur in bouts lasting a few weeks or months and during a bout the patient suffers one or several attacks, lasting from 15 minutes to several hours, each day. Not uncommonly the attacks recur at the same time of day or night and may waken the patient from sleep. There is often suffusion of the conjunctiva and blocking of the nostril on the affected side during the attacks. The aetiology of this condition, which has been variously referred to as **histamine headache, ciliary neuralgia,** or **cluster headache**, is unknown, but it has certain affinities with migraine and is probably best referred to as periodic migrainous neuralgia. Not only may typical attacks be reproduced in susceptible individuals by injections of histamine, but they are often precipitated by the ingestion of alcohol; treatment with ergotamine derivatives may be very effective (*see* Chapter 20, p. 444).

Facial Pain

Pain in the face is a common symptom which may present formidable difficulties in understanding and interpretation. Whereas it sometimes results from local causes such as maxillary sinusitis, neoplasia of the maxilla, mandible or soft tissues, caries, dental abscess, impacted wisdom teeth or parotitis, it can also be due to many pathological lesions involving the trigeminal nerve, its branches and central connexions. Thus a plaque of demyelination or a syrinx (cavity) in the brain stem can give a continuous unilateral facial ache through irritation of the central connexions of the trigeminus, as may a tumour (acoustic neuroma, meningioma, nasopharyngeal carcinoma) or aneurysm which compresses the Gasserian ganglion or the intracranial portion of the fifth cranial nerve. Similarly, herpes zoster of this ganglion, which tends to affect particularly the ophthalmic division gives severe and continuous pain in the eye and forehead. Even more frequent, however, are the syndromes of intermittent facial pain, including trigeminal neuralgia and atypical facial neuralgia. In differential diagnosis it is useful to note that pain provoked by hot or cold foods or liquids is almost invariably of dental origin, while that of paranasal sinusitis is often accentuated by stooping and there may be local tenderness over the affected sinus.

Trigeminal Neuralgia (Tic Douloureux)

Trigeminal neuralgia is an intermittent, brief, lancinating pain in the face, confined to the area innervated by one trigeminal nerve, and often evoked by facial movement or by touching the skin. It is equally common in the two sexes and is most often seen after middle-age, particularly in the elderly, though it rarely occurs in early adult life.

The aetiology of the 'idiopathic' form of the syndrome is unknown, though the condition may sometimes occur as a symptom of multiple sclerosis, resulting from a plaque of demyelination at the point of entry of the trigeminal root into the brain stem; rarely it is the first symptom of a posterior fossa tumour, such as an acoustic neuroma lying in one cerebello-pontine angle. Its increasing incidence in the elderly has given rise to the suggestion that ischaemia of the trigeminal nerve or ganglion, resulting from atherosclerosis, is the principal aetiological factor, but comparatively few cases have been studied pathologically and no consistent histological changes have been demonstrated.

The pain of tic douloureux is typically sudden, excruciating and brief, 'like the stab of a red-hot needle'; a continuous pain in the face, or one lasting for several minutes, is not tic douloureux, though some patients have a background of dull aching between paroxysms. The pain does not extend outside the area supplied by the trigeminal nerve, nor does it cross the midline. It can occur in the distribution of any one or all of the divisions of the trigeminus; if the ophthalmic division alone is involved, it is often called **supraorbital neuralgia**. Its intensity can be judged from the apparently involuntary spasm of the facial muscles on the affected side and the agonized expression which accompany each attack. The patient often holds a hand in front of the face to protect it and will not allow it to be touched as he knows that movement, as in speaking, chewing, touching the face, or in shaving or washing, may provoke an attack. Neurological examination is rarely informative, though a few patients have slight objective diminution of sensory perception on the affected side of the face.

Characteristically, tic douloureux is a periodic disorder. It occurs in bouts lasting several weeks or months, during which the pain occurs with variable frequency and severity. Long remissions of weeks, months or even years separate the bouts but these remissions tend to become progressively shorter. The condition, though intensely distressing, is essentially benign, and does not shorten life, though a few patients are driven to suicide to find relief from their agony. Fortunately, most now respond to drug treatment (*see* p. 420), but in unresponsive cases effective treatment, in the form of alcohol injection of the Gasserian ganglion, or neurosurgical division of the trigeminal sensory root, is available, at the expense of permanent facial anaesthesia.

Atypical Facial Neuralgia

Apart from the local causes of facial pain mentioned above, other painful syndromes of intermittent character can affect the face. One of these is migrainous neuralgia which has already been considered.

Costen's syndrome is a condition in which a severe shooting pain radiates down the lower jaw or into the temple whenever the patient chews. It differs from trigeminal neuralgia in that chewing is the only 'trigger' which produces the pain, and touching the face, for instance, has no effect. This condition is thought to be due to dental malocclusion with arthrosis of the temporomandibular joint, resulting in compression of branches of the auriculotemporal nerve in the neighbourhood of the joint. The pain can be relieved by building up the 'bite'.

A common form of **atypical facial pain** is an intermittent but long-lasting pain of aching character which affects the cheek and upper jaw and occurs almost without exception in young and middle-aged women. In such a case it is wise to exclude dental sepsis, sinusitis and other organic lesions, but investigations are almost always negative. This type of pain, which often responds poorly to treatment, is generally believed to be a manifestation of psychiatric illness, particularly depression or anxiety. Unquestionably the pain is sometimes improved by psychotherapy, by tranquillisers and even by electroconvulsion therapy, but in some patients it is intractable. Whereas in most cases there is positive evidence of psychiatric disturbance, the pathogenesis of this condition is poorly understood. Attempts made to relieve the pain by cervical immobilisation or by sectioning the greater auricular nerve have no rational basis, and this troublesome condition remains difficult to manage.

Glossopharyngeal Neuralgia

This rare condition resembles trigeminal neuralgia as the pain occurs in periodic bouts and is brief and lancinating. It occurs in the tonsillar fossa, back of throat and larynx and may radiate to the ear on the affected side. Swallowing is the stimulus most likely to produce the pain. Its aetiology is unknown. Like trigeminal neuralgia it may respond to drug treatment (*see* p. 420), but if intractable it can be cured by dividing the affected glossopharyngeal nerve in the posterior fossa.

Pain in the Spinal Column and Limbs

While many skeletal and ligamentous lesions produce pain in the spinal column, some lesions involving nervous tissues also give rise to spinal pain. Diffuse inflammatory conditions such as ankylosing spondylitis, or metabolic disorders producing osteoporosis, may give dull aching pain involving the greater part of the spine, while osteomyelitis of a vertebral body or a metastasis in one or more vertebrae give severe and continuous pain which is localised to the affected area. As a secondary effect of these conditions distortion and deformity of the bony architecture can occur, resulting in compression of the spinal cord (this is in general painless) or of spinal roots (giving pain in the distribution of the root concerned). Similarly, lesions of the spinal cord and its roots, whether they be intramedullary (e.g. multiple sclerosis, syringomyelia), intrathecal (meningioma, arachnoiditis) or extradural (prolapsed intravertebral disk) can irritate or compress sensory tracts or fibres or nerve roots, producing similar pain. And a neoplasm such as a neurofibroma which begins by producing pain due simply to compression of its parent spinal root, may later grow sufficiently large to erode the vertebral body, giving a dull continuous 'skeletal' type of pain in the affected spinal area. Furthermore root irritation often produces a 'protective' spasm of the overlying spinal muscles and this spasm may itself be painful, while the muscles concerned become tender. Voluntary contraction of these muscles will then increase the pain, as will nervous tension.

Nerve and Nerve-root Compression

When nerve fibres or trunks which transmit pain-carrying impulses are compressed or irritated, whether in the spinal cord, spinal roots or peripheral nerves, an intolerable, continuous, burning pain, often accompanied by unpleasant spontaneous sensations (dysaesthesiae), is produced. If fibres concerned with touch and proprioception run in the same nerve, then associated paraesthesiae (tingling, numbness, pins and needles) also occur. Some of these features may be due to direct nerve irritation, others to ischaemia. Paradoxically, vasodilatation due to warmth can so increase the volume of the nerve being compressed that its blood supply is further reduced and the pain is made worse, while excessive cold, giving vasoconstriction, will also increase ischaemia and hence the symptoms. Pain due to compression of a peripheral nerve is referred to the skin area from which it receives sensory fibres. Similarly, root pain radiates throughout the dermatome of the root concerned, but it is less well known that deep muscular pain due to the same cause may be more widespread, corresponding broadly to the muscles supplied by the homologous motor root. Root pain has other special characteristics; thus it is affected by sudden movements of the spinal column which would be likely to cause movement of the root or of the lesion which is compressing it. Similarly a sudden increase in the CSF pressure, as in coughing or straining, will cause a sharp, shooting paroxysm of pain in the appropriate distribution. When symptoms of this type are of long standing, the trunks of peripheral nerves which contribute to the sensory root or roots involved often become tender on pressure.

Causalgia

Causalgia is the name given to a peculiarly unpleasant burning type of continuous pain which may follow peripheral nerve injuries, or, much less often, root lesions, particularly those in which severance of a nerve has been incomplete and some regeneration has occurred. This type of pain is most common in the hand and arm but does occur occasionally in the leg; it is most frequent after median nerve lesions. The skin area in which this spontaneous pain occurs is usually shiny and perspires excessively; the patient will not allow the skin to be touched as this greatly accentuates the pain. Although the exact mechanism of this syndrome is not fully understood it is clear that autonomic pathways play an important role, as blocking or section of somatic sensory nerves from the skin area concerned do not relieve the pain, but sympathectomy is usually effective.

Phantom-limb Pain

After amputation of a limb (or removal of an ear or some other member), sensations may be experienced for several months or years suggesting that the part concerned is still *in situ*. Not infrequently, pain of a curiously unpleasant and intolerable nature, resembling causalgia in many respects, develops in the phantom member. Usually such patients are found to have plexiform neuromas in the amputation stump, resulting from regeneration of fibres from the severed ends of peripheral nerves, and digital compression of such a neuroma will reproduce the patient's spontaneous pain. Repeated percussion or sometimes excision of the neuroma may relieve the pain.

Post-herpetic Neuralgia

Pain in the distribution of the affected root, whether it be the ophthalmic division of the trigeminus, or a cervical, dorsal or lumbar posterior root, is a striking feature of herpes zoster. In younger patients the pain generally resolves within a few weeks, but in the elderly a severe continuous burning pain may persist for years afterwards. It seems that the pain must depend upon the reception of sensory stimuli from the skin area concerned, since in the early stages it can sometimes be relieved by subcutaneous infiltration of local anaesthetic. However, relief is usually only temporary and it seems that a progressive facilitation occurs in the central nervous system with opening of the 'gate' (*see* p. 81), for eventually the pain continues to occur apparently spontaneously, despite division of peripheral pathways. The pain can be so intolerable that some patients are driven to suicide. Eventually in most cases spontaneous improvement occurs, but nevertheless the condition is very difficult to manage (*see* p. 419).

Thalamic Pain

Mechanisms by which irritation or compression of peripheral nerves or sensory roots may give rise to pain were discussed above, and it was mentioned that spinal cord lesions which affect the spinothalamic tracts can also give rise to pain in the limbs; such pain is often accompanied by burning dysaesthesiae and by sensations of undue warmth or even coldness. Similarly, a lesion of the thalamus itself (usually an infarct) can cause severe pain in the contralateral face, arm and leg. So-called thalamic pain is intense, burning and continuous in character and has other peculiarly unpleasant qualities, often described by the patient with such adjectives as 'tearing' or 'grinding'. Typically it is felt around the angle of the mouth and cheek and in the affected hand and foot. Pain of this type is fortunately rare as it is relatively unaffected by any but the most powerful analgesics. Neurosurgical measures, occasionally utilised in such cases are mentioned in Chapter 20 (p. 420).

Conclusions

Headache and pain in the face, spine and limbs are among the most common symptoms of nervous disease. A rational approach to differential diagnosis and treatment of these manifestations must depend upon a working knowledge of the anatomy of the sensory pathways and of the pathophysiology of pain. The patient must also be assessed as an individual so that the importance of emotional factors in the genesis of his symptoms, as well as the significance of his emotional reaction to the pain he is experiencing, may be taken into account.

References

Baskin, N. H. and Appenzeller, O., 'Headache', Vol. XIX in *Major Problems in Internal Medicine*, Ed. L. H. Smith, Jr. (Philadelphia and London, W. B. Saunders, 1980).

Dalessio, D. J. (Ed.), *Wolff's Headache and other Head Pain*, 4th ed. (New York, Oxford University Press, 1980).

Hart, F. D. (Ed.), *The Treatment of Chronic Pain* (Lancaster, Medical and Technical Publishing Co., 1974).

Keele, C. A. and Smith, R. (Eds.), *The Assessment of Pain in Man and Animals* (Edinburgh, Livingstone, 1962).

Lance, J. W., *The Mechanism and Management of Headache*, 3rd ed. (London, Butterworths, 1978).

Melzack, R., *The Puzzle of Pain* (Harmondsworth, Middlesex, Penguin Education, 1973).

Pawl, R. P., *Chronic Pain Primer* (Chicago and London, Year Book Publishers, 1979).

Pearce, J., *Migraine: Clinical Features, Mechanisms and Management* (Springfield, Ill., Thomas, 1969).

5 Disorders of Speech, Apraxia and Agnosia

To understand the means by which the function of speech is developed and controlled and the ways in which it may be disordered, is an endeavour which defeats many students. Even less comprehensible to some are the functions of praxis and gnosis, the first of which is concerned with the performance of complex willed movements, the second with the recognition of sensory information (visual, auditory, and tactile). Admittedly the anatomical and physiological organisation of these functions is complex and far from being wholly understood. The many views expressed about localisation of speech function within the cerebral hemispheres, and the profusion of minutely varying disorders of speech which have been described, each with its own title, have added to the confusion. And yet, at the risk of over-simplification, it can be said that an appreciation of some simple basic principles may bring a degree of clarity to what has long been a singularly difficult field. First it is necessary to understand something of the way in which speech and other higher cerebral functions are acquired and developed and then to mention some of the ways in which they are disordered by disease.

The Organisation of Speech

Control of Speech in the Cerebral Cortex

The young infant takes his first step towards the acquisition of speech function when he begins to associate specific sounds with particular objects in his environment. These sounds are subsequently organised into words which are symbols used to identify the objects concerned. Nouns, therefore, are first acquired, and subsequently conceptual or abstract powers of thought are developed in the utilisation of adjectives, verbs and adverbs to qualify these nouns or to describe activities instead of things. As the psychological concept of a word symbol develops, so the proprioceptive sensory impulses derived from the muscles of articulation come to be unconsciously associated with the expression of the word concerned, so that the child learns that a group of movements of the larynx, lips and tongue will result in the production of this word. Gradually, as additional words are acquired, these symbols lose some importance as individual entities but acquire new significance or meaning from their association with other words. In this way meaningful phrases and sentences are built up. When the child begins to read, visual symbols take their place alongside the appropriate sounds and in writing (visual speech), these same symbols acquire new associations in proprioceptive sensations derived from the fingers of the writing hand. Similarly, in learning a new language, the words utilised in a foreign tongue develop associations with words of the same meaning in the individual's native language. Words have now acquired new and abstract meanings and are utilised not only for the communication of thoughts to others, but also for so-called 'internal speech' or the conscious logical process of abstract thought. Not all thought is verbal; some depends upon the construction of visual or auditory images within the mind, but the more complex problems are generally dealt with by the thinker in verbal form. The scientist or the musician may, by contrast, think in terms of mathematical or chemical formulae or of musical sounds, but these too are symbols, either auditory or visual, which are comparable to the written or spoken word.

It follows that many sensory and motor activities are concerned in understanding and producing words, whether spoken or written, and other auditory or visual symbols. Thus in order to speak a sentence, it is necessary first for the individual to formulate the thought he wishes to express, then to choose the appropriate words (a choice which depends upon his acquired knowledge of the significance of these symbols), and then to control the motor activity of the muscles of phonation and articulation, a process which involves the reception and correlation of proprioceptive sensory impulses from the muscles concerned. If the message is to be written rather than spoken, the motor and sensory impulses from the hand are also involved. Similarly, in understanding speech, whether spoken or written, the accurate recording of auditory or visual stimuli is essential before the significance of the symbols utilised can be appreciated.

If we then consider the parts of the brain which control speech function it can be seen that those areas of the cerebral cortex which are particularly concerned with the production or understanding of spoken or written verbal symbols must have connexions with those which control the motor activity of the muscles of articulation and writing and with those dealing with the reception of auditory and visual stimuli. These connexions are achieved by means of subcortical association fibres which not only pass between various areas of cortex in one cerebral hemisphere but also communicate, via the corpus callosum, with comparable cortical areas on the other side. The process of learning speech, as with other functions, presumably depends upon the repeated passage of impulses along stereotyped pathways in these association tracts, a process which involves progressive facilitation of synapses, so that the ease of passage of impulses is greatly increased. The function of memory and the ability to recall words or other symbols, as well as the emotional responses or visual images conjured up by particular words or phrases, presumably depend upon the reactivation, either involuntarily or at will, of association pathways in which the necessary information has been 'stored'.

It is thus apparent that the function of speech cannot be said to be 'localised' in any particular part of the brain, as so many different cortical areas and association pathways are concerned in its integration. However, in nearly all persons (93 per cent of the population) who are right-handed, the overall control of speech function is subserved by the left cerebral hemisphere. In about 60 per cent of the remaining 7 per cent who are left-handed or ambidextrous, the left hemisphere remains dominant and controls this faculty, but in others it is controlled from the right side. And it is also apparent that the area of the dominant hemisphere which lies at the posterior end of the inferior frontal convolution (Broca's area), just in front of that part of the motor cortex controlling movements of articulation, is particularly concerned with producing the spoken word. Similarly the posterior third of the superior temporal convolution on this side (Wernicke's area) is concerned with the understanding and interpretation of word symbols (Fig. 11c, p. 183). An important association pathway which connects Broca's with Wernicke's area is the arcuate fasciculus which passes around the posterior end of the Sylvian fissure and runs forward in the inferior parietal white matter; it passes deep to the angular gyrus and in this area makes connexions with visual association fibres. After division of the corpus callosum and of other commissural connexions in a right-handed man speech can deal only with conceptual information which reaches the left cerebral hemisphere. The right hemisphere is then isolated from verbal expression (the so-called disconnexion syndrome).

The Peripheral Neuromuscular Control of Speech

There are two essential processes, namely phonation and articulation, by which the voluntary musculature converts the thought conceived in the cerebral cortex into the spoken word. Phonation, or the production of sound, results from the controlled passage of a column of air across the vocal cords, and the sound so produced resonates in the sounding-box of the larynx and pharynx. The sound is then modified by movements of the lips and tongue which subserve the function of articulation. These processes can be disturbed by lesions of the motor pathways controlling the voluntary muscles concerned and the clinical features so produced will be discussed below.

Aphasia

Although the term 'aphasia', if strictly interpreted, means absence of speech, it is usually utilised instead of the more correct 'dysphasia' to identify any disorder, however mild, of the use of words as symbols. Aphasia occurs in various forms and degrees, depending upon the situation, extent and severity of the cerebral lesions which is responsible.

The principal varieties of aphasia can be classified as follows:

1 Broca's aphasia (expressive or motor aphasia, anterior aphasia)
2 Wernicke's aphasia (sensory or receptive aphasia)
3 Conduction aphasia
4 The posterior (association) aphasias
    (*a*) nominal, anomic or amnestic aphasia
    (*b*) the syndrome of the isolated speech area
5 Global or total aphasia
6 Related disorders of language: agraphia, alexia, acalculia, amusia.

Broca's motor or expressive aphasia, generally results from a lesion in the neighbourhood of Broca's area. In its severest form the patient completely loses the power to speak or may say little more than 'yes' or 'no'. He nevertheless understands fully the spoken word, and readily obeys commands. His inability to express his thoughts in words may cause severe distress and it is often apparent that he is well aware of what he wishes to say, but is unable to find the appropriate words. The writing of words, a form of motor speech, is usually similarly affected (**agraphia**). When Broca's aphasia is less severe, the patient uses far fewer words than his normal vocabulary would allow and these are utilised hesitantly and sometimes repetitively (perseveration) with slurring and long pauses; nevertheless the words which are used are appropriate to the thoughts being expressed. Occasionally in polyglots or immigrants there is loss of the ability to utilise the language of the adopted country with preservation of fluent expression in their native tongue but more often all the languages which the patient knows are equally impaired. And even when speech can no longer be utilised at will to express the patient's thoughts, emotional expression such as the use of expletives in response to an appropriate stimulus may be unimpaired. **Palilalia** is a name given to a rare syndrome characterised by an increasingly rapid repetition of stereotyped words or phrases; it is virtually limited to cases of postencephalitic Parkinsonism.

Wernicke's sensory or receptive aphasia is essentially an inability to appreciate the significance of words, whether spoken or written, as symbols. The patient with this condition, which is generally produced by a lesion in Wernicke's area of the dominant cerebral hemisphere, shows a complete failure to comprehend the meanings of words which he hears or sees. The appreciation of musical sounds may also be lost (**amusia**). The patient still has words at his command and his speech is often fluent and voluble but he uses them inappropriately so that what he says or writes may thus be agrammatic and unintelligible; this form of speech disorder has sometimes been called **jargon aphasia**. **Word-deafness** is a fractional form of receptive aphasia in which the patient is totally unable to understand the meaning of words spoken to him, but yet his own speech, reading and writing are normal and he himself is able to use words appropriately. Similarly, in **word-blindness**, he cannot recognise written words or letters. In 'pure' word-blindness it is only the ability to recognise verbal symbols which is impaired, but sometimes the patient is also unable to appreciate the significance of numbers and even of colours. These two rare sub-varieties of receptive aphasia result from subcortical lesions close to Wernicke's area.

Conduction aphasia (central aphasia) is due to a lesion of the arcuate fasciculus, dividing association fibres between Broca's and Wernicke's areas. The patient's speech is copious but paraphasic errors (use of incorrect words or sounds as a part of individual words) are common. Object-naming is impaired as in nominal aphasia (*see below*), and the patient has difficulty in reading aloud; the speech content is similar to that of Wernicke's aphasia but the patient can understand both written and spoken language.

In **nominal or amnestic aphasia** the patient cannot identify people or objects by their proper names though he is aware of their nature and significance. In other words it is the association between a particular object and a particular word which is lost; the patient, when shown a pencil, for instance, cannot recall the word 'pencil', though he will say and demon-strate that the object is used for writing and recognises that the word 'pencil' is correct when it is offered to him. This sign most often results from a lesion in the angular gyrus or the dominant superior temporal convolution. Spontaneous speech is usually fluent with only occasional paraphasic substitutions, but writing is often impaired. More severe lesions in this region which isolate Wernicke's area from the rest of the brain (with the exception of the connexion with Broca's area through the arcuate fasciculus which lies much deeper) causes impaired comprehension of speech (as in sensory aphasia), impaired writing and object-naming and many paraphasic substitutions in fluent speech (**'the syndrome of the isolated speech area'**). The patient may show rapid 'parrot-like' repetition of phrases (**echolalia**).

All of the syndromes described above are seen in clinical practice but mixed syndromes are equally common. Thus where a large lesion of the dominant hemisphere involves both Broca's and Wernicke's areas there is impairment of both the expression and comprehension of speech, so-called **global aphasia**.

Other lesions of association pathways can produce the fractional dis-orders of speech which have been called agraphia, alexia and acalculia. **Agraphia**, the inability to write, is simply a form of expressive aphasia and occurs in lesions near Broca's area, but can result from a lesion of association pathways when spoken speech is unimpaired. Similarly **alexia**, an inability to understand the written word, is a form of receptive aphasia but can occur, usually with agraphia, as a result of focal lesions in the angular or supramarginal gyri of the dominant parietal lobe. **Acalculia**, or the inability to calculate, is a closely related phenomenon; the patient cannot appreciate the symbolic significance of figures rather than of letters and words; a similar disorder may derange the understanding of musical or scientific symbols.

Hence the organisation of speech function in the dominant hemisphere is a complex mechanism, depending not so much upon 'localisation' in specific cortical areas but upon many neuronal pathways and cell stations in which patterns of speech and related functions are stored and can be recalled at will. Pathological lesions may impair these functions by destroying cell-stations or their intercommunicating pathways, and many types of speech disorder are thus produced. Hence, speech can be thought to be a function of almost the entire dominant cerebral hemisphere; nevertheless the recognition of forms of aphasia is of great assistance in the clinical localisation of cerebral lesions, for certain specific disturbances in the use or understanding of words are consistently produced by lesions in different areas of the brain.

Dysarthria

Complete loss of speech due to a disorder of the neuromuscular mechanisms controlling articulation is known as **anarthria**; it is quite different from aphasia in that the patient's understanding of speech, his reading and writing are intact, but he cannot speak because the muscles of the lips and tongue cannot so control the movements of the expired air so as to form words. Anarthria is rare, but **dysarthria**, or impaired articulation, is relatively common. The speech of a dysarthric patient is slurred and indistinct, but his use of words is appropriate and his understanding unimpaired. The muscles responsible for articulation are those of the face (supplied by the facial nerve), the larynx and pharynx (supplied by the vagus nerve), the jaw (supplied by the motor root of the trigeminal nerve) and the tongue (supplied by the hypoglossal nerve). Lesions causing dysarthria can be classified as, first, upper motor neurone lesions, secondly, disorders of co-ordination and of the extrapyramidal system, thirdly, lower motor neurone lesions, fourthly, lesions of the myoneural junction, and lastly myopathic lesions.

A unilateral lesion involving one pyramidal or corticospinal tract, say, in the motor cortex of one cerebral hemisphere, will occasionally give some degree of dysarthria, though this is not usually severe unless the lesion is very extensive. Bilateral pyramidal tract lesions are usually necessary to produce dysarthria of upper motor neurone type, as in patients with bilateral damage to the motor cortex or lesions of the upper brain stem; total anarthria and often dysphagia may occur in a patient who has a hemiplegia due to a unilateral cerebral infarct and then develops a second one on the opposite side. There is often a pathological emotional reaction, with inappropriate laughing and crying in such cases **(pseudobulbar palsy)**. Dysarthria can also result from lesions of nervous pathways which influence, without directly promoting, muscular activity. Thus disorders of the cerebellar system may give inco-ordination of the articulatory muscles, causing a jerky or explosive speech with undue separation of syllables (e.g. 'scanning' speech, which is sometimes seen in multiple sclerosis). Extrapyramidal disorders such as Parkinson's disease cause rigidity of the muscles subserving speech, which therefore becomes slow, quiet and monotonous.

Lower motor neurone lesions, as in patients with motor neurone disease affecting the bulbar musculature (progressive bulbar palsy), or in patients with polyneuritis (say, after diphtheria), bulbar poliomyelitis, or syringobulbia, can also give dysarthria. Depending upon the severity and extent of the muscular atrophy and weakness, the speech is slurred and indistinct and eventually unintelligible. Usually dysphagia, or other evidence of bulbar muscle weakness, is also present.

A similar type of dysarthria, again due to weakness of the articulatory muscles, is seen in myasthenia gravis, and here the slurring increases markedly with fatigue. In patients with myotonia, stiffness of the tongue may give a certain stiff or 'strangled' quality to the speech, while in facioscapulohumeral muscular dystrophy, inability to close the lips makes it impossible for the patient to pronounce labials, so that a characteristic type of dysarthric speech is produced.

Mutism

Mutism is a total inability to speak, sometimes seen in a person without any demonstrable organic disease of the central nervous system. It can occur in psychotic patients (e.g. schizophrenia) and is an occasional manifestation of hysteria. Mutism combined with the loss of volitional movement of the trunk and limbs occurring in a patient who nevertheless appears to be conscious (akinetic mutism) is a rare result of an upper brain stem lesion.

Aphonia

Patients with aphonia cannot phonate but are still able to articulate, so that they speak in a whisper. While aphonia may be the result of disease of the larynx (laryngitis, tumour or paralysis of the vocal cords) it is most often an hysterical manifestation, the unconscious motivation usually being an attempt to escape from stress. Thus it may occur in a young singer on the evening of her first professional engagement. Often it is necessary to inspect the vocal cords in order to establish the diagnosis of hysterical aphonia and to exclude organic disease, but apart from a history of previous hysterical manifestations or of recent stress, the most useful diagnostic pointer is that the patient can still phonate when coughing.

Speech Disorders in Childhood

Developmental disorders of speech form a small but important group of disorders in which accurate diagnosis is of great importance, since many children with this type of condition are wrongly regarded as mentally retarded and many respond to appropriate treatment.

Deafness

The totally deaf child remains completely mute unless properly trained, as the normal channel for acquiring speech (i.e. through hearing) is not available to him. Usually the diagnosis becomes apparent when it is noted that the child, who has caused concern to his parents through his failure to speak, also fails to respond to external noise of whatever character. High-tone deafness is more difficult to diagnose, as the child with this condition does acquire speech, though this is unintelligible to any but his parents as he fails to utilise those vowel sounds and consonants (e.g. *e* and *t*) which depend upon high tones for their recognition. Audiometry is usually necessary to confirm the diagnosis.

Developmental Dysarthria

Dysarthria in childhood can be a manifestation of local developmental abnormalities such as cleft palate, or of cerebral palsy, in which case there are usually other neurological signs which indicate its nature. There is, however, a small group of children in whom dysarthria, associated with inco-ordinate or clumsy movements of the tongue and palate, is the only neurological abnormality. The condition may be due to a congenital apraxia of the muscles of articulation. Cases of this type respond well to long-continued speech therapy.

Developmental Aphasia

Congenital **word-deafness** or auditory imperception is a rare form of speech defect in which the patient fails to acquire normal speech function, is not deaf, as he responds to sounds, yet shows no interest or attention when spoken to. After a number of years many patients acquire a vocabulary of their own which, though meaningful to them, is incomprehensible to all except their nearest relatives. This type of defective speech was once identified by the obsolete terms 'idioglossia' or 'lalling'; it may be difficult to distinguish from the defective speech of high-tone deafness except by audiometry.

Developmental dyslexia, or reading defect, also occurs in various degrees of severity, being commonest in left-handed children; it may occur sporadically or be inherited as a dominant trait. In broad terms it appears to be due to a defect in the establishment of speech function in one or other cerebral hemisphere, and is often associated with 'mirror-writing' (writing from right to left with reversals of words and letters, as if viewed in a mirror). The printed word is wrongly pronounced, a dictated word wrongly spelt and writing is usually abnormal. It commonly occurs in children who are in other respects intelligent. Many normal children, particularly in families in which one or other parent is left-handed or ambidextrous, pass through a temporary phase of 'mirror-writing', at least of certain letters, when first learning to write.

Dyslalia

Dyslalia is a benign and not uncommon form of speech disorder occurring in childhood. The child develops speech at the normal age and speaks fluently though at first unintelligibly, as he tends to substitute one consonant for another in many words. This is now thought to be a syndrome of multiple aetiology. Sometimes the child imitates the defective articulation of other family members, sometimes there is mild mental retardation, and in yet other cases the condition seems to be a mild and rapidly reversible form of developmental dysphasia or dysarthria. Usually these children acquire normal speech within three to 12 months of beginning speech therapy, but without treatment the abnormal speech pattern may persist for many years.

Stammering

Stammering is a disorder of articulation characterised by the repetition of sounds or syllables and by prolonged pauses which punctuate speech. It is much more common in boys than in girls. Dentals (*t, d*), labials (*p, b*) and gutturals (*k*) are the sounds which seem most difficult to pronounce, and severe facial grimacing may accompany the attempt to utter words containing these letters. While many have suggested that this condition is of psychogenic origin, the fact that it is common in left-handed children and particularly in shifted sinistrals (who are naturally left-handed but have been persuaded to write with the right) suggests that it has an organic basis and, like reading defects, it may be related to an incomplete localisation of speech function in one or other cerebral hemisphere. It can be present from the age of two or three years, but often begins at the age of six to eight when a child who has previously spoken fluently is beginning to read and write. While many stammerers seem shy and introspective, this mental attitude is most probably the result rather than the cause of their disability. Certainly there is no evidence that stammering is a result of acquired organic brain disease, though it may develop for the first time in some adults with mild Broca's aphasia. It is more properly regarded as a disorder of the organisation and establishment of speech function. It can often be controlled to some extent by the use of syllabic speech.

Apraxia

Apraxia is the inability to carry out a willed voluntary movement despite the fact that the motor and sensory pathways concerned in the control of the movement are intact. In other words no actual paralysis, ataxia or sensory loss may be present. Thus a patient who is asked to put out his tongue may be completely unable to do so on request, though a moment later he will spontaneously lick his lips. Hence the condition can be regarded as a loss of acquired motor skills, or an inability to reactivate those nervous pathways in which the memory and technique of specific movements (**praxis**) have been recorded. It can be considered to be a defect of the 'association' areas or fibres concerned with volitional motor activity. The supramarginal gyrus of the dominant parietal lobe appears to contain an important cell-station in this organisation of movement, and lesions of this area commonly produce bilateral apraxia. A lesion between this cortical area and the motor cortex of the left cerebral hemisphere will lead to an apraxia of the right limbs, while a lesion of the corpus callosum dividing those fibres which are passing to the right motor cortex will give rise to a left-sided apraxia.

Apraxia of the lips and tongue is relatively common, while in the extremities apraxic disturbances may be revealed as an inability to dress or undress (**dressing apraxia**) or to construct models from blocks or letters with matches (**constructional apraxia**). Dressing apraxia is usually associated with lesions of the non-dominant parietal lobe, constructional apraxia with dominant hemisphere lesions. Apraxia of gait occasionally results from bilateral frontal lobe lesions, especially in demented patients, and oculomotor apraxia involving eye movements has also been described.

Agnosia

Presumably visual, auditory and tactile stimuli are perceived in the occipital, temporal and postcentral areas of the cortex, respectively, as crude physical phenomena which only acquire significance when related to past sensory experiences which have been collated and 'stored' as sensory memories in the appropriate association areas of the cortex. This process of recognising the significance of sensory stimuli is known as **gnosis**.

Lesions of these association areas may impair this faculty of recognition, even though the primary sensory pathway is intact; the syndrome so produced is called **agnosia**. Visual agnosia is an inability to recognise objects seen, in a patient who is not blind; auditory agnosia is a failure to appreciate the significance of sounds in a patient who is not deaf (a condition which closely resembles Wernicke's aphasia). A patient with tactile agnosia (often called **astereognosis**) cannot identify objects which he feels. Usually an agnosic defect involves only vision or hearing or touch in isolation, so that a patient who cannot recognise a pen, and may not even see that it is an object with which to write (unlike the patient with nominal aphasia) will name it at once if it is placed in his hand, while conversely one with tactile agnosia will identify visually the object which was unrecognised when he held it.

The Body Image

A constant stream of sensory impulses from the special senses, skin, muscles, bones and joints informs us of the condition and situation of the parts of our body in relation to each other and in relation to our external environment. From these stimuli we build up almost unconsciously an image of our body which is continually varying. Certain parts of the body such as the hands and mouth play such important roles in our everyday activity, and are so well endowed with highly-developed sensory receptors, that their share of the body image is proportionally much greater than, say, the small of the back. A skilled craftsman or the driver of a motor vehicle may become so attuned to the use of his tools or vehicle that in a sense these become a part of his body image and he then unconsciously relates himself plus the tool or vehicle and not himself alone to his environment. This concept of the body image is 'stored' in the association areas of the parietal lobes, and when the performance of motor skills is included it becomes clearly related to the function of praxis mentioned above. Some lesions of the parietal lobe tend to distort the body image so that the patient is unable to distinguish right from left (**right–left disorientation**). He may neglect the opposite side of his body and the whole of extrapersonal space on that side (**autotopagnosia**) while he may even deny that the contralateral limbs are paralysed (**anosognosia**) and sometimes attempts to throw them out of bed. The term 'anosognosia' is sometimes used to describe denial of other gross neurological manifestations. Often the patient with a parietal lobe lesion will perceive normally sensory stimuli applied independently to the two sides of the body, but if bilateral stimuli are simultaneously applied, one may be ignored (**tactile inattention**).

It has been said that disorders of the body image occur only with lesions of the non-dominant parietal lobe, but this may be due to the fact that in lesions of the dominant hemisphere they are obscured by aphasic, apraxic or other defects. Commonly, because of the contiguity of important association areas in the dominant parietal lobe, multiple defects occur; thus **Gerstmann's syndrome** is a combination of right–left disorientation, finger agnosia (an inability to identify individual fingers) and constructional apraxia. Acalculia and/or dyslexia are also common in such cases and the lesion responsible usually involves the angular gyrus.

Developmental Apraxia and Agnosia

Specific learning defects other than developmental dyslexia (p. 102) have been recognised increasingly in recent years and appear to be the result of either minimal brain damage due to birth injury or defective physiological organisation of cerebral dominance. The term 'minimal cerebral dysfunction' is sometimes applied to this group of syndromes. In contradistinction to the dyslexics, these 'clumsy children', who are often wrongly regarded as being mentally retarded, and who often demonstrate minor choreiform involuntary movements, generally show a higher verbal than performance level on the Wechsler intelligence scale for children. Defects of sensory perception as well as of skilled motor activity may be recognised in these children who often improve to some extent as they grow older; but many require patient individual tuition in the particular skills (e.g. writing) in which they are defective.

Conclusions

It can be concluded that an understanding of the many complex disorders of speech, of movement and of recognition which occur in patients with cerebral lesions must depend upon a working knowledge of the means by which these functions are organised and controlled in the brain. If it is recognised that these functions depend not upon the activity of isolated specific cortical areas but upon a complex network of association fibres joining a series of cortical cell-stations, it then is evident why lesions in varying situations affect these individual functions in different ways, often giving fractional disorders of function to which certain specific names have been applied. It is, however, necessary to understand the whole before identifying the particular, and from this understanding, information of considerable value in the localisation of cerebral lesions may be derived. In considering disorders of the peripheral neuromuscular mechanisms subserving speech it is also clear that systematic analysis of the patient's symptoms and signs helps to identify the situation and nature of the lesion or lesions responsible.

References

Brain, Lord, *Speech Disorders,* 2nd ed. (London, Butterworth, 1965).
Critchley, M., *Aphasiology* (London, Arnold, 1970).
Critchley, M., *Developmental Dyslexia* (London, Heinemann, 1964).
Critchley, M., *The Parietal Lobes* (London, Arnold, 1953).
Critchley, M., *Silent Language* (London, Butterworth, 1975).
Geschwind, N., *Selected Papers on Language and the Brain* (Dordrecht, Holland and Boston, D. Reidel Publishing Co., 1974).
Gubbay, S. S., *Clumsy Children* (London, Saunders, 1976).
Morley, N., *The Development and Disorders of Speech in Childhood,* 3rd ed. (Edinburgh, Livingstone, 1972).
Penfield, W. and Roberts, L., *Speech and Brain Mechanisms* (Princeton, N.J., Princeton University Press; London, Oxford University Press, 1959).
Vinken, P. J., Bruyn, G. W., Critchley, M. and Frederiks, J. A. M. (Eds.), 'Disorders of Speech, Perception and Symbolic Behaviour', Vol. 4 of *Handbook of Clinical Neurology* (Amsterdam, North-Holland Publishing Company, 1969).
Walton, J. N., *Brain's Diseases of the Nervous System,* 8th ed. (London, Oxford University Press, 1977).

6 Disorders of Consciousness

Consciousness is a state or faculty which almost defies definition. It implies a state of awareness of one's self and of one's surroundings, and its contents include a variety of recurring sensory experiences combined with emotions, ideas and memories which are the product of thought processes. While it is clear that the cerebral cortex plays an important role in maintaining and determining the content of the conscious state, cortical mechanisms of motor or sensory activity are by no means autonomous and can be activated or suppressed through the activity of the reticular substance and by hypothalamic mechanisms. This reticular–hypothalamic complex exercises important influences upon the state of awareness and it is now evident that disturbances of consciousness which are observed in clinical neurological practice are largely dependent upon lesions, either functional or structural, of these areas of the brain or the pathways which connect them to the cerebral cortex.

The term **arousal** refers to a state of wakefulness which is simply the converse of **sleep**, while various disorders of consciousness are labelled **clouding of consciousness** (or confusion), **stupor** and **coma**. In this chapter we shall consider briefly the pathophysiology of consciousness and normal and pathological variations in the conscious state.

The thalamo-cortical projection system consists of specific thalamic nuclei which project to specific sensory cortical areas, but in addition there are non-specific thalamic nuclei (the intralaminar, septal or midline and ventricular thalamic nuclei) which act as pacemakers of cortical activity. These in turn are controlled by neurones of the **reticular activating system** (Fig. 2) which are situated in the **reticular formation** in the core of the pons and midbrain, extending into the posterior hypothalamus. A downward projection of this system into the medulla includes the centres which control respiration and vasomotor tone, and yet other parts of it are concerned with control of temperature and gastrointestinal secretion. Experimental work in animals has shown that electrical stimulation of this system causes arousal, while destructive lesions cause unconsciousness. Similarly, anaesthetic and hypnotic drugs selectively depress its activity, while stimulant drugs have the opposite, facilitatory effect upon it.

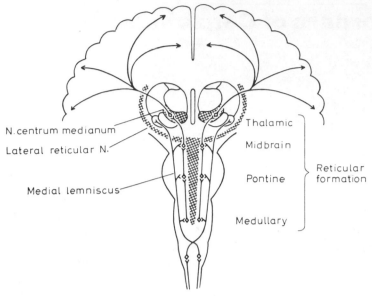

Fig. 2. The ascending reticular activating system. The reticular formation extends rostrally to include the lateral reticular nucleus of the thalamus, the midline and intralaminar nuclei, and part of the centrum medianum, which project diffusely to the cerebral cortex as the unspecific afferent system, responsible for the maintenance of consciousness. The reticular formation of medulla, pons and midbrain receives collaterals from ascending specific sensory pathways.

(Reproduced from *A Physiological Approach to Clinical Neurology*, 3rd edition, by Lance and McLeod, by kind permission of the authors and publishers.)

Plum and Posner (1980) summarised certain principles of importance in the pathophysiology of consciousness as follows:

1 Lesions which destroy the reticular formation below the lower third of the pons do not produce coma.
2 Above this level a lesion must destroy both sides of the paramedian reticulum to interrupt consciousness.
3 The arousal effects of reticular stimulation upon behaviour and the EEG are separable in that bilateral lesions of the pontine tegmentum producing coma may be associated with a normal 'waking' EEG.
4 Sleep is an active physiological process, not a mere failure of arousal and is clearly separable from stupor and coma.
5 Sleeping and waking can occur in man even after total bilateral destruction of the cerebral hemispheres.

Hence a lesion or dysfunction of the reticular system will only produce stupor or coma if it

(*a*) affects both sides of the brain stem;

(*b*) is located between the lower third of the pons and the posterior diencephalon; and

(*c*) is either of acute onset or large in its extent.

Sleep

Sleep can be regarded as a periodical physiological depression of function of the parts of the brain controlling consciousness. The EEG shows that as sleep deepens there is a transition from normal alpha waves to a phase of bursts of more rapid waves (spindles) and then the development of slow random waves. Four stages have been recognised of this so-called **'slow-wave or orthodox sleep'**. In addition, an important part of normal sleep is the so-called **'rapid eye-movement'** (**REM**) phase of paradoxical sleep during which most dreams occur. This phase occurs shortly after falling asleep and again shortly before waking and seems to be the most important stage in relieving fatigue. It also occurs about every 90 minutes throughout the night and occupies in total about 20–25 per cent of a night's sleep in the healthy adult. While severe nightmares usually occur during paradoxical sleep, sleep walking, enuresis and night terrors in childhood more often occur during orthodox sleep. The term 'paradoxical' is used because the individual seems to be in relatively light sleep, but in fact REM sleep is deeper than the deepest stage of orthodox or 'slow-wave' sleep, as measured by the arousal threshold. A disordered relationship between the REM and non-REM phases of sleep occurs in various disorders of brain function. Insomnia, particularly in the elderly, is usually associated with brief awakenings and with a reduced proportion of paradoxical sleep. In drug withdrawal syndromes (e.g. delirium tremens), the patient alternates between wakefulness and fitful sleep of which up to 100 per cent is paradoxical. Barbiturate anaesthetics produce EEG changes similar to those accompanying normal sleep. Though sleep-like states can be induced by electrical stimulation of an area in the diencephalon, it is an oversimplification to regard this as a 'sleep centre'.

During sleep not only is consciousness lost, but certain bodily changes occur. The pulse rate, blood pressure and the respiratory rate fall in orthodox sleep but rise in the paradoxical phase; the eyes usually deviate upwards (but show rapid bursts of conjugate movement in the paradoxical phase), the pupils are contracted, but usually react to light, though slowly; the tendon reflexes are abolished and the plantar reflexes may become extensor.

Recent neuropharmacological studies are also relevant. Neurones of the brain stem median raphe contain large quantities of 5-hydroxytryptamine (5-HT) and lesions here in animals give insomnia which can be reversed by giving a 5-HT precursor. Drugs such as p-chlorphenylalanine which block 5-HT synthesis decrease both REM and 'slow-wave' sleep. Destruction of norepinephrine (NE)-containing neurones of the locus coeruleus suppresses REM but not 'slow-wave' sleep, while reserpine, which depletes both 5-HT and NE, gives insomnia, but if a 5-HT precursor is then given 'slow-wave' sleep is re-established but REM sleep is not.

Many disorders of sleep are known, some of which are semi-physiological and of no serious significance, while others are due to organic lesions involving the mid-brain and hypothalamus. Several can be regarded as resulting from 'uneven' activity of the various parts of the reticular–hypothalamic complex so that in a sense the activity of one part of the brain is suppressed or reactivated before another.

Thus **sleep paralysis** is a condition in which the patient, when falling asleep, or more often on waking, finds himself unable to move a muscle, though motor activity returns immediately if he is touched. This experience can be very alarming, but movement generally returns within a minute and the condition is of no serious significance. So-called **night-nurse's paralysis**, which some believed to be a psychogenic or fear reaction, is probably closely related. Another related disorder may take the form of so-called **hypnagogic hallucinations**, a series of visual or other hallucinations which are of brief duration, though often terrifying in character, and which occur as the patient is falling asleep. Presumably this condition is due to persisting activation of cortical association areas; **night terrors** in children are probably similar. **Nocturnal myoclonus**, a sudden jerk of the musculature which occurs as the patient is drifting into sleep, is also physiological and results from a sudden transient reactivation of the motor system. Myoclonic jerks occurring repeatedly in sleep, however, must often be regarded as pathological, as some such patients develop epileptic seizures; but it is often difficult to know where to draw the line between the physiological and the pathological.

Insomnia occurs so frequently in the elderly that it is again difficult to know when it becomes pathological. In younger patients it is usually the result of anxiety, an emotional disturbance which clearly influences the reticular–hypothalamic system. **Somnambulism** or sleep-walking is also related to emotional stress and can be regarded as a reactivation of complex co-ordinated muscular movements occurring while consciousness remains impaired.

Narcolepsy is another relatively common disorder which results from a functional disturbance within the reticular–hypothalamic system. Patients with this condition experience attacks of almost irresistible sleep which develop during the day, most often in the afternoons. Such sleep is usually immediately of the REM type and in many such patients the REM/non-REM ratio of nocturnal sleep is abnormal. The desire to sleep can be resisted if the patient moves around, but if he sits down the somnolence is overwhelming and he falls asleep, usually only for a few minutes, but sometimes for several hours. He can, however, be aroused with ease, as from normal sleep. Males are affected more often than females and the condition usually begins in adolescence or early adult life; it is generally benign, and represents an exaggeration of physiological drowsiness developing under appropriate circumstances. Many patients who experience such attacks also suffer from **cataplexy**, a name given to episodes of sudden loss of power in the voluntary muscles, which cause the patient to go 'weak at the knees' and even to slump suddenly to the ground; he may be unable to move for several seconds or even for as long as a minute. These attacks are commonly precipitated by sudden emotion such as laughing, crying, fear or excitement. The condition can be regarded as a transient inactivation of that part of the reticular substance controlling motor activity and is again an exaggeration of the physiological, as normal people sometimes become 'weak with laughter'.

Organic lesions, whether neoplastic or inflammatory, in the region of the third ventricle and hypothalamus or upper brain stem, rarely give rise to symptomatic narcolepsy, but more often they produce **hypersomnia**, in which the patient sleeps for long periods, is difficult to rouse and may then be confused for some time. Periodic hypersomnia with megaphagia (excessive appetite) is a disorder of unknown aetiology (the Kleine–Levin syndrome) most often seen in adolescent males and often associated with hypersexuality; it is thought to be due to hypothalamic dysfunction (*see* p. 233). **Akinetic mutism** is a syndrome which can follow injury to the upper brain stem, and in which the patient is apparently asleep, with relaxed musculature; although his eyes may open and follow objects moved in his field of vision, or he may respond to sounds, he cannot speak or be aroused by powerful sensory stimuli. It must be distinguished from the **'locked-in syndrome'** in which the patient is alert and wakeful but mute and tetraplegic due to a low or midpontine lesion; these patients can communicate meaningfully by means of eye movements. Certain other lesions of the mid-brain and contiguous areas, and particularly those of encephalitis lethargica, produce **reversal of the sleep rhythm**, so that the patient sleeps by day but is awake and restless at night. These disorders cease to be physiological variants and are closely related to the pathological states of stupor and coma which result from structural or metabolic disorders affecting similar areas of the brain.

Stupor

Stupor is a disorder of consciousness in which the patient seems to be asleep but from which he cannot be fully aroused; he may open his eyes and on vigorous stimulation will show some responses indicating some awareness of his surroundings.

Lethargy is a state of drowsiness and indifference in which greater than normal stimulation is required to produce a response, while in stupor the subject is only aroused by vigorous and continuous stimulation. **Parasom-**

nia is stupor in which the patient remains confused when aroused. In akinetic mutism as mentioned above (sometimes called 'coma vigil') the patient retains cycles of self-sustained arousal, seeming vigilant but nevertheless immobile and incontinent, making only rudimentary movements in response to noxious stimuli and being in a state of 'motionless, mindless wakefulness'.

While stupor sometimes results from injury, compression or disease of the upper brain stem and hypothalamus, it can also occur as an effect of drug intoxication, metabolic disorders, anoxia, or severe infections such as typhoid fever, although in these conditions delirium, to be described below, is more common. Subdural haematoma is a common cause of a stuporous state.

Coma

Coma was once defined as complete unconsciousness with no reflex response to painful stimuli, while a semicomatose patient, while seeming

Table 3   The Common Causes of Stupor and Coma*

Supratentorial lesions (causing upper brain stem dysfunction)
  Cerebral haemorrhage
  Massive cerebral infarction
  Extradural haematoma
  Subdural haematoma
  Cerebral tumour
  Cerebral abscess

Infratentorial lesions (compressing or destroying the reticular formation)
  Pontine haemorrhage
  Cerebellar haemorrhage
  Brain stem infarction
  Posterior fossa tumour
  Cerebellar abscess

Metabolic processes or other diffuse lesions
  Anoxia
  Hypoglycaemia
  Deficiency disorders
  Renal or hepatic failure
  Disorders of electrolytes and/or ionic equilibrium
  Poisoning, intoxications
  Infectious or autoimmune disorders
    Meningitis
    Encephalitis
  Head injury, including concussion and contusion
  Post-epileptic states

* Reproduced from Section X by J. N. Walton in *The International Text-Book of Medicine*, Ed. J. H. Smith and S. Thier (Philadelphia, W. B. Saunders, 1981).

completely unconscious with no awareness of his surroundings, was accepted as one who responded to painful stimuli by groaning or by withdrawing the affected part. Less severe disturbances of consciousness were described as severe, moderate or mild confusion, or simply as 'clouding of consciousness'. It is now more usual to regard all such disorders of consciousness as different grades of coma. The Glasgow coma scale, in which four grades of eye opening, five of the 'best verbal response' and five of the 'best motor response' are charted, has been found to be of considerable practical value. The commoner causes of stupor and coma are listed in Table 3.

Mechanisms of Stupor and Coma

While coma can result from many conditions, some of which are lesions or diseases of the brain, while others are generalised metabolic disorders, the disturbance of consciousness, whether due to a structural or a biochemical lesion, is produced by disordered function in the reticular system.

There are certain important principles, however, which govern the production of stupor or coma as a result of supratentorial or infratentorial mass lesions (Fig. 3). While diffuse cerebral oedema can cause compress-

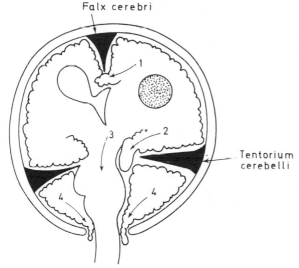

Fig. 3. Effect of expanding supratentorial lesions on cerebral structures. The cingulate gyrus may be herniated beneath the falx cerebri (cingulate herniation) (1), a portion of the temporal lobe may be compressed between brain-stem and margin of tentorial notch (2), or the brain-stem may be displaced downwards through the tentorial opening (central herniation) (3). In expanding infratentorial lesions, or after injudicious lumbar puncture in the presence of raised intracranial pressure, the cerebellar tonsils may herniate through the foramen magnum (4).

(Reproduced from *A Physiological Approach to Clinical Neurology*, 3rd ed., by Lance and McLeod, by kind permission of the authors and publishers.)

ion of the upper brain stem through symmetrical downward pressure, a localised space-occupying lesion or unilateral oedema (say after extensive infarction) produces a similar effect upon the reticular substance either as a consequence of uncal herniation through the tentorial hiatus or, less often, as a result of herniation of cerebellar tonsils through the foramen magnum. Cingulate gyrus herniation beneath the falx cerebri, by contrast, produces its effects by compressing the anterior cerebral vessels, thus increasing frontal lobe oedema. In uncal herniation, compression of the trunk of the third nerve against the free edge of the tentorium often gives unilateral pupillary dilatation, followed by ptosis and ultimately a complete third nerve palsy. Persisting uncal herniation can give rise to haemorrhages in the median raphe of the brain stem causing irreversible coma. Subtentorial lesions, by contrast, may compress the brain stem directly or else may cause either upward displacement of the midbrain and cerebellum through the tentorial notch or downward cerebellar tonsillar herniation. Any form of herniation may be accentuated, with disastrous effects, if cerebrospinal fluid is removed by lumbar puncture. Destructive brain stem lesions (e.g. infarction), on the other hand, cause coma through direct damage to the reticular formation, as do inflammatory processes such as encephalitis, while meningitis combines with the effects of inflammation to give a marked increase in intracranial pressure. Ischaemia and hypoxia also affect the reticular substance directly, while post-epileptic stupor depends upon a temporary suppression of synaptic transmission in this system and/or in the pathways connecting it to the cortex.

Some Specific Causes of Stupor and Coma and their Recognition

In examining and investigating the comatose patient **the head** should be examined for signs of recent or past injury and **the tongue** for scars resulting from previous fits. The smell of alcohol on **the breath** or of acetone (in diabetic coma) or foetor (in uraemic or hepatic coma) may be of diagnostic value. **Cervical rigidity** will suggest either meningitis or intracranial haemorrhage, while **a bruit** over the cranium or in the neck may indicate a vascular malformation or arterial stenosis. In **the skin** cyanosis (in respiratory insufficiency), a cherry-red colour (in carbon monoxide poisoning), purpura (in various blood diseases), the typical changes of Addison's disease or hypothyroidism or scars of previous injections (in drug addicts) may give clues to the cause of the coma.

Changes in the **respiratory rate** and volume should also be noted. Periodic (Cheyne-Stokes) respiration in which hyperpnoea alternates with apnoea usually indicates a central cerebral or high brain stem lesion. Brain stem lesions can also give central neurogenic hyperventilation, apneustic breathing (a pause at full inspiration) or ataxic respiration in which random deep and shallow breaths occur; the latter type of breathing is most often found in medullary lesions.

Examining the **pupils** is also important. Thus mid-brain lesions may give pupils of medium size which react neither to light nor other stimuli, while lesions of the pontine tegmentum more often give small fixed pupils which may be pinpoint in pontine haemorrhage. Pinpoint pupils also result from opiate intoxication while atropine-like drugs and cerebral anoxia cause pupillary dilatation. A fixed dilated pupil on one side as indicated above, often in the comatose patient, indicates herniation of the medial temporal lobe through the tentorial hiatus.

Examination of the **ocular movements** is also useful. Thus, in lesions of the cerebral hemispheres oculocephalic reflexes (*see* p. 24) are normal and caloric stimulation of the ears (say with cold water) gives normal evoked nystagmus. These reflexes are lost when there is an extensive brain stem lesion involving the pons. A massive frontal lesion may, however, give deviation of the eyes towards the side of the lesion, while a pontine lesion can cause conjugate deviation of the eyes to the opposite side with absence of oculocephalic and caloric responses. Skew deviation of the eyes results from a pontine or cerebellar lesion while downward conjugate deviation implies damage to the mid-brain.

Clearly examination of other systems to exclude disease in the heart, lungs, liver and kidneys is obligatory in any comatose patient, and routine estimations of the blood sugar, urea, electrolytes and pO_2 and pCo_2 are usually indicated. A CAT scan, when available, may be invaluable, but if not then an EEG or echo-encephalogram can be helpful. Cerebral angiography and other invasive radiological investigations should only be performed after very careful consideration as they may be dangerous in deep coma.

The **differential diagnosis** of the causes of coma is a difficult but common clinical problem. Where an adequate history is available from friends or relatives the diagnostic problem is often eased, but when a patient is found comatose and no accurate history of the onset is available, diagnosis may bristle with difficulties. Thus **head injury**, an important cause, is generally identified by the history; even if this is lacking there is usually some external evidence of laceration or contusion. In cases of **subdural haematoma**, however, the causal injury may have been trivial and the patient may gradually have become increasingly drowsy over a period of weeks or months. Some such patients are stuporose rather than comatose. In **subarachnoid haemorrhage** a history of sudden onset with headache and neck stiffness, and the presence of blood-stained CSF are revealing; however, the clinical picture of **primary cerebral haemorrhage** is not dissimilar, though in such cases a profound hemiplegia is usually present from the onset. When **cerebral thrombosis** is the cause, the onset is generally more gradual with less severe clouding of consciousness, though if the infarct is extensive, the patient can be comatose and hemiplegic, a clinical picture which differs little from that of cerebral haemorrhage. The onset of **cerebral embolism** is of course abrupt, and there is often clinical evidence of a source of emboli, generally in the heart (mitral stenosis, bacterial endocarditis, cardiac infarction). **Encephalitis** and **meningitis** are usually accompanied by fever, and the patient's comatose state is usually the end-result of an illness which has lasted for a day or two or longer, with headache, neck stiffness (in meningitis particularly), drowsiness and confusion. In such individuals, CSF examination is of the greatest importance. Similarly, sudden coma is uncommon in patients suffering from **cerebral tumour**, many of whom have experienced previous headache, focal fits or the gradual development of paralysis, and papilloedema will often be present. In patients with **cerebral abscess**, too, the onset is generally gradual and there will often be an evident focus of infection in the middle ear, nasal sinuses, skin or lung. The relatively uncommon **hypertensive encephalopathy** is generally recognised through the retinal changes of malignant hypertension combined with the blood pressure reading. Recognition of the stupor or coma which follows an attack of **epilepsy** rests upon a history of previous fits.

Turning to toxic and metabolic causes of coma, **anoxia** will generally be identified by a history of carbon-monoxide poisoning, whether from coal gas, a coke brazier or exhaust fumes, or by a history of partial drowning, difficult general anaesthesia or chronic pulmonary insufficiency. **Acute alcoholism** will be suspected from the smell of alcohol on the breath and confirmed by urine or blood-alcohol estimation. However, intoxicated patients are particularly liable to suffer head injury, while cerebral vascular catastrophes sometimes occur during an alcoholic debauch. Deep, hissing, 'acidotic' respiration with acetone in the breath, glycosuria and ketonuria, will usually establish a diagnosis of **diabetic coma**, while a pale, sweating and flaccid patient with bilateral extensor responses may be shown by blood–sugar estimation to be suffering from **hypoglycaemia** due either to insulin administration or to a tumour of the pancreatic islet cells. Patients with **uraemia** tend to have a deep acidotic breathing like that of diabetic coma, but the breath has a uriniferous smell, and hypertension, retinal changes and albuminuria are usually present. **Liver disease** is easily overlooked as a cause of coma, but the patient will often have shown the characteristic 'flapping' tremor of the outstretched hands, and there may be jaundice, dark urine and stigmata of hepatic cirrhosis such as 'liver palms' and cutaneous spider naevi.

Other rare causes of a comatose state include **malaria, heat stroke** (as in athletes competing in hot countries), **Addison's disease, myxoedema** and **hypopituitarism**. In the latter two conditions, **hypothermia** is a common cause of coma and the rectal temperature may be less than 36°C. Finally, **drug intoxication** must also be remembered as an increasingly common cause of a type of coma which may show no specific clinical features, especially if **barbiturates, psychotropic drugs or anticonvulsants** have been taken, say, in an attempt to commit suicide. **Salicylates**, by contrast, tend to produce a characteristic deep cyanosis with acidotic breathing, while

opiates give characteristic pin-point pupils and paracetamol usually gives liver damage. However, in any patient with coma of unknown cause, when no history is available, poisoning should be considered and the patient's belongings should be searched for a container which may have held the offending tablets, while it will sometimes be necessary to wash out the stomach or to examine the blood or urine for the presence of drugs.

The Diagnosis of Brain Death

This problem has assumed increasing importance in recent years, first because of the increasing difficulty of deciding in patients with brain damage whether it is justifiable to maintain life indefinitely with assisted respiration and other supportive measures, and secondly because of the difficult question of deciding when it may be concluded that the cerebral lesion is irreversible, that cardiac arrest is imminent, and that preparations may be made to remove viable organs for subsequent transplantation.

This topic has been a fertile source of national and international dispute, but there is now reasonably general agreement that the British criteria adopted by the Departments of Health on the advice of the Conference of Royal Colleges and Faculties of the United Kingdom are reliable, and these are given below. It is recommended that in any individual case diagnosis according to the criteria should be confirmed by two experienced doctors acting independently and that the tests should be repeated after a 24-hour interval before the decision is made to discontinue life support systems and to remove organs when appropriate. It is now regarded as unnecessary to carry out an EEG since this may show normal waking rhythms in the presence of an irreversible brain stem lesion.

The following are the conditions and criteria laid down:

Conditions under which the diagnosis of brain death should be considered.

1 The patient is deeply comatose.
  (*a*) There should be no suspicion that this state is due to depressant drugs.
  (*b*) Primary hypothermia as a cause of coma should have been excluded.
  (*c*) Metabolic and endocrine disturbances which can be responsible for or can contribute to coma should have been excluded.
2 The patient is being maintained on a ventilator because spontaneous respiration had previously become inadequate or had ceased altogether.
  (*a*) Relaxants (neuromuscular blocking agents) and other drugs should have been excluded as a cause of respiratory inadequacy or failure.
3 There should be no doubt that the patient's condition is due to

irremediable structural brain damage. The diagnosis of a disorder which can lead to brain death should have been fully established.

Diagnostic tests for the confirmation of brain death

All brain stem reflexes are absent:

(i) The pupils are fixed in diameter and do not respond to sharp changes in the intensity of incident light.
(ii) There is no corneal reflex.
(iii) The vestibulo-ocular reflexes are absent.
(iv) No motor responses within the cranial nerve distribution can be elicited by adequate stimulation of any somatic area.
(v) There is no gag reflex or reflex response to bronchial stimulation by a suction catheter passed down the trachea.
(vi) No respiratory movements occur when the patient is disconnected from the mechanical ventilator for long enough to ensure that the arterial carbon dioxide tension rises above the threshold for stimulation of respiration.

Delirium and Confusion

There are many physical illnesses which are accompanied by mental symptoms of varying degree, most of which present as **clouding of consciousness**, with or without other more specific manifestations. These disorders are the **symptomatic psychoses**. They occur not only as a result of cerebral lesions but also in many infective and metabolic disorders. These are not primarily diseases of the nervous system but they may affect profoundly its function, even without producing histological changes in the brain identifiable by present techniques. The lack of awareness which results may be no more than the minimal disinterest and 'fuzziness' in the head which accompanies mild influenza, but it can take the form of a severe psychotic reaction with grossly disturbed consciousness and bizarre disorders of thought. There is evidence that the type of reaction an individual shows may depend partly upon his previous personality and emotional constitution.

Delirium is a term used to identify a state of severely clouded consciousness in which the patient is disorientated in time and place, and his attention-span is brief. His thought processes are disordered so that he cannot appreciate his present circumstances and relate them to past experience; he may be living in a fantasy world peopled by the products of his imagining. Hence delusions or false imaginary ideas are frequent, as are hallucinations, usually visual, which can be vividly real and may result in an intense fear reaction with restless or even violent behaviour. Fluctuation in the mental and physical state is common, so that periods of shouting and restlessness alternate with others of apparent somnolence, punctuated by muttering. Commonly speech is slurred. Drowsiness is often worst during the day, while the patient becomes excited, hallucinated and uncontrollable at night. The stage of true delirium is often preceded by one of restlessness and irritability, insomnia, lack of concentration and pathological brightness or euphoria, a stage which may last for hours or days, depending upon the cause. Often there are also motor manifestations; the patient is tremulous, and spontaneous twitching or jerking of the voluntary musculature occurs, even in sleep. A return to restful sleep may be the first sign of resolution of the delirium, but even after apparent recovery, delusions may persist and often have a paranoid character, encompassing ideas of persecution or ill-treatment.

Delirium classically occurs in patients with chronic alcoholism after a debauch or after alcohol withdrawal and is then known as **delirium tremens**. The condition which follows withdrawal of barbiturates or amphetamine in patients habituated to these drugs is similar, and is also characterised by the occurrence of drug-withdrawal convulsions. Less severe delirious states, differing only in detail but not in overall pattern, are seen in patients with encephalitis or meningitis, in severe infections such as septicaemia or typhoid fever, in metabolic disorders such as liver disease and pernicious anaemia, in some cases of bronchogenic carcinoma without cerebral metastases, after treatment with ACTH or steroids and in many other disorders. Mild delirium is common in febrile illness in childhood, particularly at night.

When mental disturbances are less striking but yet the patient shows fluctuations in awareness, with incoherence of thought and variable disorientation ('where am I'), but usually without frank delusions or hallucinations, the condition is often called **confusion** or a **confusional state**, of mild, moderate or severe degree. This differs from delirium only in detail and indeed these disorders merge with one another so that the delirious patient generally passes through a phase of confusion during recovery. In recovery from a head injury causing coma, for instance, the patient may be delirious and later confused as consciousness slowly returns. Hence some authorities have suggested that the term confusion should be dropped and the condition referred to as **subacute delirium**. Other terms utilised to identify these disorders include toxic-infective psychosis, metabolic or exhaustion psychosis, or organic reaction state, as these disorders are essentially mental reactions resulting from organic disease which is disordering brain function. From the standpoint of convenient clinical usage it is probably justifiable to retain the term 'delirium' to identify the severe disturbance and 'confusion' the less severe, provided it is appreciated that there is no essential difference between the two.

Memory and its Disorders

The limbic system of the brain, which includes the amygdala and hippo-campus in the mesial temporal lobe, with the cingulate gyrus and orbito-frontal cortex and the fornix, mammillary bodies and anterior thalamic nuclei, clearly plays a crucial role in the control of memory and of the emotions.

Sensory memory is the ability to retain recorded signals in the sensory (receptive) areas of the brain for a very short period of time after the sensory experience. Short-term (or primary) memory is the ability to retain facts, words, numbers or letters (such as telephone numbers or a name and address) for a few seconds or minutes combined with ability to recall the information at will. Long-term memory is the storage in the brain of information which can be recalled minutes, hours, days, months or years later. Secondary memories are those long-term memories which are stored in the form of relatively weak memory traces so that the information can only be recalled for a few days or is difficult to remember at all. Tertiary memories, by contrast, are so deeply imprinted (such as the individual's name, the letters of the alphabet) that they can be recalled at will throughout life. The recall mechanism is attributed to activity in precisely defined reverberating neuronal circuits, long-term memory to progressive synaptic facilitation; repetition of information (rehearsal) and the codify-ing of sensory stimuli into different classes of information assist in the consolidation of long-term memories and the transfer of sensory into long-term memory.

Derangement of memory is a feature of many of the disorders of consciousness referred to above and accounts for some of the associated spatial and temporal disorientation. Presumably, the structural or metabolic abnormalities concerned produce their effects by impairing the efficiency of the cerebral pathways upon which our memory of objects, of events and of language depends. Hallucinations may result from fractional reactiva-tion of some parts of these pathways. A syndrome which is frequently identified as a specific entity, though it has some affinities with confusion and even delirium, is **Korsakoff's syndrome**, or the so-called 'amnestic syndrome'. Its salient feature is that the patient loses the ability to record and retain new impressions. At one minute he appears alert and his conversation is lucid, but within a moment or two he has forgotten the interview completely. The memory of his remote past may be intact. As a result he becomes disorientated, certainly in time and often in place, and in order to conceal this memory defect he confabulates; thus he may describe in detail fantastic activities which he claims to have carried out hours or days earlier, though in that time he may not have left his bed. Usually his descriptions have some basis in fact in the remote past but he utilises these previous experiences to fill gaps in the period for which his memory is defective. Though Korsakoff's syndrome occurs most often in patients with alcoholism and polyneuropathy and in association with Wernicke's encephalopathy (*see* p. 392), it sometimes complicates other metabolic and infective illnesses; it may develop during recovery from head injury or subarachnoid haemorrhage or indeed in patients recovering from delirium resulting from many causes. Lesions of the corpora mammillaria are often found in patients with this clinical picture. Severe loss of memory has also been found to follow resection or disease of the anterior portions of both temporal lobes. Rarely a unilateral temporal lobe tumour has a similar effect. Severe memory impairment also occurs in the various cerebral degenerative processes which cause dementia, and may follow severe head injury, whilst transient amnesia can follow toxic confusional states, anoxic episodes, meningitis, encephalitis, and drug intoxication.

A syndrome of **transient global amnesia**, thought to be due to transient ischaemia in one or both temporal lobes, may occur in middle-aged or elderly individuals with evidence of arterial disease. The disorder develops acutely with memory loss for recent events; patients retain their personal identity but are usually deeply anxious about their memory loss into which they have considerable insight. Attacks often follow exposure to cold. Recovery is usually complete within a few hours but the patient remains amnesic for events occurring in the attack itself.

That psychological as well as physical causes can seriously impair memory is apparent from the occurrence of **hysterical amnesia**, a syndrome in which the patient, who is apparently alert, may have no recollection of his identity, his address or of any other details concerning himself. The condition, which is usually of acute onset, so that the patient is found wandering aimlessly, is presumably due to some process of psychological inhibition resulting in an inability to reopen voluntarily the pathways where memories are retained. Usually it develops as a method of escape from undue stress. Hysterical amnesia may be feigned as a defence against a criminal charge and can then be difficult to distinguish from the genuine disorder.

Cerebral Irritation

In addition to the manifestations of delirium or confusion which occur in patients with diffuse brain disease such as meningitis, encephalitis and subarachnoid haemorrhage, these individuals often show a typical behaviour pattern which is characteristic of so-called 'cerebral irritation'. They lie curled up on one side in bed, often with their eyes away from the light, and resent being disturbed, so that they may pull back the bedclothes when the doctor attempts to remove them. If the meninges are inflamed, neck stiffness will generally be apparent as well.

Transient Disorders of Consciousness

One of the commonest problems which a doctor is asked to solve is to determine the significance of brief disorders of consciousness, often referred to as 'blackouts'. Are these fits or faints, that is, are they epileptic or syncopal or, less commonly, of metabolic or emotional origin? No distinction can be more important for social and occupational reasons and, at times, none can be more difficult to make with confidence.

Epilepsy

Epilepsy is difficult to define in view of the many guises which it may assume. Many definitions have been offered, varying from the frankly mechanistic (a recurrent cerebral dysrhythmia) to the unrealistically psychoanalytical (a manifestation of an unconscious desire for unconsciousness). Though no definition can be sufficiently broad and at the same time exclusive of disturbances of consciousness which are essentially different, it is possible to regard epilepsy as a recurrent disorder of consciousness which is typically transient, ceases spontaneously, and is often preceded or accompanied by motor or sensory phenomena. Though such a definition used would embrace most cases of epilepsy it could unfortunately also be used to describe certain cases of syncope and other conditions which are certainly not epilepsy and must be distinguished from it. Furthermore, loss of consciousness is not invariable in some attacks which are undoubtedly epileptic.

In considering the **pathophysiology** of epilepsy, it is notable that application to the cerebral cortex of acetylcholine (ACh) can precipitate depolarisation of groups of neurones giving localised uncontrolled discharge and clinical manifestations of focal epilepsy. By contrast, gamma-aminobutyric acid (GABA) increases the concentration gradient of sodium across the neuronal cell membrane to give hyperpolarisation and reduced excitability. Thus GABA acts as a natural anticonvulsant and any disorder which upsets the ACh/GABA ratio (such as deficiency of pyridoxine, which is essential in the synthesis of GABA) could predispose to epilepsy. Many circumstances which alter cerebral metabolism, including metabolic disease, toxins, drugs and drug withdrawal, may have a similar effect.

In considering **aetiology** it is possible to divide cases of epilepsy into two broad groups, namely so-called *idiopathic* and *symptomatic* epilepsy. In cases of idiopathic epilepsy there is no evidence of any organic brain lesion which is responsible for the attacks, nor do these usually have a focal onset. Because idiopathic attacks are believed to result from a functional disturbance in the basal areas of the brain which exercise control over cortical activity (such as the reticular substance), they are often referred to as 'central', 'centrencephalic', or 'cryptogenic' epilepsy (Fig. 4). In symptomatic epilepsy, the attacks are a symptom of organic brain disease,

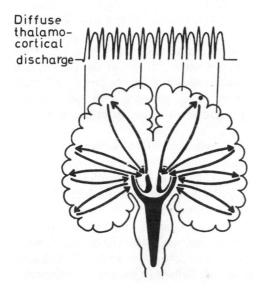

Diffuse
thalamo-
cortical
discharge

Fig. 4. Diffuse thalamocortical discharge, associated with impairment of consciousness. This may be triggered by extension of epileptic activity from a cortical focus
(secondary centrencephalic epilepsy) or may occur spontaneously in patients with
the centrencephalic trait of petit mal epilepsy.
(Reproduced from *A Physiological Approach to Clinical Neurology*, 3rd edition, by Lance and McLeod, by kind permission
of the authors and publisher.)

whether it be the effects of fever (febrile convulsions), diffuse degenerative
brain disease, an infarct, encephalitis or abscess, a cerebral tumour or a
scar following head injury (post-traumatic epilepsy), anoxia, toxaemia,
hypoglycaemia, hypocalcaemia or drug withdrawal. Some suggest that
seizures occurring as a result of overt brain disease should not be regarded
as epilepsy, and that this term should be reserved for the 'idiopathic'
condition. This view is untenable as the nature of the attacks may be the
same in the two types of case and more and more cases previously
considered to be suffering from idiopathic epilepsy are being found to be
cases of the symptomatic variety, in which unsuspected cerebral lesions
account for the attacks. Many apparently normal individuals would have
fits if their brains were subject to a pathological or biochemical insult of
sufficient degree, but this tendency is a variable one which is probably
specific to the individual. The so-called 'convulsive threshold' shows
marked variation from one person to another. Those with a very high
threshold would never suffer a convulsion, no matter how severe the
stimulus, while those in whom it is low are the 'idiopathic' epileptics who
have attacks without apparent cause. But it is difficult to draw a clear line
of demarcation between the epileptic and non-epileptic in those whose
'convulsive threshold' falls between these two extremes. Thus not more
than 50 per cent of patients with penetrating brain injuries develop

post-traumatic epilepsy. Hence it is reasonable to regard all epileptiform seizures as epilepsy, but always to look for an organic cause and only to accept a diagnosis of idiopathic epilepsy if the search is negative. How assiduous this search should be depends upon the age of the patient and many other factors which will be considered in Chapter 20 (*see* p. 422). With present investigative techniques many patients with symptomatic epilepsy are probably wrongly diagnosed as suffering from the idiopathic variety.

The convulsive threshold is clearly constitutional and a hereditary factor is important as many epileptics have epileptic relatives. Even so, no clear pattern of inheritance emerges and the chances that an epileptic may have a child who is similarly affected are not very great statistically if the other partner of the marriage is normal. Although certain analeptic drugs (picrotoxin, leptazole, bemegride) may precipitate epileptic seizures, as may fluid retention in the body, no consistent biochemical or other abnormality has been found in patients with idiopathic seizures. Although attacks are common in some women just before or during the menstrual period (*catamenial epilepsy*), endocrine factors seem unimportant.

A further factor to be considered is the resistance of the brain to the spread of the epileptic discharge, a property which may be independent of the convulsive threshold. If this resistance is low and spread is rapid, a focal lesion will give a generalised convulsion with immediate loss of consciousness and no localising features (Fig. 4), while if it is high, the epileptic manifestations will remain localised to the appropriate area of the body (*focal* or *Jacksonian epilepsy*) and consciousness may be unimpaired throughout the attack. Where resistance is intermediate between these two extremes the onset of the fit may be focal but it then develops into a generalised seizure.

Hence one satisfactory method of classifying cases of epilepsy is on an aetiological basis, but this can only be done with confidence in a comparatively small proportion of cases. Some important causes of symptomatic epilepsy are listed in Table 4. However, for practical purposes relating to diagnosis and management it is necessary to rely upon a clinical classification depending upon the character of the attacks, as outlined in Table 5. Traditionally such attacks, whether idiopathic or symptomatic, have been divided into minor epilepsy (petit mal), major epilepsy (grand mal), focal or Jacksonian epilepsy, temporal lobe epilepsy (psychomotor epilepsy) and myoclonic attacks. However, as Table 5 indicates, this descriptive classification is unsatisfactory, first because there are many forms of minor epilepsy which are not true petit mal, while temporal lobe epilepsy is now recognised to be no more than a specific variety of focal epilepsy, commonly called nowadays complex partial epilepsy. The description given below will deal successively with the different clinical varieties of attacks, indicating how each of these stands in relation to the more modern classification outlined in Table 5.

Table 4   Some Important Causes of Symptomatic Epilepsy*

Local Causes

(*a*) Focal intracranial lesions sometimes associated with increased intracranial pressure:
  Intracranial tumour; cerebral abscess; subdural haematoma; angioma or haematoma.
(*b*) Inflammatory and demyelinating conditions:
  Meningitis; all forms of acute and subacute encephalitis; toxoplasmosis; neurosyphilis; multiple sclerosis; cerebral cysticercosis.
(*c*) Trauma:
  Perinatal brain injury and/or haemorrhage; head injuries of later life.
(*d*) Congenital abnormalities:
  Congenital diplegia; tuberous sclerosis; porencephaly.
(*e*) Degenerations and inborn errors of metabolism:
  The cerebral lipidoses; diffuse sclerosis and the leukodystrophies; encephalopathies of infancy and childhood, including 'infantile spasms'; phenylketonuria and other inborn errors; Pick's disease; Alzheimer's disease; progressive myoclonic epilepsy; subacute spongiform encephalopathy; Creutzfeldt-Jakob disease.
(*f*) Vascular disorders:
  Cerebral atheroma, intracranial haemorrhage, thrombosis, embolism; eclampsia; hypertensive encephalopathy; cerebral complications of 'connective tissue' or 'collagen' diseases; polycythaemia; intracranial aneurysm; acute cerebral ischaemia from any cause.

General Causes

(*a*) Exogenous poisons:
  Alcohol; absinthe; thujone; cocaine; strychnine; lead; chloroform; ether; insulin; amphetamine; camphor; *Metrazol*, organophosphorus and organochlorine compounds used as insecticides, and fluoracetic acid derivatives; amine-oxidase inhibitors, imipramine and its derivatives; and *withdrawal* of alcohol, barbiturates and other drugs.
(*b*) Anoxia:
  Asphyxia; carbon monoxide poisoning; nitrous oxide anaesthesia; profound anaemia.
(*c*) Disordered metabolism:
  Uraemia; hepatic failure; hypo-adrenalism; water intoxication; porphyria; hypoglycaemia; hyperpyrexia; alkalosis; hyperkalaemia; pyridoxine deficiency.
(*d*) Endocrine disorders:
  Parathyroid tetany; idiopathic hypoparathyroidism and pseudohypoparathyroidism.
(*e*) Conditions associated particularly with childhood:
  Rickets; acute infections ('febrile convulsions').

---

* Modified from *Brain's Diseases of the Nervous System*, 8th edition (Walton, 1977) by kind permission of the publishers.

Table 5   The Clinical Classification of Epileptic Seizures*

Generalised Seizures
   Bilaterally symmetrical seizures without local onset:
   (*a*) Absences (petit mal)
   (*b*) Bilateral myoclonus
   (*c*) Infantile spasms
   (*d*) Clonic seizures
   (*e*) Tonic seizures
   (*f*) Tonic-clonic seizures (grand mal)
   (*g*) Akinetic seizures

Partial Seizures
   Seizures beginning locally with:
   (*a*) Elementary symptomatology
         motor   ⎫
         sensory ⎬ Jacksonian epilepsy
         autonomic ⎭
   (*b*) Complex symptomatology
         impaired consciousness ⎫
         complex hallucinations ⎬ temporal lobe epilepsy
         affective symptoms   ⎪
         automatism   ⎭
   (*c*) Partial seizures becoming generalised tonic-clonic seizures

Unclassified Seizures
   Seizures which cannot be classified because of incomplete data.

* Modified from *Brain's Diseases of the Nervous System*, 8th edition (Walton, 1977) by kind permission of the publishers.

Generalised Seizures

Minor Epilepsy

Attacks of true **petit mal** (absence seizures) begin only in childhood, occur in either sex and sometimes continue into adult life, but often cease in adolescence. Often patients with this type of epilepsy also have occasional major seizures and in others when petit mal ceases it is replaced by major attacks. True petit mal can be regarded as the classical form of idiopathic epilepsy; it is practically never symptomatic, although attacks which are clinically identical may be observed in children with diffuse brain disease or cerebral birth injury; in such cases there are also major attacks as a rule. Petit mal can often be identified by the typical generalised spike-and-wave discharge in the EEG.

An attack of petit mal is usually momentary, lasting only a few seconds; the child's expression suddenly becomes blank, his eyes roll upwards and there may be a brief spasmodic jerk of the limbs (**myoclonus**); within a moment he is normal again. The loss of consciousness is so transient that the child does not fall, and his attention span is so briefly disrupted that he may, for instance, continue to read aloud after an almost imperceptible pause. In very occasional cases the attack is sufficiently prolonged for the child to fall to the ground, only to pick himself up again immediately (**akinetic epilepsy**—a purely descriptive term implying loss of consciousness without spasmodic movements). However, attacks of the latter type are variable in aetiology and are more often episodes of major epilepsy. Attacks of petit mal can occur as often as 20 to 30 times daily and are sometimes increased by emotional stress. This form of epilepsy usually has a good prognosis as many sufferers lose their attacks in adolescence and remain well, but others go on to develop major seizures, while in a few cases, attacks of petit mal, having begun in childhood continue, usually with diminished frequency, in adult life.

The rare condition of so-called *tonic epilepsy* is one in which one or more limbs suddenly become extended and rigid but there are no clonic movements; consciousness may or may not be lost. Usually such attacks result from organic brain disease. Focal tonic fits have been described in multiple sclerosis.

A type of attack which develops suddenly in infants and is characterised by momentary flexion of the head, neck and trunk with drawing up of the knees (salaam attacks) has been identified by the name of *infantile spasms*. The attacks may occur many times in the day and most affected infants eventually become spastic and severely retarded mentally even after the attacks cease, as they usually do after some months. The EEG usually shows hypsarrhythmia (*see* p. 53). The cause is unknown but a few cases are due to tuberous sclerosis and these attacks rarely occur in patients with phenylketonuria. Anticonvulsants are relatively ineffective in such cases but steroid drugs may arrest the process.

Major Seizures (Clonic and Tonic-Clonic Seizures)

A major convulsion or grand mal attack (Fig. 5) will result from a focal cerebral lesion, in the temporal lobe or elsewhere, if the spread of the epileptic discharge occurs rapidly throughout the cerebral hemispheres. It can also be a symptom of diffuse brain disease, but in many cases no cause can be found and the attacks are presumed to be idiopathic or 'centrencephalic' in origin. The younger the patient, the more likely this is. Most patients with idiopathic major epilepsy first develop attacks in childhood or early adult life, whereas in middle age the number found to have cerebral tumours or vascular disease as a cause of the fits is much greater; however, even in late life no cause is demonstrable in many cases.

The typical major attack may begin with an aura or warning which indicates the situation of onset of the discharge but often this sensation is indefinable and little more than a 'sinking feeling' or an 'odd sensation in the head'. It is rare for an aura to last for more than a second or two and very often there is no warning at all. Consciousness is lost, the patient falls and may injure himself in the process, as when falling on to a fire. Cuts

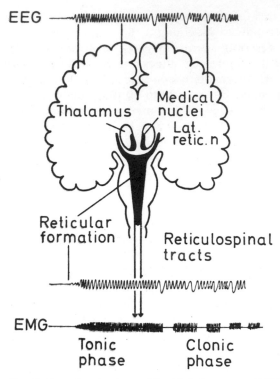

EEG

Thalamus

Medical nuclei

Lat. retic. n

Reticular formation

Reticulospinal tracts

EMG

Tonic phase

Clonic phase

Fig. 5. Grand mal seizure. The high-frequency EEG discharge of the tonic phase is later interrupted by slow waves which inhibit cerebral activity and permit brief periods of muscular relaxation, responsible for the clonic phase of the seizure.
(Reproduced from *A Physiological Approach to Clinical Neurology*, 3rd edition, by Lance and McLeod, by kind permission of the authors and publisher.)

and bruises and falls downstairs are relatively common. The muscles then go rigid (the tonic phase), the teeth are clenched, the tongue is often bitten, the patient becomes cyanosed, and salivates at the mouth (frothing). Within a few seconds, the musculature relaxes and rhythmical repetitive jerking of the limbs and trunk occurs (the clonic phase). The patient is often incontinent of urine and occasionally of faeces. Sometimes the clonic phase is absent and the attack is so brief that the patient falls and then jumps up almost immediately (akinetic seizures). More frequently the jerking continues for a minute or two and is followed by relaxation. Often the patient falls into a deep sleep, but if roused he is briefly confused, or confusion may even last for several minutes or hours. In other cases he is lucid and co-operative almost at once. Often there is a headache and muscular aching which persists for some hours and vomiting occasionally occurs.

Death in a major convulsion is a very rare complication if the airway is kept clear, but if repeated convulsions occur without recovery of consciousness between them (*status epilepticus*) there is some danger to life and treatment is an urgent matter.

It was once thought that mental disease may be a sequel of long-continued epileptic seizures. While some patients with temporal lobe epilepsy become psychotic, it is questionable whether it is the epilepsy itself or the primary pathological changes in the temporal lobe which are responsible. Similarly there is no evidence that epilepsy itself influences the mentality, but many diffuse cerebral disorders which give rise to dementia can produce symptomatic epileptic seizures. Diffuse brain damage resulting from anoxia occurring in repeated attacks of severe major epilepsy can, however, cause progressive dementia.

Myoclonic Epilepsy

Myoclonus, a momentary shock-like contraction of a group of voluntary muscles, can accompany attacks of petit mal, but similar manifestations occur sporadically and repetitively in some cases without apparent impairment of consciousness. Occasional myoclonic jerks occurring when falling asleep are physiological, but frequent nocturnal myoclonic jerks are often an epileptic manifestation and many such patients also have major seizures. Repeated myoclonic jerking can also be a symptom of diffuse progressive brain disease, in such conditions as cerebral lipidosis (when it occurs particularly on startle), subacute sclerosing panencephalitis (when there is also progressive dementia) and the rare condition of progressive myoclonic epilepsy of Unverricht (in which the myoclonus becomes progressively more frequent and severe, dementia also occurs and the patient eventually dies from exhaustion and inanition). In such cases degenerative changes and intranuclear inclusions (Lafora bodies) may be found in the dentate nucleus of the cerebellum and abnormal mucopolysaccharides may be found in the serum.

Myoclonic jerking is also common in some cases of rapidly progressive degenerative brain disease (e.g. Creutzfeldt–Jakob disease) which give rise to progressive dementia and paralysis in middle or late life. Paramyoclonus multiplex is a name which has been given to a relatively benign disorder in which widespread myoclonic jerks of distressing frequency develop in adult life and involve facial and limb muscles to a variable extent but major fits and dementia do not occur. The condition may be familial (hereditary essential myoclonus) and is similar to another uncommon condition (hyperekplexia) in which severe sudden jerks resembling myoclonus occur only on startle (e.g. sudden noise).

Partial Seizures

This group embraces a great variety of epileptic manifestations, including most forms of **focal** or **Jacksonian epilepsy** in which the spread of epileptic discharge is not sufficiently rapid to give a major convulsion. The pattern of the seizures depends upon the area of the brain which is being irritated by the organic lesion whether it be a tumour, a scar of previous injury, or any other pathological change, and upon the direction of spread of the epileptic discharge. Focal epilepsy always implies the presence of a localised cerebral lesion, even though in some cases techniques of investigation at present available are inadequate to demonstrate its nature. In such cases, the EEG may show focal spike or sharp-wave discharges, or localised slow activity.

If the lesion lies in or near the motor cortex, then the attack usually consists of intermittent rhythmical (clonic) jerking of a hand and arm and this may spread to the face or leg, depending upon which part of the cortex is involved. If the discharge continues for hours or even days, these manifestations can be prolonged (*epilepsia partialis continua*), but more often the attack subsides in seconds or minutes. It may be followed by transient weakness of the affected member (Todd's paralysis). Though consciousness is often clouded during the attack it is sometimes unimpaired throughout. So-called *adversive attacks* with turning of the head and eyes and even of the whole body to the opposite side, can result from lesions in the frontal eye field anterior to the precentral gyrus. *Sensory epilepsy* will result from lesions near the sensory cortex, when paraesthesiae rather than jerking are the primary manifestation, though the latter may develop if spread to the motor cortex follows. When epileptic discharges begin in the occipital lobe, crude visual phenomena result (bright lines or flashes of light), while if visual association areas are involved the patient can experience formed visual hallucinations of people or of past events. Similarly a lesion near the speech areas may give transient aphasia and one near the auditory cortex auditory hallucinations, either crude or highly organised, depending upon whether the actual cortex or its association areas are primarily affected. Should the spread of the epileptic discharge be rapid, any of these manifestations can constitute the brief aura of a major seizure and will give useful information concerning the situation of onset of the epileptic discharge.

The commonest and most important form of focal epilepsy is **temporal lobe epilepsy**, which has been variously referred to as psychomotor epilepsy, 'epileptic equivalents' or complex partial seizures. Many patients with both minor and major seizures have foci of epileptic discharge in one or other temporal lobe, a fact which may be indicated either by the content of the seizure or by the aura or sequelae of a major attack. The high incidence of this form of epilepsy is due to the frequency with which pathological changes occur in the anterior and medial parts of the temporal lobes (uncus, hippocampus, amygdaloid nucleus, Ammon's horn). These changes can result from birth injury, with 'moulding' of the head and herniation of the medial part of the temporal lobe through the tentorial hiatus, or from cerebral anoxia, however caused. Transient anoxia occurring in repeated attacks of major epilepsy may increase such changes.

Although the lesions responsible are often present from birth, and some attacks of temporal lobe epilepsy begin in childhood, these seizures sometimes do not develop until adolescence or adult life, though acquired lesions (such as vascular malformations or neoplasms) are responsible in some older patients. The number of clinical manifestations which may be noted in such cases is legion and is clearly dependent upon the many important physiological functions which are subserved by the temporal lobes. Thus the attack may embrace intense *emotional experiences* (fear, depression, anxiety), feelings of unreality (*depersonalisation* or *jamais vu*) or a sensation of intense familiarity as if the patient were living through a vivid past experience (*déjà vu*). There may also be unpleasant hallucinations of smell or taste (*uncinate seizures*), *vasomotor manifestations* (sweating, salivation, palpitation and 'butterflies in the stomach'), or *vertigo,* while *irrational speech or behaviour* (automatism, such as undressing in public) or even episodes of *violent rage* can occur. It is, however, exceptional for crimes of violence to be committed in such attacks, although such a mechanism is sometimes postulated in epileptic patients charged with murder. *Gelastic epilepsy* (uncontrolled laughing during the attack) and *cursive epilepsy* (running or 'circling' as an epileptic phenomenon) are forms of automatism.

It is in occasional cases of this type that *permanent mental changes* of psychotic type may develop. The negativism and paranoid delusions which occur in some patients with severe and longstanding temporal lobe epilepsy can often be confused with schizophrenia. Contrary to views once expressed in the past, however, there is no evidence that there is a specific 'epileptic personality'. Sometimes when there is spread of discharge to the lower end of the motor cortex, smacking of the lips or twitching of the corner of the mouth occurs, while if epileptic discharge spreads more posteriorly there may be distortion of visual images so that objects look smaller (*micropsia*) or larger (*macropsia*) or appear to be fading into the distance. Any such manifestations occurring episodically, without warning, either in isolation or in succession, should suggest a diagnosis of temporal lobe epilepsy, particularly if there is associated clouding of consciousness and certainly if they are followed by a major convulsion. Nevertheless, it may be difficult to distinguish between temporal lobe seizures on the one hand and episodes of phobic anxiety (with panic and depersonalisation) on the other, as fainting can result from the hyperventilation which often occurs in panic attacks. Any irritative focal lesion in the temporal lobe can produce the features described and while this may be a scar of long standing, it is sometimes an expanding lesion such as a tumour.

It is of interest that powerful sensory stimuli can sometimes provoke focal epileptic discharges in patients who have foci in the appropriate area of the brain. Thus activation of epileptic seizures by music (*musicogenic epilepsy*) or intermittent light flashes (photic stimulation) has been observed and some children with '*self-induced*' epilepsy find that they can produce petit mal attacks by passing their open fingers rapidly between their eyes and a bright light. Other forms of **'reflex epilepsy'** include *television epilepsy* (attacks of minor or major type induced by watching television, particularly when the set is poorly adjusted), *reading epilepsy* (attacks induced by reading), and seizures (which are usually focal) precipitated by movement of the part of the body in which the fit begins (*kinesogenic epilepsy*). So-called 'drop' attacks (sudden falling without loss of consciousness) are rarely due to akinetic or inhibitory epilepsy; such episodes occurring in adolescents may be hysterical whereas in elderly patients they may be due to brain stem ischaemia but are more often unexplained. In contrast to reflex epilepsy, it is sometimes possible to abort an epileptic seizure by applying sensory stimuli which presumably compete for the occupancy of the fibre pathways along which the epileptic discharge is spreading. Some patients find that they can shorten minor attacks by means of powerful concentration, while others, for instance, who experience seizures with an aura of uncinate type (*see above*) can stop the attack by sniffing a substance with a powerful odour.

While it is impossible to describe all the possible manifestations of partial epilepsy, the principles outlined indicate that almost any symptom of disordered cerebral function can occur as a manifestation of this condition.

Conclusions

Epilepsy may thus be classified from the aetiological standpoint into idiopathic and symptomatic varieties and the idiopathic group is clearly one which is diminishing steadily, as newer techniques reveal more organic disorders of the brain which produce epilepsy as a symptom. Clinically true petit mal (absence seizures) is to be distinguished as a separate entity, at present of unknown aetiology; in many patients with major seizures, too, the condition must still be regarded as 'idiopathic'. Many patients with grand mal, however, and most of those with partial seizures, are suffering from focal organic brain disease, frequently affecting the temporal lobe. As we shall see in Chapter 20 (pp. 422–427), accurate diagnosis is of great importance from the point of view of treatment.

Syncope and Other Brief Disorders of Consciousness

It is sometimes very difficult to differentiate clinically between simple faints or syncopal attacks and epileptic seizures. Syncope is most common in young patients, particularly adolescent girls, and is often produced by long periods of standing in one position (as in church, on parade or in morning school assembly), by an emotional shock ('the sight of blood'), or by 'stuffy' atmospheres. It is particularly liable to occur in early pregnancy, can develop at any age in patients with uraemia or blood loss, or with heart block (**the Stokes–Adams syndrome**). In the latter condition, syncope with pallor occurs during a period of cardiac asystole, and when the circulation is restored, the patient's face flushes and there may even be convulsive movements. Indeed, syncope however caused can rarely result in transient epileptic manifestations, including transient twitching of the limbs and urinary incontinence, if cerebral anoxia is sufficiently prolonged. Cardiac lesions other than heart block, which diminish cardiac output (e.g. aortic stenosis, auricular fibrillation or paroxysmal tachycardia) can be associated with recurrent fainting. So too are chronic bronchitis and emphysema in that severe bouts of coughing with fixation of the chest wall in expansion may so impair venous return to the heart as to result in episodes of **cough syncope**. **Carotid sinus syncope** occurs in those in whom turning of the head or pressure upon the neck causes abnormal slowing of the heart rate or even asystole due to increased sensitivity of the carotid sinus. Rarely, fainting occurs in patients with stenotic lesions of the carotid and vertebral vessels which reduce cerebral blood flow. **Micturition syncope** is not uncommon, particularly in the elderly male patient who gets up during the night with a full bladder and loses his senses in the toilet.

In general terms, syncope is due to cerebral ischaemia, resulting usually from pooling of blood in the skin and viscera. Generally the patient feels a 'swimming in the head' and a sensation of heat; he then perspires and can usually reach a place of safety before consciousness is lost (unless he is standing on parade). The loss of consciousness is usually brief, the patient's skin is deathly pale, cold and clammy, and his pulse is often thin and rapid, but occasionally slow. The aura of a syncopal attack is usually considerably longer than that of an epileptic seizure, there are often emotional or physical precipitants, and injury in attacks is uncommon, while convulsive movements and incontinence are rare. The attacks usually occur when standing and not when sitting or lying. Often they are brought on by standing up abruptly. These are the principal points upon which differential diagnosis is based. Syncope due to transient postural hypotension is particularly likely to occur after a hot bath, over-indulgence in alcohol, after sympathectomy, in patients with spinal cord lesions impairing pressor reflexes (as in tabes dorsalis) and in those taking hypotensive drugs or some tranquillisers (especially phenothiazines).

In the uncommon condition of **chronic orthostatic hypotension** (the Shy–Drager syndrome), which is often familial and is due to degeneration in the autonomic nervous system, the blood pressure falls when the patient assumes the upright position and as the compensatory reflexes are impaired there is no pallor, sweating or tachycardia and consciousness is lost; recovery occurs as soon as the patient lies down. In many cases dysarthria and cerebellar ataxia eventually develop; at autopsy, degeneration of cells in the intermediolateral grey column of the spinal cord is usually found. Some patients develop progressive Parkinsonian features, dementia and impotence, even occasionally incontinence (so-called **progressive multi-system degeneration**).

So-called **vaso-vagal attacks** have been described in which the patient becomes flushed and his pulse is slowed, while gastric or cardiac discomfort may occur. There is considerable doubt as to whether stereotyped attacks of this nature are at all common, and it now seems that they should not be afforded separate identification, being merely one form of syncopal attack.

Drop attacks are episodes in which the patient's legs give way and he falls but does not lose consciousness. They are commonest in elderly women and are either due to transient brain stem ischaemia or to an inhibitory mechanism of unknown cause involving the brain stem reticular substance.

Hysterical convulsions are generally bizarre and florid with more violent and varied and less stereotyped movements than occur in epilepsy, while tongue-biting, injury and incontinence do not generally occur and the patient shows other manifestations of hysteria. In some patients tongue-biting and/or incontinence may eventually be produced in the attacks when the patient has been repeatedly questioned about these symptoms. In young women, hysterical attacks may also take the form of sudden falling with, apparently, transient loss of consciousness and without convulsive movements. Similar attacks are seen in some male patients who develop a so-called accident neurosis after minor injury. When these attacks occur in young females who have also had genuine attacks of epilepsy, differential diagnosis can be very difficult. Hysterical hyperventilation (rapid panting respiration) which is often accompanied by panic and which leads to paraesthesiae in the lips and tongue and even to tetany, may also give rise to syncope and is often misdiagnosed. The **tetany** which occurs as a result of hyperventilation is due to alkalosis resulting from loss of CO_2 in the expired air. Other disorders associated with tetany which reduce the serum ionised calcium (repeated vomiting, dietary alkalosis, rickets and osteomalacia, hypoparathyroidism and malabsorption) do not usually give rise to attacks of loss of consciousness. However, in idiopathic hypoparathyroidism attacks of epilepsy are common. The typical carpopedal spasms of tetany with other evidence of neuromuscular excitability (positive Cvostek's and Trousseau's signs) usually ensure that attacks of this nature are not confused with focal epilepsy and estimation of the serum calcium will be diagnostic.

Spontaneous hypoglycaemia can give rise to attacks of light-headedness, fatigue, sweating, paraesthesiae, giddiness and even confused and irrational behaviour. Rarely, major epileptic convulsions result, particularly in those patients who have a tumour of the islets of Langerhans, with excessive insulin production (organic hyperinsulinism). When reactive or functional hyperinsulinism is the cause, due to an excessive fall in blood sugar following the peak produced by a high carbohydrate meal, or after rapid gastric emptying (such as may follow gastrectomy or gastroenterostomy), the symptoms are as a rule less severe. Nevertheless this condition, too, must be considered in determining the cause of transient disturbances of consciousness.

References

Adams, R. D. and Victor, M., *Principles of Neurology*, 2nd ed. (New York, McGraw Hill, 1981).

Critchley, M., O'Leary, J. L. and Jennett, B. (Eds.), *Scientific Foundations of Neurology* (London, Heinemann, 1972).

Jackson, J. H., *Selected Writings of John Hughlings Jackson,* Ed. Taylor, J., Vol. 1 (London, Staples, 1958).

Laidlaw, J. and Richens, A., *A Textbook of Epilepsy*, 2nd ed. (Edinburgh, London, New York, Churchill Livingstone, 1981).

Lance, J. W. and McLeod, J. G., *A Physiological Approach to Clinical Neurology,* 3rd ed. (London, Butterworth, 1981).

Matthews, W. B., *Practical Neurology,* Chapters 3–4, 3rd ed. (Oxford, Blackwell, 1975).

Mayer-Gross, W., Slater, E. and Roth, M., *Clinical Psychiatry,* 3rd ed., 291–318 (London, Cassell, 1969).

Penfield, W. and Jasper, H., *Epilepsy and the Functional Anatomy of the Human Brain* (London, Churchill, 1954).

Plum, F. and Posner, J. B., *Diagnosis of Stupor and Coma,* 3rd ed. (Oxford, Blackwell and Philadelphia, Davis, 1980).

Patton, H. D., Sundsten, J. W., Crill, W. E. and Swanson, P. D., *Introduction to Basic Neurology* (Philadelphia, W. B. Saunders, 1976).

Smythies, J. R., *Brain Mechanisms and Behaviour* (New York, Academic Press, 1970).

Sutherland, J. M., Tait, H. and Eadie, M. J., *The Epilepsies: Modern Diagnosis and Treatment,* 3rd ed. (Edinburgh and London, Churchill Livingstone, 1980).

Walton, J. N., *Brain's Diseases of the Nervous System,* 8th ed. (London, Oxford University Press, 1977).

Walton, J. N., Section X on Neurological pathophysiology, in *International Textbook of Medicine*, Ed. Smith, J. H. and Thier, S. (Philadelphia and London, W. B. Saunders, 1981).

7 Disorders of the Mind

A complete appreciation of the brain–mind relationship has defied the understanding of philosophers and physicians for centuries and is likely to do so for many years to come. Though much has been learned concerning the disorders of thought processes which result from brain disease, and the Freudian discipline of psychopathology has cast light upon some factors which may be responsible in part for mental disease, we still know little of the means by which cerebral activity subserves and controls human thought. It is this lack of fundamental knowledge concerning the physiology of thought which has led to the wide divergence of opinion between groups of psychiatrists, some of whom believe that virtually all mental disorder can be accounted for by physical changes, some as yet unidentified, which affect the functioning of the brain, while others, and particularly the psychoanalysts, consider that psychological influences are all-important. In fact, it seems probable that it is a combination of factors, psychological, physical and constitutional, which generally account for symptoms of mental disorder in any individual case. So many varieties of mental disease (in the broadest sense) can result from the interplay of these aetiological factors that the concept of specific mental diseases is gradually disappearing, to be replaced by a more flexible terminology which takes account of psychiatric syndromes, their variability and their interrelationship. Thus it was once agreed that a **neurosis**, characterised usually by anxiety and related symptoms, and resulting from psychological causes, was different aetiologically and prognostically from a **psychosis**, a term generally implying insanity, and typified by serious derangement of thought processes. It is now apparent that the distinction between these two disorders is not absolute and that neurotic or psychotic reactions may occur in response to organic disease.

A detailed survey of the minutiae of psychiatric classification and differential diagnosis would be out of place in a work on neurology, and for this information the reader must turn to a textbook of psychiatry. However, so many mental symptoms can accompany or simulate brain disease that a brief survey of some common psychiatric syndromes is essential in order to assist in the identification of neurological disorders which may be complicated or imitated in this way.

As disorders of consciousness and of memory, including the symptomatic psychoses, were considered in the preceding chapter, it will be convenient to consider first developmental or constitutional disorders such as mental retardation or handicap (**amentia** or **oligophrenia**), which can be considered to be a disorder of physical development, then **abnormalities of personality and character**, disorders which are primarily abnormalities of psychological development. Secondly we must discuss **dementia**, which is a diffuse disintegration of mental function, involving intellect, memory, thought, emotions and behaviour, and is usually due to organic brain disease. Next we shall consider a number of **fundamental psychiatric reactions** which occur in response to various physical or mental stimuli, some of which are known, others unknown. Commonest of these are **disorders of mood or affect**, sometimes called the affective disorders, of which the most prominent symptoms are anxiety and/or depression. **Hysteria** is another common psychiatric reaction, in which there are symptoms of mental or physical type, unaccounted for by organic disease, but activated by the desire to gain profit from the symptom or to escape from stress. Another type of neurotic reaction is the **obsessive-compulsive** variety, in which insistent thoughts so occupy the patient's mind that they may compel him to carry out actions which he knows are foolish or unnecessary but which he cannot resist. The **schizophrenic** reaction is characterised particularly by introversion, severe distortion of thought processes and by paranoid features which imply ideas of persecution; this disorder is essentially constitutional and is not usually the result of exogenous factors. Finally, brief mention must be made of some so-called **psychosomatic disorders,** a group of physical conditions in which psychological factors clearly play an important aetiological role.

Mental Retardation

Mental retardation implies an intellectual deficit which is present from birth and can be confirmed by psychometric testing, by means of which the intelligence quotient (I.Q.) and 'mental age' of the patient are assessed. In the past, low-grade mental defectives were divided into the idiots (mental age of up to three in an adult) and imbeciles (mental age of up to seven). Nowadays the terms 'severe' and 'moderate' retardation or handicap are preferred. The severely retarded are incapable of guarding themselves against common dangers and must usually be confined in institutions. Moderately retarded individuals are also incapable of managing themselves or their affairs, but are occasionally able to live satisfactorily in a protected domestic environment and may even be able to do work of a low-grade nature. The group which used to be called high-grade mental defectives or morons, now known as cases of mild mental retardation, some of whom have IQs approaching the lower normal limit of 80, are common and mostly live outside institutions. Some can be educated in ordinary schools but others must attend schools for the educationally subnormal. The diagnosis of mild retardation can readily be overlooked and the patient is often regarded as being 'rather stupid', 'incapable of giving a reasonable history', 'hypochondriacal'. Character defects are common in such retarded patients and many habitual petty criminals, prostitutes, sexual offenders and murderers fall into this group.

In many severely and moderately retarded individuals, as well as in some of those less severely affected, there are associated congenital abnormalities involving other organs, while epilepsy or signs of 'cerebral palsy' may coexist. In **mongolism** (Down's syndrome), there is a characteristic facial appearance and disorders of skeletal development are also seen. The epicanthal folds are wide, the palpebral fissures oblique, the mouth is usually open with a protruding tongue, the bridge of the nose is broad, the ears are square, and the facial profile is flattened; muscular hypotonia and congenital heart disease are often present and mental retardation is moderate or mild. This condition is now known to result from a disorder of chromosomal constitution in that an extra chromosome may be attached to the 21st pair ('trisomy 21'). Occasionally it results from a chromosomal translocation or mosaic. Sometimes mental retardation is a result of an inborn error of metabolism affecting the nervous system as in **amaurotic family idiocy** (Tay-Sachs form of cerebral lipidosis) or **phenylpyruvic oligophrenia** (a disorder of phenylalanine metabolism), but more often it appears to be due to a combination of genetic influences and not to a single factor or to any definable physical or metabolic disease. Mongolism in the fetus and many of the inborn errors of metabolism can now be detected, when their presence is suspected, by examining amniotic cells (obtained by amniocentesis at about the 12th–14th week of pregnancy) in culture. Selective abortion of affected fetuses then becomes possible.

However it is notable that more than 50 metabolic disorders, some common and some rare, and many involving amino acid metabolism, have now been described in association with mental retardation. In phenylpyruvic oligophrenia (phenylketonuria) the children, who are usually fair-haired and blue-eyed and may suffer from infantile convulsions, become severely retarded if untreated. The diagnosis can be made in the first few days of life by detecting phenylpyruvic acid in the urine with the ferric chloride test. A simple paper-strip test is now used for routine screening of all newborn infants. Treatment with a diet low in phenylalanine may result in normal mental development. Of the many other enzyme defects causing retardation (including Hartnup disease, oculo-cerebral dystrophy, maple-syrup urine disease, galactosaemia, fructosuria, and nephrogenic diabetes insipidus, to quote only a few) few can yet be controlled by dietary or other methods. Nevertheless, careful biochemical screening of infants with suspected retardation is paying increasing dividends, although approximately 50 per cent of cases remain unexplained (non-specific mental retardation).

Abnormalities of Personality and Character

We can recognise in the shy, introverted and absent-minded idealist, or in the fanatical adherent of outlandish cults or causes, differences in personality which distinguish him from his fellows though he may not necessarily be regarded as abnormal. Such an individual is often referred to as **schizoid**, as this type of personality is common in relatives of schizophrenic patients. We shall consider the **hysterical** and **obsessional** characters and the **cyclothymic** personality below. Here, however, **psychopathy** must be mentioned. Psychopaths are persons who, though not insane or mentally defective, behave in a socially abnormal manner. This appears to be a constitutional defect of personality, in which genetic influences play a considerable part. That structural abnormalities of the brain cannot be entirely excluded as a possible cause of psychopathy is indicated by the fact that similar defects of moral sense can occur as a sequel of encephalitis lethargica, but no consistent pathological changes have been found in most psychopaths. A common type of psychopath is the unstable or constitutionally inadequate individual, lacking in determination and diffuse in his efforts, who is incapable of holding down any job for more than a short period. Many such patients are socially irresponsible, and become embezzlers, alcoholics or petty criminals. Flagrant antisocial behaviour is common in other psychopathic individuals and some are inherently aggressive, being liable to sudden outbursts of temper in which they may commit crimes of violence. Education, discipline and punishment have little effect upon these patients, who are essentially lacking in conscience and moral sense, but as they are not insane or mentally retarded their management presents a formidable problem to society.

Dementia

Dementia, or progressive disintegration of the intellect, of memory and of the powers of abstract thought, is a mental disorder which results from organic disease and generally from physical or metabolic disturbances affecting the brain. The first sign of a dementing process may be an error of judgement incompatible with the patient's previous ability, or a failure to grasp all facets of a difficult situation. It may simply be felt that Mr X is 'losing his grip'. Subsequently, memory, particularly for recent events, becomes impaired, so that the patient is forgetful, unable to concentrate and his attention wanders freely. Increasing emotional lability with inappropriate laughing or crying or with irritability and irrational impulsive acts may follow, with striking changes in mood, presenting as elation in some cases and apathy in others. By the time the patient becomes neglectful of his personal appearance and dirty in his habits, the diagnosis is usually obvious, but in the earlier stages it is much more difficult to make. Increasing unpunctuality, neglect of detail, and longer periods spent alone in the bathroom may be useful pointers. Aphasia, apraxia and/or agnosia occur in some cases. It is nevertheless remarkable how often patients with severe dementia continue to hold responsible jobs, despite increasing 'eccentricity', until some major error of judgement or *faux pas* brings matters to a head. In the late stages, delusions occasionally occur, in the form of grandiose imaginings ('I am the King of Spain') or ideas of hostility or persecution towards relatives or business associates. Progressive dementing processes must be distinguished from reversible toxic confusional states, due to metabolic disorders or subdural haematoma, and from the pseudodementia (due to psychomotor retardation) which may be seen in severe endogenous depression or, rarely, in hysteria.

Many forms of organic brain disease give rise to progressive dementia. Most of these disorders are progressive and incurable, but others are eminently treatable and may show no very specific clinical features so that remediable causes should always be borne in mind. The first of these is **neurosyphilis** (particularly general paresis), in which a fatuous euphoric dementia is common and there may also be Argyll Robertson pupils and rarely spastic paresis of the limbs. Diagnosis can be made by cerebrospinal fluid examination. Another possible cause is **intracranial tumour**, either primary or secondary, and involving particularly the frontal lobes. In such cases memory and intellect are often severely affected when other aspects of behaviour and personality are reasonably well preserved, while there may be features (headache, vomiting and papilloedema) to indicate raised intracranial pressure. Recent evidence suggests that a communicating **'low-pressure' hydrocephalus** can sometimes cause a fluctuating confusional state and later progressive dementia, often associated with increased unsteadiness in walking; diagnosis may be made by air encephalography and isotope ventriculography, and in some cases improvement has followed continuous ventricular drainage through a valve inserted into a ventricle with drainage by catheter into the venous circulation (an atrioventricular 'shunt'). A number of **toxic and metabolic disorders** can also result in a progressive dementia; **drug intoxication** and **alcoholism** are usually self-evident causes if the history is adequate, but **pernicious anaemia** and **myxoedema** are other treatable conditions which are easily overlooked and in which the dementia may be reversible with appropriate treatment. When intellectual deterioration follows upon severe diffuse **head injury, anoxia, inflammatory disease**, such as encephalitis or meningitis, **multiple sclerosis, Parkinsonism**, long-standing **temporal lobe epilepsy** or a **chronic psychosis**, the cause is generally apparent and little can usually be done. This also applies to cases of cerebral lipidosis, diffuse cerebral sclerosis and other **degenerative disorders** which cause dementia in childhood. The same is unfortunately true of cases of **cerebral atherosclerosis** in which, however, the dementia, though progressive, is usually step-like, rather than insidious in its advance, being accompanied by transient episodes of confusion, aphasia and/or motor or sensory disturbance, indicating minor 'strokes' due to focal cerebral ischaemia (**multi-infarct dementia**).

Another group of conditions in which progressive deterioration of personality and intellect occurs insidiously and which are unfortunately uninfluenced by treatment, are the group of degenerative cerebral disorders of unknown aetiology known as the **presenile and senile dementias**. Of these, Alzheimer's disease is by far the commonest, and the pathology is the same whether the patient is in the presenile (under 65 years) or senile (over 65) age group. No distinction is now made between presenile and senile dementia. In **Alzheimer's disease** and in **Pick's disease**, there is degeneration of cortical neurones and deposition of argyrophilic material in the form of plaques ('senile plaques') in the cerebral cortex. Granulo-vacuolar degeneration in hippocampal neurones is also found, along with neurofibrillary tangles within the cytoplasm of neurones. Senile plaques occur as a result of normal ageing processes but their number and density is greatly increased above the normal range in demented patients. Along with these changes there is microscopic shrinkage of cortical gyri with dilatation of the cerebral ventricles, changes which are generally demonstrable by CAT scanning. In senile cases, the patient is usually in the seventh or eighth decade, the intellect and personality deteriorate hand in hand and very often there is characteristic nocturnal restlessness, so that the patient wanders about in the middle of the night. Alzheimer's disease may, however, cause progressive dementia in the 40 to 60 age group. In the late stages, aphasia and spasticity of the limbs may develop (what used to be called presenile dementia). Recent research has demonstrated a deficiency of acetylcholine (ACh) and of choline acetyl transferase in the cerebral cortex of such patients and attempts have been made to treat the condition with choline or lecithin which are acetylcholine precursors. In Pick's disease, again a condition of late middle life, there is often affection of more than one member of a family and the pathological changes are more circumscribed, often beginning in one or other frontal lobe. As the changes are initially focal, epilepsy or neurological signs suggesting a localised brain lesion are occasionally seen, while aphasia and defective memory are common at a time when the personality remains reasonably well-preserved; eventually, however, a global dementia supervenes.

Huntington's chorea must also be mentioned as a cause of presenile dementia of relatively non-specific type. In such cases there is generally a clear-cut family history of the condition and the characteristic involuntary movements of the limbs and face are seen though rarely dementia alone is the first manifestation. In the rare degenerative condition sometimes known as **cortico-striato-nigral degeneration**, a disorder which is sometimes familial and has sometimes been called erroneously Creutzfeldt–Jakob disease, a presenile dementia is associated with signs of bilateral pyramidal tract dysfunction, with clinical features suggesting Parkinson's disease, and often with weakness and wasting of peripheral limb muscles. This condition shows some resemblances to the so-called **Parkinsonism-dementia complex** which is endemic in the Chamorro people in the Mariana islands of the South Pacific. It is also well recognised that progressive dementia occurs more often in the later stages of idiopathic Parkinsonism (**paralysis agitans**) than was once thought, and it is also a feature of **progressive multisystem degeneration** (the Shy-Drager syndrome, *see* p. 133) and of some of the hereditary ataxias. True **Creutzfeldt–Jakob disease** (often called also subacute spongiform encephalopathy) is a rapidly-progressive form of dementia accompanied by myoclonic jerking and progressive paralysis in most cases and by a characteristic irregular spike-and-wave discharge in the EEG; the condition is usually fatal in a few months. It is now known to be due to a transmissible agent (a 'slow virus') and has been transferred from one human subject to another by corneal transplantation. It shows several clinical and pathological resemblances to scrapie in sheep.

Hence many possible causes must be considered in any case of dementia; accurate diagnosis is of considerable importance, for in some conditions the prognosis is grave, while in others (neurosyphilis, intoxication, pernicious anaemia, myxoedema and benign intracranial neoplasms) the condition may be reversible with appropriate treatment.

Disorders of Mood (Affective Disorders)

An individual's mood at any moment can broadly be considered to be synonymous with his emotional state. As the hypothalamus and limbic brain (p. 225) exercise considerable control over the emotions it is apparent that disorders of mood may result from certain organic cerebral lesions. It is equally true, however, that the prevailing mood or mood changes may also be substantially influenced, not by physical disease, but by the patient's emotional constitution and by many psychological factors.

The principal mood disturbances which result from organic cerebral disease are emotional liability, apathy, euphoria, excitement, depression and anxiety; those of psychogenic origin are similar but include mania, hypomania and depression (manic-depressive psychosis) and anxiety (anxiety neurosis). **Emotional lability**, characterised by laughing or crying in response to minor or inappropriate emotional stimuli, and by rapid alternation of these emotional responses, is seen usually in patients with extensive bilateral cerebral lesions, particularly when both frontal lobes are involved. It rarely occurs as a result of unilateral lesions and is most often observed in patients with diffuse cerebral vascular disease giving the syndrome of 'pseudobulbar palsy'. **Apathy**, or progressive loss of interest in one's surroundings, leading sometimes to stupor, is an emotional state which generally results from lesions in the hypothalamic region. It occurs in patients with severe postencephalitic Parkinsonism and in diffuse degenerative cerebral disorders, including the presenile dementias, while a similar mental state is also seen in certain psychoses such as severe endogenous depression and schizophrenia. **Euphoria** is a feeling of cheerful well-being, verging sometimes on elation. It occurs in some patients with general paresis and in some with multiple sclerosis, who remain excessively cheerful, sometimes fatuously so, despite their disability; transient euphoria may also result from drugs such as amphetamine and alcohol. **Excitement,** or mental over-activity, which can take the form of elation, rage or excessive volubility, is related to euphoria on the one hand and mania on the other and is often accompanied by agitation and physical restlessness. It is often a feature of the delirious state, and may rarely result from hypothalamic lesions. **Depression** is probably more often psychogenic than due to organic disease, but can be seen in patients with head injury, general paresis, temporal lobe lesions, bronchogenic carcinoma and also in multiple sclerosis. Although this mood disorder can occur as a psychogenic reaction to the presence of incurable illness, there is little doubt that severe depression may also be physically determined, as in that which typically follows severe influenza. **Anxiety**, too, is a natural reaction to many physical illnesses but it too may occasionally be a direct result of organic pathological change, as in the fear and apprehension which may colour delirious states or that which occurs during recovery from severe head injury. A sensation of **angor animi**, or fear of impending doom, typically accompanies an episode of cardiac infarction and a similar sensation or alternatively depression or apprehension amounting to panic can occur as a part of the aura of temporal lobe epilepsy.

Turning to the more serious disorders of mood, the **manic-depressive psychoses** are essentially endogenous, that is, they develop primarily as a result of constitutional or other influences arising within the subject. Recent neuropharmacological studies and work on the biochemistry of depression have suggested that disturbances involving 5-hydroxy-tryptamine (serotonin) and various other neurotransmitters may be involved in the aetiology of depressive illness. Anxiety, on the other hand, is usually a result of exogenous stress, though constitution has a profound influence upon the development of this symptom. Depression, too, may be the result of exogenous factors, in which case it is known as **reactive depression**.

The true manic-depressive fluctuates between a state of mania on the one hand and intense depression on the other. This disorder is constitutional; when similar but less florid mood swings occur the condition is called **cyclothymia**. The **manic patient** is initially gay, talkative, cheerful and elated, restless and excitable. As the state of mania develops he may become increasingly distressed, aggressive and even violent, and his mind flies from one idea to another without obvious connexion between the two ('flight of ideas'). A less severe degree of mania, or hypomania, is evident in the vigorous, active and voluble extravert who is 'the life and soul of the party' and hypomania may be compatible with successful social adaptation and material gain. In true mania, however, if the patient is not sedated, exhaustion supervenes.

The depressive, by contrast, is slow, retarded and lacking interest. In **severe melancholia** the patient retires to bed in a state of utter apathy and may lie staring fixedly at the ceiling, taking no account of all that goes on around him. There is severe constipation, motor activity is slowly and lethargically performed and the pulse is slow. Less severe endogenous depression is much more common, particularly in middle age, as in post-menopausal women, and in patients who have never previously shown severe mood disorders; this is often referred to as **involutional depression**. The patient passes his days in a state of gloom and dejection; everything is viewed with a pessimistic air and he looks at the world 'through grey-coloured spectacles'. Interest in home, family and hobbies is lost and he may spend long hours in silence, sitting gazing into space. There is often a desire for solitude, friends are shunned, work neglected, and ideas of guilt, unworthiness and inadequacy are common. Suicidal ruminations are frequent, as joy in living is lost, and suicide is a serious potential hazard in this disease. Physical symptoms (headache, giddiness, indigestion and aching pains in the limb muscles) are common and there is a typical form of insomnia in that patients tend to wake in the early morning after falling asleep quickly on retiring. Mild forms of depression are difficult to recognise and are easily confused with an anxiety state by the uninitiated. The distinction is important, for treatment of the two conditions is different. Prolonged lethargy, undue fatigue and feelings of vague ill-health and lack of interest and energy in those past middle-age are often due to masked depression. They may say, 'Things which I once took in my stride now seem to be an intolerable burden and minor problems seem insurmountable'. Paradoxically, some patients with severe depressive states become agitated and tears flow readily.

Anxiety is a common emotional disturbance which can be a normal reaction under stressful conditions. It is when the feeling of anxiety or apprehension is not clearly related to any specific object or thought that it becomes pathological and may then be thought to constitute an anxiety neurosis. Physical concomitants of anxiety are frequent and include sweating, feelings of suffocation or choking, sighing, restlessness, fatigue, 'dizzy bouts', and tension headaches. The anxious patient is often unable to rest or to relax. Whereas anxiety is common in many psychiatric syndromes and may accompany depression or even psychosis, it is those individuals who are constitutionally predisposed to developing severe anxiety symptoms as a result of minor stress who become neurotic. In such individuals episodes of anxiety may occur acutely as 'panic attacks', or may present with episodes of tension and with physical symptoms of the type outlined above, but with intervening periods when life is lived on a relatively even keel. In a chronic anxiety state, the patient exists in a state of continual worry and is irritable and unhappy. Often symptoms are focused upon one particular organ; for instance the patient with a cardiac neurosis or 'effort syndrome' complains of breathlessness, palpitation and precordial pain. Reactive depression frequently coexists with anxiety but self-reproach and suicidal ideas are much less common than in the endogenous variety and patients with this type of depression have difficulty in getting to sleep but do not usually wake early in the morning.

Depersonalisation, or a feeling of unreality of the self, can coexist with either depression or anxiety. Patients can feel so intensely unreal or detached from the world about them that they feel themselves to be 'floating in air' and may even have delusional ideas that they are soon to die or that their bodies are shrinking. When depersonalisation is severe and combined with panic attacks and phobias (unreasoning fear of heights, of people, of enclosed places, or of crossing the road) this syndrome has been called a 'phobic anxiety state'. Agoraphobia (fear of open spaces) is common in such cases and the patient is afraid of leaving the house alone ('the house-bound housewife'). A feeling of chronic instability, with associated light-headedness and faintness, often confused with true vertigo unless the history is carefully taken, is often due to depersonalisation and is typically more troublesome out-of-doors than in the home.

Obsessional Neurosis

Obsessions are thoughts which intrude compulsively into the mind, even though, on reflection, the sufferer is aware that they are unreasonable or irrational. Many normal individuals have a few obsessions so that they are ritualistic in their habits. The child who walks on the lines of the pavement, the housewife who repeatedly straightens minutely crooked pictures on the wall is somewhat obsessional, as are many excessively tidy and rigidly conscientious people. Obsessional features are common in childhood but often disappear with increasing maturity. The obsessional personality is not always abnormal; it is when compulsive thoughts impose a senseless ritual that the borderline of normality is crossed. Thus it is normal to wash one's hands several times in the day but the person who does so every few minutes may be obsessed with fear of dirt, of germs, or of disease. Similarly obsessed is the patient who checks that the doors and windows are locked at night, not once, but five or six times. Though minor obsessional traits are compatible with reasonable adjustment to life and often occur, in fact, in those whose attention to detail makes them successful, the patient with a severe obsessional neurosis is so occupied with his compulsive thoughts that any other occupation than thought is impossible and he retires into a life of seclusion.

An obsessional neurosis is different in aetiology, nature and prognosis from a simple anxiety state, though many obsessionals are neurotic and many anxiety neurotics have obsessional ideas. A disorder which has affinities with both these forms of neurosis is **hypochondriasis**, a state of mind in which the patient is intensely introspective and excessively occupied with his own bodily symptoms, so that his only topic of conversation is his own illnesses, whether imaginary or real. In so-called malignant hypochondriasis the patient's ideas may assume a frankly delusional quality. An example is the patient who is so firmly convinced, say, that he has an abscess in the skull or in the throat that he goes from doctor to doctor in search of one who will operate to remove the offending but imaginary infective focus.

Hysteria

The differential diagnosis between hysteria and organic disease is one of the most difficult in medicine. In neurology the problem is particularly common and has been the graveyard of many a professional reputation; for although hysterical symptoms can simulate almost any physical disease, disorders of the nervous system are most often imitated. The most important point in the diagnosis of hysteria is that this condition must not be diagnosed by exclusion, as a label casually applied when clinical examination and ancillary tests fail to reveal organic disease. On the contrary, there must be positive evidence of hysteria, for hysterical symptoms are purposive, arising in order to obtain for the patient some real or imagined gain, either to fulfil an ambition, to realise a fantasy, or to escape from stress. To lose a job or to fail an examination through illness is more respectable than to do so through inefficiency; whereas such motivations may not be wholly conscious, the end desired by the patient is usually revealed on careful enquiry.

Patients with hysterical symptoms often have characteristic personality traits. They commonly deceive themselves that they are more able or important than they really are, they are emotionally shallow, easily influenced and unreliable and often utilise hysterical symptoms in order to draw attention or sympathy upon themselves or to dominate relatives and friends. Hysteria may occur in both sexes but is commoner in females; as the basic abnormality is constitutional, symptoms usually appear first in adolescence or early adult life, though much depends upon the severity of the stress to which the individual is subjected. Unfortunately there is no objective test available to distinguish between hysteria (subconscious motivation) and malingering, in which motivation is wholly conscious. This problem in differential diagnosis often arises when manifestations suggestive of hysteria arise against a background of industrial injury or in any other situation where prospects of financial compensation are involved.

Anxiety symptoms are often prominent in hysterical reactions, but relatively few neurotic patients exhibit frankly hysterical manifestations. A typical group of mental symptoms due to hysteria results from an ability to dissociate one part of the personality from another. Thus, hysterical 'twilight states', trances, or simulation of insanity (Ganser states) may occur, but most common is the **hysterical amnesia** or **fugue**, in which the patient wanders away from home for hours or days, having lost all sense of his identity.

As a rule, hysterical symptoms are a result either of suggestion or of an idea or fantasy in the patient's mind. Suggestion is of particular importance; thus a hysteric may become paralysed because her mother had a stroke, or a symptom develops in response to a leading question asked by a doctor, which the patient then endeavours to justify. It is from discrepancies between the patient's idea of a physical illness and the signs of the organic disorder itself that most diagnostic assistance is obtained. Motivation is also important; thus a patient with 'stage-fright' loses her voice, while another who is dreading forthcoming examinations develops hysterical blindness and is then unable to study. In hysterical **aphonia** the patient is able to cough on demand, while the individual with **hysterical blindness** blinks on threat or avoids obstacles in his path. **Hysterical convulsions** are staged for their histrionic effect and invariably occur with an audience; the patient is careful not to injure himself and tongue-biting and incontinence do not occur unless the patient who has often been asked about these features decides to oblige by providing them. The convulsion is often preceded by **hyperventilation** and actual tetany may develop through respiratory alkalosis. In **hysterical paralysis**, a single limb is usually involved, though hemiplegia or paraplegia are seen. There are generally discrepancies between the clinical findings and those resulting from organic nervous disease in particular, the reflexes are generally normal or show slight but symmetrical exaggeration, and the plantar responses are flexor. Typically, when the patient tries to move the affected limb, there is a massive apparent expenditure of effort with little result, and palpation of the muscles involved reveals that agonists and antagonists contract simultaneously. Hysterical disorders of **gait** are seen in some patients who claim to have paresis of the lower limbs, but in others there is no abnormality at all on examining the patient in bed, although the gait is bizarre, and unlike that associated with any organic nervous disease. Falling may be frequent, but significantly without injury. One must be sure to exclude the broad-based gait of truncal ataxia due to a midline cerebellar lesion, in which, too, signs of cerebellar dysfunction are conspicuously absent in the recumbent patient. Hysterical **sensory loss** is common; it frequently occurs in 'glove and stocking' distribution, with a clear-cut upper margin (unlike polyneuropathy where the transition is gradual) or there may be a total hemianaesthesia affecting all forms of sensation. Loss of vibration sense over one half of the skull or sternum is invariably hysterical. Co-ordinated movements are also good in such patients despite apparent complete loss of position and joint sense. In a limb showing hysterical weakness or paralysis the sensory impairment often ends at the elbow, knee, groin or shoulder, giving a pattern of sensory impairment which could not be produced by an organic lesion. These patients are very suggestible and 'islands' of normal sensation can sometimes be induced by suggestion in anaesthetic areas. In any event, the sensory impairment never corresponds to the cutaneous distribution of any peripheral nerve, sensory root or tract. Other less common hysterical manifestations include **dermatitis artefacta**, produced by self-inflicted cutaneous trauma, and hysterical **pyrexia**, which is commonest in nurses and is usually an artefact produced by cups of tea, cigarettes or hot water bottles or by substituting thermometers. Some patients even produce subcutaneous or intra-articular abscesses by injecting themselves with bath water, in which case the infecting organism is generally *E. coli*. Related to hysteria, but psychiatrically more complex, is the condition often called **'von Munchausen's syndrome'**; these patients become skilled at feigning organic disease and seek admission to one hospital after another. Some few are drug addicts but others simply demonstrate 'a desire to be ill'. Along with all the features described there is, in hysteria, a characteristic **belle indifférence** or seeming unconcern about what, if physically determined, would be a serious disability.

From this description it may be asked why the differential diagnosis from organic disease should sometimes be so difficult. Unfortunately the clinical picture is not always clear-cut. For example, the early manifestations of extrapyramidal disorders such as dystonia musculorum deformans can produce abnormalities of gait which initially look hysterical. Furthermore, hysterical manifestations arise in patients with organic disease and it may be difficult to determine how much is overlay and how much genuine. In multiple sclerosis, for instance, early manifestations of hysterical type are common even before distinctive physical signs have appeared. In many such patients the hysterical manifestations seem to develop as a means of impressing the doctor who may, inadvertently or deliberately, have given the impression to the patient that he does not understand the significance of the symptoms. Hysterical manifestations developing for the first time late in life can be the first symptoms of an endogenous depression or organic dementia. The most important principles to follow in establishing the diagnosis are first to seek assiduously for any motivation, unconscious or otherwise, which may be responsible for the symptoms and secondly to look for sources of suggestion which could be determining the pattern of the illness. Even when all clinical evidence suggests a diagnosis of hysteria the possibility of underlying organic disease or of more serious psychiatric illness should invariably be considered. It is in just this setting that such disorders are often overlooked when the hysterical overtones cloud the clinical picture.

Schizophrenia

Schizophrenia is a psychosis or psychotic reaction which is so common and yet so variable in its manifestations that the reader must turn to a textbook of psychiatry for an adequate description of its clinical features. And yet it is a disorder which occasionally mimics organic nervous disease; for this reason its most common features will be mentioned briefly.

The disease typically occurs in young adults, often those of shy, dreamy and introverted personality. Emotional disturbances may occur early, in the form of apathy and disinterest, with shallowness or incongruity of affect; nothing is felt deeply and inappropriate giggling is common. Indecision and lack of initiative are frequent. Gradually the patient becomes more and more withdrawn, with self-neglect and eventual stupor. In the **catatonic** schizophrenic, stupor is accompanied by a curious waxy flexibility of the limbs, which may be placed in bizarre positions and remain there. Lack of ideas is accompanied by a sudden stoppage or block in conscious thought and the patient may yet have sufficient insight to realise that he is unable to think logically. Thought disorders of this type with deterioration in personality and work performance are the salient features of the simple or **hebephrenic** form of schizophrenia. Hallucinations often occur and are usually auditory in character, so that the patient hears imaginary voices which may be so vivid that he answers their remarks. Delusions are also frequent; the patient may believe that he is being influenced by electricity or by radio waves. In the **paranoid** schizophrenic these delusions have a flavour of intense suspicion and the patient believes that he is being persecuted, often by a religious group or sect. Such a paranoid psychosis developing comparatively late in life is often referred to as **paraphrenia,** and in this condition the personality is relatively well-preserved.

Physical abnormalities, of which cyanosis of the extremities is the most constant, are relatively frequent in patients with schizophrenia, and there is some increasing evidence from neuropharmacological studies suggesting that this will ultimately prove to be an organic disease. It is also apparent that inherited traits are important. Whereas the fully-developed case is not difficult to recognise, in the early stages the condition is difficult to distinguish from depression, anxiety with depersonalisation, chronic hypochondriasis, delirium and organic dementia, although the age incidence and natural history of many of these disorders are generally quite different.

Puerperal Psychosis

Many forms of psychotic reaction can occur during the puerperium. Some of these illnesses show features of endogenous depression, many have close affinities with schizophrenia. Whereas the illness is often short and recovery complete, particularly with appropriate treatment, the psychosis persists in some cases.

Occupational Neurosis

Of the many 'craft palsies' which have been described, writer's cramp is the commonest and is believed to be, like other disorders in this group, of emotional origin. It is, however, typical that the affected hand can be used normally for all activities other than writing and it is difficult to see how this could be explained by an organic lesion in the basal ganglia or elsewhere. Typically as the patient begins to write the thumb and fingers grip the pen more and more tightly so that writing ceases and the pen may even be driven through the paper. If the patient learns to write with the other hand or to type, these activities may subsequently be affected. While tranquillising drugs and deconditioning techniques sometimes help, in many cases the prognosis is poor and the patient is eventually compelled to avoid writing. Similar problems affecting the specific movements involved in the craft concerned are well known to occur in typists, violinists, professional players of wind instruments, needleworkers and in many more occupations, making it difficult for the individual to continue in his or her normal employment.

Psychosomatic Disorders

That somatic symptoms can be the most prominent or indeed the only manifestations of a mental disorder is now clearly apparent. Many patients with endogenous depression, for instance, seek medical advice because of headaches or other symptoms which seem to be physically determined. It is equally clear that many organic diseases are powerfully influenced by psychological factors. Thus thyrotoxicosis may develop after emotional shock, the symptoms of peptic ulcer, migraine and ulcerative colitis may be greatly increased by anxiety, and there is some correlation between chronic nervous tension and raised blood pressure. The means by which psychological factors produce their effects in these disorders is unclear; many of them are consistently more frequent in individuals with certain types of emotional and physical constitution. By dividing humanity into different constitutional types or somatotypes, on the basis of physical characteristics, it is sometimes possible to predict the mental or physical disorders to which they are likely to be subject. Although our understanding of the mechanism by which psychological factors influence organic disease is incomplete, any physician who attempts to treat disease without taking into account all relevant emotional influences and without attempting to alleviate those which appear to be significant, is failing in his duty to his patient.

References

Allison, R. D., *The Senile Brain* (London, Arnold, 1962).

Crome, L. C. and Stern, J., *Pathology of Mental Retardation*, 2nd ed. (Edinburgh and London, Churchill-Livingstone, 1972).

Curran, D. and Partridge, M., *Psychological Medicine*, 9th ed. (Edinburgh, Livingstone, 1981).

Gellis, S. S. and Feingold, M., *Atlas of Mental Retardation Syndromes* (Washington, DC, US Department of Health, 1968).

Henderson, D. K. and Gillespie, R. D., *Textbook of Psychiatry*, 10th ed., revised by I. R. C. Batchelor (London, Oxford University Press, 1969).

Mayer-Gross, W., Slater, E. and Roth, M., *Clinical Psychiatry*, 3rd ed. (London, Cassell, 1969).

Pearce, J. M. S. and Miller, E., *Clinical Aspects of Dementia* (London, Baillière Tindall, 1973).

Sim, M. and Gordon, E. B., *Basic Psychiatry*, 3rd ed. (Edinburgh, Churchill-Livingstone, 1976).

8 The Special Senses

The special senses include the faculties of smell, vision, hearing and taste. Closely related to hearing, at least in an anatomical sense, is the maintenance of equilibrium (vestibular function). These functions are mediated by those cranial nerves which convey the sensory impulses concerned in appreciating these sensations to the appropriate areas of the cerebral cortex. Thus the first or olfactory nerve contains the peripheral pathway for the sense of smell, while the second or optic nerve carries visual impulses. The ability to see is closely related to mechanisms subserving binocular vision and ocular movement, so that in considering visual processes one must also discuss the functions of the third (oculomotor), fourth (trochlear) and sixth (abducens) cranial nerves which control external ocular movement. The third nerve, along with sympathetic fibres derived from the autonomic nervous system also influences those intrinsic ocular muscles controlling the size of the pupils as well as the process of accommodation. Hearing and the control of bodily equilibrium are respectively mediated through the cochlear and labyrinthine divisions of the eighth or auditory nerve, while taste sensations from the anterior two-thirds of the tongue travel in the chorda tympani along with the seventh or facial nerve and those from the posterior one-third are conveyed by the ninth or glossopharyngeal nerve. Disorders of function of the special senses, produced by lesions of the primary sensory receptors, of the cranial nerves concerned, or of their central connexions, are common in patients with neurological disease, and an adequate understanding of the means by which lesions produce their clinical effects is essential for accurate diagnosis.

Smell

The olfactory receptors are bipolar nerve cells situated in the upper part of the mucous membrane on either side of the nasal cavity. Inhaled gases given off by all odorous materials become dissolved in the nasal secretions which continually bathe the surface of these sensitive cells. Impulses so produced are conveyed by nerve fibres through the cribriform plate of the ethmoid bone into the cranial cavity to join the olfactory bulb which lies on the under-surface of the ipsilateral frontal lobe. Thence impulses travel posteriorly to the olfactory tracts to reach the prepyriform cortex and uncus in the parahippocampal gyrus of the temporal lobe which is the primary rhinencephalic (olfactory) area of the cerebral cortex. The anterior commissure unites the cortical olfactory regions of the two hemispheres, carrying fibres from each olfactory tract to the opposite side.

There is a strong relationship between the faculties of smell and taste, which combined give the sensation of flavour. Thus if either faculty is impaired so too may be the ability to appreciate flavours; in such a patient it is not sufficient to test taste sensation alone, as an inability to perceive olfactory sensations may be the primary abnormality. Furthermore, disease of the nasal mucosa such as rhinitis, a severe coryza, or sometimes excessive smoking, can so impair the sensitivity of the olfactory nerve cells that the sensation of smell is lost or greatly impaired (**anosmia**). Bilateral loss is thus not always significant, though it may follow a head injury with tearing of the olfactory nerve fibres as they traverse the ethmoid bone. Unilateral impairment of the sense of smell is, however, an important physical sign, since in the absence of a primary nasal abnormality it may indicate compression of one olfactory bulb or tract, possibly by a tumour underlying the ipsilateral frontal lobe. Total anosmia can also be hysterical or feigned and in such cases the patient may deny that he can appreciate concentrated ammonia which stimulates trigeminal rather than olfactory nerve endings. Olfactory hallucinations, as previously mentioned, sometimes occur in schizophrenia and in patients with lesions in one or other temporal lobe, as in some cases of temporal lobe epilepsy (**uncinate seizures**) and are presumably due to abnormal discharges arising in the anterior temporal cortex. **Parosmia** is an abnormal or perverted sense of smell, rarely due to organic lesions but more often occurring in mental illness (e.g. severe depression).

Taste

Taste fibres from the anterior two-thirds of the tongue travel through the lingual nerve to the chorda tympani, joining the facial nerve at the geniculate ganglion and proceeding to the pons in the pars intermedia which lies alongside the facial nerve. Taste sensations from the posterior one-third of the tongue are conveyed by the glossopharyngeal nerve. In the pons the fibres of these nerves enter the tractus solitarius, cross the midline and proceed in the gustatory fillet to the optic thalamus whence they are conveyed to the lower end of the postcentral gyrus.

Loss of taste (**ageusia**) on the anterior two-thirds of the tongue can result from lesions of the geniculate ganglion. A facial paralysis due to a lesion at or proximal to this point is usually associated therefore with unilateral loss of taste, while one resulting from a more distally-situated lesion is not. A lesion of the glossopharyngeal nerve will result in loss of taste on the posterior third of the tongue on the same side, but taste sensation is so difficult to test with even a reasonable degree of accuracy, that disorders of this sense have little value in clinical neurological diagnosis. Bilateral loss of taste sensation can rarely follow head injury; much more often the head-injured patient who complains of loss of taste sensation is found to be suffering from anosmia with resultant impairment of the sense of flavour, but on testing, the primary taste sensations (sweet, salt, bitter, and sour) are found to be intact. **Parageusia**, an abnormal or perverted sense of taste, is rarely the result of organic lesions and is more often due to depressive illness.

Vision

The Visual Pathways

Visual impulses recorded upon the retina are conveyed by the optic (second cranial) nerves through the optic chiasm. In the chiasm, fibres from the nasal half of each retina decussate, whereas temporal fibres do not. Hence each optic tract carries fibres from the temporal half of the ipsilateral retina and from the nasal half of the contralateral one (Fig. 6). This means that impulses from the right half-field of both eyes are carried in the left optic tract and vice versa. The tract continues to the lateral geniculate body where its axons synapse with nerve cells which give origin to the optic radiation. The optic radiation then travels backwards through the temporal lobe, hooking around the tip of the temporal horn of the lateral ventricle, and onwards to that part of the cerebral cortex which lies in the lips and in the depth of the calcarine fissure of the occipital lobe. This is the primary visual receptive area and has profuse connexions with the surrounding association areas in which, it appears, visual sensations are recognised and interpreted.

The light-sensitive receptors in the retina itself are the rods which are found diffusely throughout the retina except in the fovea centralis or macular area, and the cones which are concentrated largely in the region of the fovea but are scanty elsewhere. The cones have a high stimulus threshold, function mainly in daylight or conditions of high illumination **(photopic illumination)** and are responsible for high-acuity vision and colour vision. The rods, by contrast, have very low thresholds of stimulation, are insensitive to colour and relatively to fine visual detail and subserve vision in conditions of poor illumination (night vision, **scotopic illumination**). For detailed information about the physiology of vision, including the anatomy and electrophysiology of the retinal ganglion cells and the respective roles of light-sensitive pigments such as rhodopsin or visual purple in the rods and iodopsin and other pigments in the cones, the reader is referred to textbooks of physiology. It is clear, however, that

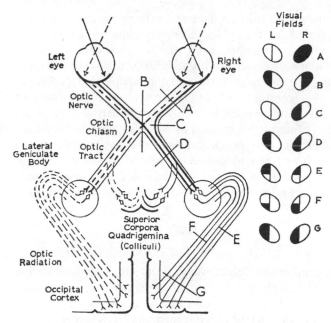

Fig. 6. A diagram of the visual pathways. On the right are examples of visual field defects produced by lesions interrupting these pathways at the points signified by the letters *A* to *G*.

information recorded by the rods and cones passes to the retinal ganglion cells which lie in its superficial layers and whose axons form the fibres of the optic nerve and come together in the optic disk or nerve-head.

In the optic nerve there also travel afferent fibres from the retina and from the muscles of accommodation, which influence pupil size; these synapse in the lateral geniculate body and in the superior corpora quadrigemina (colliculi) of the upper mid-brain, whence fibres arise which travel to the third, fourth and sixth nerve nuclei and to a sympathetic centre in the hypothalamus. These pathways are responsible for constriction of the pupil in response to light or fixation on near objects, and dilatation when the visual field is darkened or when distant objects are observed. A similar reflex pathway, controlled by visual impulses from the retina, influences the ocular movements necessary for ocular convergence and fixation and for following objects with the eyes.

Visual Acuity

The visual acuity in each eye can be measured independently by means of test-types of the Snellen and Jaeger type (*see* p. 18). The acuity is essentially a measurement of the efficiency of macular or central vision as it depends largely upon normal functioning of this part of the retina and of its nervous connexions, provided the mechanism for focusing light upon the retina is intact. Thus peripheral retinal lesions rarely influence acuity, but a small lesion of the macula or of optic nerve fibres which come from the macular area may seriously affect the ability to read or to distinguish small objects. This is seen particularly in retrobulbar neuropathy (*see below*) which often produces a central field defect or scotoma. Disorders of refraction (myopia, presbyopia, astigmatism) can seriously impair visual acuity as may other primary abnormalities of the eye (iridocyclitis, cataract, vitreous haemorrhages) which influence the passage of light to the retina, as well as disorders which damage retinal sensitivity (retinal detachment, glaucoma, etc.), but these local causes are usually self-evident and refractive errors can be corrected by the use of appropriate lenses.

Colour Blindness

Colour blindness is an inherited defect which occurs in 8 per cent of the male population and in less than 0.5 per cent of females. It is generally inherited as a sex-linked (X-linked) recessive character; though it occurs in many forms, the commonest variety is red–green blindness, either partial or complete, in which the affected individual finds it difficult to distinguish reds from greens. Many complex defects of colour vision occur. **Trichromats** (three-colour vision) include normal individuals but also some with weak red vision (protanomaly) or weak green vision (deuteranomaly). **Dichromats** are those who cannot perceive red (protanopia) or green (deuteranopia). **Monochromats** (with total colour blindness) are very rare and also have severe photophobia. Many such patients are unaware of their colour blindness, as they recognise 'colours' by their brightness, but the diagnosis can be confirmed with the Ishihara charts. The defect is of no serious significance except in those occupations where the recognition of coloured lights or signals, say, is important. However in patients with minimal lesions of the visual pathways, field defects for coloured objects (red is commonly used) can be demonstrated at a time when the field for white objects is complete. The field for red is normally smaller than that for white.

The Visual Fields

Defects of the peripheral visual fields as charted by perimetry, or of the central fields as recorded with the Bjerrum screen, may be of great value in neurological diagnosis (Fig. 6). From a knowledge of the anatomy of the visual pathways it is generally possible to localise with reasonable accuracy the site of the lesion which is responsible. Circumscribed defects of the central fields are referred to as scotomas. In each central field there is a normal 'scotoma', medial to the fixation point; this is the caecum or 'blind spot', corresponding to the optic disk in which there are no visual receptors. A scotoma which surrounds the fixation point or macular area is called a **central scotoma**, and gives marked impairment of visual acuity. It is most commonly seen as a sequel of **retrobulbar neuritis**, an inflammatory lesion of the optic nerve which is often due to multiple sclerosis. A central scotoma can rarely result from **compression of one optic nerve**, presumably because macular nerve fibres are very sensitive to pressure ischaemia, in patients with a tumour (usually a meningioma) behind the orbit. It may also be observed in **pernicious anaemia**, or in **neuromyelitis optica**, an acute demyelinating disorder related to multiple sclerosis, and in retrobulbar neuropathy due to many toxic and metabolic causes, of which **methyl alcohol poisoning** is a good example. **Tobacco amblyopia**, which is a cause of progressive visual failure in smokers of certain brands of pipe tobacco and which may be related to the effect of cyanide in the tobacco upon vitamin B_{12} utilisation, usually gives a **centrocaecal scotoma**, joining the fixation point to the blind spot.

A severe lesion of one optic nerve gives, of course, complete blindness of the ipsilateral eye, while the peripheral field of the other eye is full. This may be seen, for instance, after severe head injury or occlusion of the central retinal artery due to embolism, atherosclerosis, cranial arteritis, or even severe papilloedema. Lesions of the optic chiasm can give a variety of field defects, depending upon the character and situation of the causal lesion. Atherosclerotic ischaemia of the chiasm is occasionally responsible, but the lesions in this area which most often cause field defects are those which compress the chiasm, namely **parasellar neoplasms** and **aneurysms**. **Tumours of the pituitary gland**, as they protrude from the sella turcica, compress first of all the decussating fibres from the lower nasal portions of the retinae, producing defects in the upper temporal fields of both eyes, and eventually a **bitemporal hemianopia**. A lesion which compresses the chiasm asymmetrically from above, such as a suprasellar meningioma, a craniopharyngioma or a suprasellar aneurysm of the internal carotid or anterior communicating artery, may produce first a defect in the nasal field of one eye, progressing to complete unilateral blindness and followed by a defect in the temporal field of the other eye. Other variations can readily be deduced on anatomical grounds.

A complete lesion of one **optic tract** gives rise to a contralateral **homonymous hemianopia**, that is loss of the nasal field of the ipsilateral eye and of the temporal field of the contralateral eye. Thus in a lesion of the left optic tract, which can be produced by lesions like those which compress the chiasm, the right half-field of both eyes is lost. However, since optic tract compression is frequently asymmetrical, a progressive increase in size of the defects in these half-fields may develop slowly and the defect may initially be larger in one field than in the other until the hemianopia is complete. When homonymous defects in the two fields are unequal in size and shape they are said to be **incongruous**.

Lesions of one **optic radiation**, whether in the internal capsule, temporal lobe, or occipital lobe, and whether of vascular (infarction, haemorrhage), neoplastic or inflammatory (encephalitis, diffuse sclerosis) aetiology, also cause homonymous defects. A large lesion will give a complete homonymous hemianopia, but a smaller one, say in the temporal lobe affecting the lower fibres of the radiation, may give a contralateral upper quadrantic homonymous defect. As the nerve fibres from the retina are closely intermixed in the radiation, so that those from homologous portions of the two retinae lie alongside one another, field defects due to radiation lesions are **congruous**, i.e. they are the same in both eyes. It has been suggested that there is bilateral representation of the macula in the two occipital lobes, so that in a homonymous hemianopia resulting from an occipital lobe lesion the macular area of the blind half-field is spared. This finding is now known to be an artefact due to poor fixation during charting of the fields, and in such a case the macular field is actually split. Visual acuity is unimpaired in a patient with a complete homonymous hemianopia, but reading is difficult, as in normal reading words are read in groups of two or three and in a patient with a hemianopia ability to see only half the words in the group can cause great difficulty, so that he must learn again to read word by word.

Abnormalities of the visual fields may also result from local ocular conditions such as glaucoma and retinal detachment, but these disorders are generally apparent on examining the eye and rarely give diagnostic difficulty. Some **concentric diminution** of the fields with enlargement of the blind spot is seen in severe papilloedema and less often in optic atrophy due to syphilis or constriction of the optic nerve due to arachnoiditis. Loss of the peripheral field with retention of only a small central area (**tubular vision**) is usually an hysterical phenomenon but can occur in retinitis pigmentosa.

The Optic Fundus and its Abnormalities

Ophthalmoscopic examination of the optic disk, of the retinal vessels, and of the retina itself is an essential and often revealing part of a neurological examination. The optic disk is normally slightly pink in colour, but its temporal half is generally paler than the nasal, while some lack of definition of its nasal margin is common. In the centre of the disk, or slightly more towards its temporal margin, is the physiological cup into which the vessels dip; this cup is often much paler than the rest of the disk and its appearance must not be confused with that of optic atrophy. Excessive cupping is, of course, seen in glaucoma. Sometimes a leash of pale fibres is seen spreading for a short distance across the retina, in fan-like manner, from one part of the edge of the disk; these **medullated nerve fibres** are common and have no pathological significance.

The two most frequent abnormalities of the optic disk are swelling (papilloedema) and excessive pallor (optic atrophy).

Papilloedema generally results from obstruction to the venous return from the retina, so that the first sign may be distension of the retinal veins, which look unusually tumid. This is followed by obliteration of the physiological cup, and later the centre of the disk becomes raised above the level of the surrounding retina, while its margins become progressively more blurred and indistinct. When swelling is severe, haemorrhages and sometimes patches of white exudate develop around the disk margins in a radial manner. A star-shaped patch of white exudate ('macular star') may also develop in the macular area, which is normally a relatively avascular area of the retina, lying about two disk-breadths lateral to the disk. The two principal causes of papilloedema are first, **increased intracranial pressure**, transmitted to the optic nerve sheath and so compressing the veins, as in cases of intracranial tumour, abscess, haemorrhage, hydrocephalus or meningitis; and secondly, much less commonly, **optic** or **retrobulbar neuritis**. The latter is an 'inflammatory' neuritis of the optic nerve, due most often to a demyelinating lesion of multiple sclerosis or the related neuromyelitis optica, but rarely resulting from syphilis or from toxic, nutritional and metabolic disorders. These two causes of disk swelling can generally be distinguished by the fact that visual acuity is seriously impaired at an early stage in retrobulbar neuritis. Furthermore, disk swelling is rarely as great in retrobulbar neuritis as in true papilloedema, while haemorrhages and exudates are uncommon; indeed the disk may look surprisingly normal even in the acute stage when visual acuity is severely impaired. The typical history is one of progressive failure of vision in one eye, often associated with local pain, and usually leading to partial or total monocular blindness within a few hours or days. There is often complete recovery from this condition after several weeks or months, although a central scotoma may persist. Nowadays the condition is presumed to be due to multiple sclerosis unless some other cause is clearly apparent; however it may be many months or years before other neurological manifestations develop, and in some cases they never do so. Severe papilloedema due to increased intracranial pressure is often present, by contrast, without loss of visual acuity, though there may be some concentric diminution of the fields with enlargement of the blind spot, and the patient sees flashes of light or 'haloes' around lights, symptoms which may presage impending visual failure. These symptoms indicate that urgent measures to reduce the intracranial pressure are needed, since if visual loss occurs as a result of papilloedema it is due to compression of the central retinal artery and is usually complete and irreversible. Transient episodes of visual loss in patients with papilloedema, provoked often by stooping, are due to retinal ischaemia and give warning of impending occlusion. Papilloedema can also be due to severe arterial disease, as in **chronic nephritis** and **malignant hypertension**, to local lesions giving venous obstruction in the orbit or elsewhere (**central retinal vein thrombosis, cavernous sinus thrombosis, cor pulmonale**), or to **polycythaemia vera**.

Occasionally, congenital hyaline bodies lying on or in relation to the optic disk can give sufficient blurring of its margins (**pseudopapilloedema**) to make diagnosis from true papilloedema difficult. Fluorescein retinal angiography may then be diagnostic.

The optic disk in patients with **optic atrophy** is chalky-white or grey in colour, its pallor contrasting with the surrounding retina. The edges of the disk are clear-cut and often irregular. The form of optic atrophy seen in **multiple sclerosis** which typically follows an attack of retrobulbar neuritis, although no history of such an episode may be obtained, affects the temporal half of the disk much more than the nasal, as the fibres from the macular area of the retina enter this part of the disk. This so-called **temporal pallor**, which may be difficult to distinguish from the normal comparative pallor of the temporal part of the disk, except through experience, is almost diagnostic of multiple sclerosis. Optic atrophy may also be inherited; it is a feature of **cerebral lipidosis** of the Tay–Sachs type (cerebromacular degeneration), in which case there may also be a cherry-red spot at the macula; it is a common accompaniment of diseases in the **hereditary ataxia** group (*see* pp. 245–248). It also occurs in **retinitis pigmentosa**, a genetically-determined disorder which causes progressive bilateral visual failure, usually in early adult life, and in which there is also spidery pigmentation of the periphery of the retina and narrowing of the retinal vessels.

Leber's optic atrophy is another inherited condition (usually due to a sex-linked (X-linked) recessive gene) in which bilateral optic atrophy often develops rapidly in young adult males. The history is often reminiscent of that of retrobulbar neuritis but vision recovers only temporarily, if at all. The condition may be due to an inherited defect of cyanide metabolism and in occasional cases hydroxocobalamin may have produced temporary improvement. **Syphilis** is also an important cause; up to 15 per cent of patients with tabes dorsalis, particularly of the congenital type, have pale disks and the visual fields show peripheral constriction with enlargement of the blind spot. Of more immediate consequence as a cause of optic atrophy is **compression of the optic nerve**, whether by a tumour of the nerve itself or of its sheath, or by a meningioma, pituitary neoplasm or aneurysm which lies in relation to the nerve in its intracranial course. Less commonly a **head injury** will injure one optic nerve with a similar result, while severe papilloedema, glaucoma, choroidoretinitis and occlusion of the central retinal artery may all in time give rise to optic atrophy. When this occurs as a sequel of long-standing papilloedema, it is referred to as **secondary** or **consecutive optic atrophy**. Various **metabolic, toxic and nutritional disorders** may also damage the optic nerves. Thus, blindness can result from methyl alcohol poisoning while quinine, arsenical drugs and chloroquine have all been known to produce such an effect, as may the dietary ingestion of cyanide in cassava root in cases of tropical ataxic neuropathy with amblyopia. It is uncertain whether nutritional amblyopia (as observed in some prisoners of war) is due to Vitamin B_1 deficiency or to lack of other B vitamins, while pyridoxine deficiency (as in patients taking isoniazid) rarely, and B_{12} deficiency (pernicious anaemia or dietary deficiency in vegans) more commonly, can cause optic atrophy.

Changes in **retinal vessels** are also of considerable diagnostic value. The venous engorgement of papilloedema has already been mentioned. In subarachnoid haemorrhage, the rapid inflow of blood into the optic nerve sheath can give such severe venous obstruction that a large brick-red **subhyaloid haemorrhage** may be seen extending from the edge of the optic disk. Early changes of **atherosclerosis** and **hypertension** may take the form of slight 'silver-wiring' of retinal arteries (Grade I retinopathy) with subsequent narrowing of veins where the arteries cross them (Grade II); when the changes are more severe, flame-shaped haemorrhages and patches of hard white exudate appear in the retina (Grade III) and eventually papilloedema develops (Grade IV). In **diabetic** patients, small micro-aneurysms are sometimes found on peripheral retinal arteries. **Occlusion of the central retinal artery** may give sudden unilateral blindness; the arteries are seen to be reduced in calibre and optic atrophy follows. While this syndrome can result from atherosclerosis, in elderly patients it is often due to **cranial arteritis**, and thickening of the temporal arteries with other features of this disease are generally found. Transient unilateral blindness is often due to embolism of the artery, and occurs most commonly in patients with internal carotid artery stenosis: emboli of platelets or cholesterol may be seen in retinal arteries during attacks ('amaurosis fugax').

Among other retinal abnormalities of diagnostic value are **retinal angiomas** (tangles of abnormal blood vessels) found in patients with haemangioblastoma of the cerebellum (Lindau–von Hippel disease), **retinal tubercles** (yellowish nodules, often about half the size of the optic disk) which help to confirm a diagnosis of tuberculous meningitis or miliary tuberculosis and flat yellow plaques or **phakomas** which may be seen in tuberous sclerosis or neurofibromatosis.

The Cornea and Lens

A cloudy 'ground-glass' opacity of the cornea, due to interstitial keratitis consequent upon congenital syphilis, may help to confirm that a patient's neurological symptoms are due to neurosyphilis. Arcus senilis may occur prematurely in patients with hypercholesterolaemia and atherosclerosis, but a paler white rim around the periphery of the cornea (marginal keratitis) is usually indicative of hypercalcaemia. Of even greater diagnostic value, though rare, is the golden-brown peripheral rim of pigmentation (the Kayser–Fleischer ring) of Wilson's disease, which may only be visible on examination with a slit-lamp. The latter instrument may also be needed to detect the early cataract of dystrophia myotonica and the lens opacities seen in some rare storage disorders (such as the mucopolysaccharidoses) of childhood.

The Pupils

The parasympathetic nerve fibres which innervate the constrictor of the pupil travel in the third cranial (oculomotor) nerve, while sympathetic fibres responsible for pupillary dilatation arise in the hypothalamus and traverse the tegmentum of the brain stem and the cervical cord to the lateral horn of grey matter in the eighth cervical and first and second dorsal segments. They leave the cord in the anterior roots to reach the superior cervical ganglion, from which postganglionic fibres arise which enter the skull in the plexus in the wall of the internal carotid artery. Some then pass to the ophthalmic division of the fifth (trigeminal) nerve and enter the orbit with its branches, while others go from the carotid plexus directly to the ciliary ganglion in the orbit, giving rise to the short ciliary nerves.

Both pupils normally constrict when a light is shone upon one retina; the reaction in the illuminated eye is called the direct reaction, that in the opposite eye the consensual one. The afferent pathway for the light reflex travels in the optic nerve to the lateral geniculate body and superior corpora quadrigemina (colliculi) and thence to the third nerve nuclei, whence efferent constrictor fibres arise. Hence a lesion on the afferent side of the pathway (e.g. optic atrophy) impairs both the direct and the consensual reaction to light, while a lesion in the efferent pathway (e.g. third-nerve paralysis) to the eye being stimulated will affect the direct but not the consensual reaction. Constriction of the pupil also occurs when vision is focused upon a near object, a procedure which involves both accommodation (through contraction of the ciliary muscle) and convergence, and which is subserved by a series of reflexes involving the oculomotor nuclei. Both the light and accommodation reactions are impaired by a lesion of the third nerve. Paralysis of the pupillary reaction to accommodation with preservation of the light reflex is rare, though it can occur occasionally in lesions of the mid-brain and may seem to be present when ocular convergence is impaired, as may be seen with ageing or in post-encephalitic Parkinsonism. Loss of the light reflex with retention of that to accommodation-convergence is, however, one feature of the **Argyll Robertson pupil** of tabes dorsalis, which is also sometimes present in general paresis. Additional features are that the pupils are small, irregular and unequal; there is atrophy of the iris, and loss of the ciliospinal reflex (pupillary dilatation on pinching the skin of the neck). There is some controversy about the location of the lesion responsible for the Argyll Robertson pupil; some believe it to be in the peri-aqueductal region of the mid-brain, others in the ciliary ganglion. In congenital syphilis, the light reflex may be lost, but the pupils are usually large and are not therefore of typical Argyll Robertson type.

A lesion of the **third-nerve nucleus** or of the nerve in its intracranial course can paralyse the pupillo-constrictor muscles, so that the pupil becomes dilated and fixed. As the parasympathetic fibres lie relatively superficially in the nerve trunk, along with those innervating the levator palpebrae superioris, this pupillary change may be the first sign of a third-nerve lesion, being followed by ptosis and later by external ophthalmoplegia. Pressure upon the nerve by an aneurysm or pituitary neoplasm, and ischaemia or infarction of the nerve in diabetes mellitus, are common causes of a unilateral third-nerve palsy. A similar effect can result from herniation of the temporal lobe through the tentorial hiatus so that a unilateral fixed dilated pupil may be an early sign of a space-occupying lesion in or overlying one cerebral hemisphere (such as an extradural or subdural haematoma).

A lesion of the sympathetic pathway gives a constricted pupil (myosis) and usually the other features of **Horner's syndrome** (myosis, ptosis, enophthalmos and loss of sweating on the affected side of the face). The lesion responsible may lie in the descending pathway in the brain stem (as in certain cases of brain stem infarction, e.g. posterior inferior cerebellar artery thrombosis), in the neck, involving one of the cervical sympathetic ganglia, or in the internal carotid artery, damaging sympathetic fibres which run in the wall of the vessel (e.g. aneurysm). In the latter case, facial sweating, mediated by fibres in the coat of the external carotid artery, is unimpaired (**Raeder's paratrigeminal syndrome**). Sympathetic overactivity, due for instance to fright, dilates the pupils. Lesions in the brain stem often affect the size and reactivity of the pupils; changes of localising value in comatose patients and in identifying the site of brain stem lesions are described on p. 115.

Drugs have a profound influence upon pupillary size and activity. Myotics, which cause pupillary constriction, include morphine, pilocarpine, neostigmine and eserine, while mydriatics or dilators include the long-acting atropine, homatropine which is used to dilate the pupil for ophthalmoscopy, and cocaine. When examining the pupils it should also be remembered that **local ocular conditions** can influence their shape and size. Iridocyclitis, for instance, often gives irregularities of the iris and adhesions to the lens (synechiae), which may restrict the range of pupillary movement. **Hippus** is a phenomenon of intermittent rhythmical pupillary contraction and dilatation; though sometimes observed in patients with neurological disease it has no diagnostic value. Of greater value is the **retrobulbar pupil reaction**; there is loss of the direct light reaction in the affected eye with a brisk consensual reaction when the other eye is stimulated.

Another interesting pupillary abnormality is that known as the **myotonic pupil**. When this pupillary abnormality is associated with sluggishness or absence of the tendon reflexes, the condition is referred to as the **Adie** or **Holmes–Adie syndrome**. Characteristically it occurs in young women, though it is occasionally seen in males. The patient may notice a sudden onset of blurring of vision in one eye or alternatively she observes on looking into the mirror that one pupil is dilated. On examination the pupil is widely dilated and shows a sluggish, delayed reaction to light. The reaction to accommodation is usually better but this too may be impaired and indeed it may be impossible to produce pupillary constriction with either stimulus. The condition is benign but its aetiology is unknown and it is uninfluenced by treatment. The lesion responsible is a loss of cells in the ciliary ganglion.

The Eyelids and Orbital Muscles

That part of the levator palpebrae superioris consisting of voluntary muscle is innervated by the third cranial nerve but there is also a smooth muscle component (Muller's muscle) innervated by the sympathetic. Hence paresis of the third nerve or of the sympathetic can give rise to **ptosis**. Ptosis can also be congenital and is then either unilateral or bilateral; it also occurs in myasthenia gravis when it typically worsens as the day wears on, in tabes dorsalis, and in myopathic degeneration of the external ocular muscles (ocular myopathy). **Blepharospasm**, a prolonged or intermittent spasm of the orbicularis oculi, causing eye closure, is often due to habit spasm or hysteria but is sometimes seen in Parkinsonism and other extrapyramidal disorders.

Lid retraction, or a failure of the upper lid to follow the globe on downward movement of the eye, is typically seen in thyrotoxicosis in which **exophthalmos**, or protrusion of the eye, is also common. The term **proptosis** is sometimes used to identify a unilateral exophthalmos, particularly when asymmetrical. Severe exophthalmos, sometimes unilateral, but more often bilateral, can result from excessive output of the exophthalmos-producing substance, which is neither LATS nor thyrotropic hormone, by the anterior pituitary. In this condition there is swelling of the external ocular muscles and orbital tissues, and ophthalmoplegia is common (**exophthalmic ophthalmoplegia, thyrotropic ophthalmopathy** or **ophthalmic Graves' disease**). Sometimes the condition begins with minimal exophthalmos on one side only and often with weakness limited to one superior rectus muscle. By contrast, severe painful exophthalmos with total paralysis of all ocular movement and severe conjunctival chemosis can develop in acute cases within a few days and papilloedema may ensue, so that urgent surgical decompression may be needed. Other conditions which may cause exophthalmos include orbital tumour, 'pseudotumour' (*see below*) other inflammatory lesions in the orbit or paranasal sinuses, retro-orbital intracranial tumours (meningiomas in particular) and thrombosis of, or arteriovenous aneurysm in, the cavernous sinus. Intermittent exophthalmos, occurring particularly on coughing or stooping, may be due to an orbital venous angioma; that due to an arteriovenous fistula in the cavernous sinus may pulsate and a systolic bruit will be heard over the globe of the eye. A painless exophthalmos, often unilateral, is rarely due to an orbital pseudotumour resulting from autoimmune orbital myositis in which the histology of the ocular muscles resembles that of polyarteritis nodosa or polymyositis. This condition, too, may require surgical decompression, but in many cases there is a good response to treatment with steroid drugs. A mucocele of the ethmoid sinus, by contrast, usually gives unilateral proptosis with lateral deviation and protrusion of the globe of the eye.

External Ocular Movement and its Abnormalities

The Nature and Control of Ocular Movements

The ocular movements include horizontal movement outwards (abduction); horizontal movement inwards (adduction); vertical movement upwards (elevation); vertical movement downwards (depression). The eye is capable of diagonal movements at any intermediate angle. The term 'rotation' should be reserved for wheel-like movements around an imaginary pivot passing through the centre of the pupil; such movements of rotation are not normal but only occur as a result of the unbalanced action of certain muscles. Inward rotation is a movement like that of a wheel rolling towards the nose, outward rotation the opposite. Normally the movements of the two eyes are harmoniously symmetrical constituting conjugate ocular movement, whether horizontal or lateral, upward or downward. Conjugate adduction of the two eyes is known as convergence. Other varieties of ocular movement will be considered below.

The Nuclei of the Ocular Muscles

The lower motor neurones which innervate the ocular muscles originate in the nuclei of the third, fourth and sixth cranial nerves. The first two lie in the midbrain just anterior to the cerebral aqueduct at the level of the superior and inferior colliculi. The nuclei of the sixth nerve lie in the pons beneath the floor of the fourth ventricle and partly encircled by the fibres of the seventh nerve (Fig. 7). Figure 8 is a diagram of the anatomy of the third nerve nucleus. The median, unpaired nucleus of Perlia is the centre for convergence and accommodation, while the lateral, paired nucleus of Edinger–Westphal innervates the parasympathetic constrictor of the pupil. The remainder of the nucleus is the paired, large-celled, lateral nucleus in which the muscles are represented from above downwards as follows: levator palpebrae, superior rectus, inferior oblique, medial rectus, inferior rectus. Decussating fibres unite the lower parts of the nuclei. Immediately below the third nerve nucleus lies that of the fourth nerve which innervates the opposite superior oblique. This nucleus and the adjacent lowest part of the third nerve nucleus innervate the two muscles concerned in depression of the eye, and the two elevating muscles are innervated by mutually adjacent portions of the upper half of the nucleus.

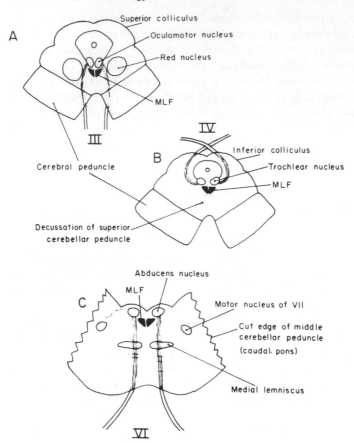

Fig. 7. Diagrammatic cross sections at the levels of the nuclei for the (A) oculomotor nerve (III), (B) trochlear nerve (IV), and (C) abducens nerve (VI). MLF locates the medial longitudinal fasciculus.

(Reproduced from *Introduction to Basic Neurology* by Patton *et al.*, by kind permission of the authors and publisher.)

The Extrinsic Ocular Muscles

The extrinsic ocular muscles are the four recti, superior and inferior, lateral and medial, and the two obliques, superior and inferior. The action of each of these muscles is shown in Fig. 9. Only the lateral and medial recti act in a single plane. The other muscles always act in concert; thus when the two obliques aid the lateral rectus in abduction their vertical and rotatory forces cancel out; and when the superior rectus and inferior oblique contract together to elevate the eye their horizontal and rotatory components also cancel. But owing to the anatomy of the superior and inferior recti and the obliques, their actions are influenced by the position of the eye in the orbit. When it is rotated outwards 23° the superior rectus is a pure elevator and the inferior rectus a pure depressor. The more it is

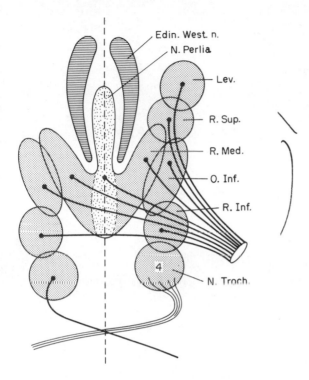

Fig. 8. Diagram of the oculomotor nucleus.
(Reproduced from *Brain's Diseases of the Nervous System*, 8th edition, by Walton, by kind permission of the publisher.)

turned inwards the more they act as internal and external rotators. The converse is true of the obliques. In conjugate deviation there is a harmonious contraction of the appropriate muscles of the two eyes. In lateral conjugate deviation the lateral rectus of one eye and the medial rectus of the other are associated; in conjugate deviation upwards and downwards, the elevators and depressors of the two eyes respectively; and in convergence, the medial recti. Graded contraction and relaxation of their antagonists play an important part in orderly movement.

Paralysis of Individual Ocular Muscles
The more important results of paralysis of an ocular muscle are: (1) defective ocular movement; (2) squint; (3) erroneous projection of the visual field; and (4) diplopia.

Defective ocular movement is demonstrated by asking the patient to fix his gaze on an object, such as the observer's finger, which is then moved upwards and downwards and to either side, convergence being tested by bringing it towards the patient. The movement is defective in the direction in which the eye is normally moved by the muscle which is paralysed.

Squint, or **strabismus,** is the term applied to a failure of the normal

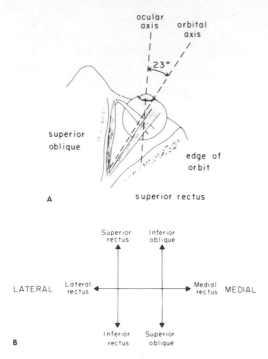

Fig. 9. A: Dorsal view of the orbit, globe, superior rectus muscle, and superior oblique muscle. Note the relationship of the ocular axis to the orbital axis with regard to insertion of each muscle. B: Primary direction of pull by each of the six extra-ocular muscles.
(Reproduced from *Introduction to Basic Neurology* by Patton *et al.*, by kind permission of the authors and publisher.)

co-ordination of the ocular axes. Paralytic squint must be distinguished from concomitant squint. Paralytic squint may be present when the eyes are at rest, due to the unbalanced action of the normal antagonist of the paralysed muscle; for example, the affected eye may be slightly adducted when the lateral rectus is paralysed. More often it is seen only when the eyes move in the direction in which the eye should be pulled by the paralysed muscle, or squint present at rest is increased by this movement. Concomitant squint, however, is present at rest and is equal for all positions of the eyes; if the fixing eye is covered, the movements of the squinting eye are full. Concomitant squint is not usually associated with diplopia; paralytic squint, at least in the early stages, usually is. However, when there is long-standing ocular muscle imbalance (latent concomitant squint or heterophoria) the patient may be able for many years to contract the ocular muscles so as to fuse the images from the two eyes; as he becomes older the effort is no longer possible so that the latent squint breaks down and diplopia may result. Similarly, in long-standing paralytic squint, one image may ultimately be suppressed so that diplopia disappears; suppression of this type often results in one eye becoming amblyopic as a result of untreated concomitant squint in early childhood. When the lateral rectus is paralysed the ocular axes converge and the squint is said to be convergent. Paralysis of the medial rectus causes divergent squint.

Erroneous Projection of the Visual Field
If we look at a light in any position of the eyes, the image of the light falls upon the macula. When the right lateral rectus is paralysed, on conjugate deviation to the right the left eye moves normally but the right eye remains directed forwards. The image of the object falls in the left eye upon the macula, in the right eye upon the nasal half of the retina. The patient is accustomed to regard an object, the image of which falls upon the nasal half of the right retina, as being situated to the right of one of which the image falls upon the macula. Consequently he sees two images and projects the false image perceived by his affected eye to the right of the true image perceived by his normal eye. If now his normal eye is covered and he is asked to touch the object, he will direct his finger to the right of its true position. The erroneous projection is always in the normal direction of action of the affected muscle. Hess's screen can be used to record the position of the false image. Erroneous projection of the visual field of the affected eye is thus responsible for **double vision** or **diplopia**. When both eyes are used, two images are seen, one correctly and one erroneously projected, the true and the false image. From the facts outlined, three simple rules about diplopia can be deduced:

1 The separation of the images increases the further the eyes are moved in the normal direction of pull of the paralysed muscle.
2 The false image is displaced in the direction of the plane of action of the paralysed muscle.
3 The diplopia is said to be simple, or uncrossed, when the false image lies on the same side of the true image as the affected eye, and crossed when it lies on the opposite side. The true and false images can also be identified by placing coloured glasses over each eye.

From these facts it is a relatively easy matter to deduce which muscle or muscles are involved in a patient with paralytic squint.

Nuclear and Infranuclear Lesions which Affect Ocular Movement
Having confirmed which muscle or muscles are affected and hence which nerve is diseased, it is then necessary to decide the nature of the lesion responsible. Rarely, an isolated paralysis of abduction of one eye simulating a sixth nerve lesion is congenital and often familial (Duane's syndrome) and is due to fibrosis of the lateral rectus muscle. Many traumatic, inflammatory, neoplastic and degenerative disorders arising in the brain stem or in the basal cisterns or orbital foramina can give rise to paralysis of

one or more of the oculomotor nerves. In the brain stem itself, **infarcts**, **gliomas** and **Wernicke's disease** are the most common, while in the basal cisterns, the third, fourth or sixth nerves may be damaged by **trauma**, **meningitis**, **meningovascular syphilis**, **subarachnoid haemorrhage** or **tumour**. A third or sixth nerve palsy of sudden onset in an elderly person may result from compression of the trunk of the nerve by an **atherosclerotic artery**, or from actual infarction of the nerve trunk itself, and these palsies generally clear up spontaneously in from three to six months. They are particularly common in patients with **diabetes mellitus**. The third nerve in particular is also vulnerable in patients with basal **arterial aneurysms** or **pituitary tumours**, while it can be paralysed as a result of a cerebral hemisphere lesion giving **tentorial herniation.** When complete third, fourth and sixth nerve palsies develop and are associated with sensory loss in the upper face, then an **aneurysm in the cavernous sinus**, compressing also the first and second divisions of the trigeminal nerve, which accompany these nerves within the sinus, may be present. A similar syndrome results from lesions in the neighbourhood of the **superior orbital fissure**; one such is so-called orbital apicitis or 'painful ophthalmoplegia' (the Tolosa–Hunt syndrome) resulting from a steroid-responsive inflammatory process of unknown aetiology at the apex of the orbit. Pain behind the eye often precedes the ophthalmoplegia in such cases.

Lesions of the myoneural junction and of the ocular muscles themselves can also give rise to ptosis, strabismus and diplopia. In **myasthenia gravis**, for instance, drooping of the eyelids towards the end of the day and intermittent or fluctuant squint and diplopia are common. An uncommon condition in which there is a slowly progressive bilateral ptosis, with, eventually, impairment of ocular movement in all directions, is **ocular myopathy**. Most cases of this type were previously referred to as **progressive nuclear ophthalmoplegia** on the assumption that the disease was one of the oculomotor nuclei, but it is now recognised that the process responsible is only occasionally nuclear and is more often a progressive dystrophy of the external ocular muscles. In some such cases there are associated retinal pigmentation and cerebellar degeneration with abnormal mitochondria in the ocular muscles and cerebellum (the Kearns–Sayre syndrome).

The Supranuclear and Internuclear control of Ocular Movement

During **conjugate** or **version** movements of the eyes the visual axes remain parallel, while during **disconjugate** or **vergence** movements the axes intersect. Version movements are of two types: in one (**saccades** or **saccadic movements**) the eyes jump rapidly and successively from one point of fixation to another, while in the other (**smooth-pursuit movements**) the eyes follow smoothly a moving object. All voluntary eye movements (except when viewing a moving object) take the form of fast saccades; thus in reading a line of print the eyes read one to four words in the course of a single fixation and then jump to the next series of words. Speed and efficiency of reading depend upon the number of words read during each fixation. Smooth pursuit movements, used to track moving objects, are much slower than saccades and cannot be performed at will without the stimulus of a moving target. By contrast, vergence movements, which are slow, track approaching (convergence) or receding (divergence) objects, and during these the eyes move in opposite directions.

Supranuclear and Internuclear Pathways
The supranuclear pathway concerned with voluntary conjugate eye movement (saccades) in a lateral direction originates in the frontal eye field in the contralateral middle frontal gyrus (Brodmann's area 8). Stimulation in this area gives contralateral saccades, while destructive lesions give difficulty in carrying out voluntary version movements of the eyes to the opposite side. The pathway from this cortical area descends through the corona radiata, internal capsule and cerebral peduncle, subsequently decussating in the midbrain and descending in the pons to join the medial longitudinal fasciculus at about the level of the sixth nerve nucleus. Thus stimulation in the pons, below the decussation of this pathway, causes conjugate deviation of the eyes towards the lesion or point of stimulation, while a unilateral lesion of the ponto-mesencephalic reticular formation may cause paralysis of conjugate gaze towards the affected side. Another important cortical centre controlling ocular movements lies in or near the visual cortex in the occipital lobe and is probably concerned especially with smooth pursuit movements and with vergence.

Because co-ordination of the movement of the two eyes is essential for binocular vision, the nuclei of the individual third, fourth and sixth cranial nerves are linked together in the medial longitudinal fasciculus which is the principal internuclear pathway controlling ocular movement. Supranuclear pathways as described above all feed into this fasciculus. Cerebellar lesions often cause over- or undershoot of saccadic movements and/or the breaking down of smooth-pursuit movements into saccades.

Reflex Ocular Movement
In voluntary conjugate deviation of the eyes the patient may turn his eyes spontaneously or on command, but some ocular movements are reflexly induced. Visual stimuli usually result in movement of the head or eyes in order to keep the image upon the macula. Continuous movement of a series of objects or lines in one direction evokes optokinetic nystagmus (*see below*). Similarly, auditory stimulation may give deviation of the eyes towards the origin of the sound, while caloric or electrical excitation of one labyrinth evokes conjugate ocular deviation and nystagmus (*see below*). If the patient fixes his gaze upon an object and the head is then flexed, rotated or extended at the neck, reflex ocular deviation occurs in an attempt to keep the image of the object upon the macula. This oculocephalic reflex (the doll's head manoeuvre) is dependent upon the integrity of

the medial longitudinal fasciculus and of its connexions with the vestibular system, and is thus valuable in determining whether pontine vestibulo-ocular connexions are intact in patients in coma.

Supranuclear and Internuclear Lesions

Spasmodic conjugate lateral movement of the eyes may occur in focal attacks of epilepsy due to lesions involving the contralateral frontal eye field. **Paralysis of conjugate lateral movement** may occur as the result of a lesion at any point in the supranuclear pathway, but this effect is always transient in lesions situated above the pons, though one involving the decussation of the pathways at the ponto-mesencephalic junction can give paralysis of conjugate gaze to both sides. However, a unilateral pontine lesion may give long-lasting paralysis of both voluntary and reflex conjugate gaze to the affected side. This can result from encephalomyelitis or Wernicke's disease but is more often due to brain stem infarction. **Dissociation of conjugate lateral movement** is usually a consequence of a lesion of the medial longitudinal fasciculus (an internuclear lesion). Much the commonest effect is the so-called **anterior internuclear ophthalmoplegia** (Harris' sign or **'ataxic nystagmus'**) in which there is phasic nystagmus confined to the abducting eye associated with failure of medial movement of the adducting eye. While this sign can rarely be a consequence of brain stem tumour or infarction, it is much more often due to multiple sclerosis and can be unilateral or bilateral.

Skew deviation of the eyes, in which one eye is deviated upwards and outwards, the other downwards and out, is a rare consequence of an acute cerebellar or pontine lesion. **Spasmodic conjugate vertical movement** of the eyes upwards is a rare phenomenon, occasionally occurring in an attack of epilepsy, especially petit mal, but it is also seen in the oculogyric crises of post-encephalitic Parkinsonism. **Paralysis of conjugate vertical deviation** in an upward direction is not uncommon, but paralysis of downward movement is excessively rare. In midbrain lesions involving the region of the superior colliculus, voluntary upward deviation can be lost even though the movement can still be excited reflexly. The term 'Parinaud's syndrome' is often applied to isolated defects of upward conjugate gaze, which can rarely be congenital, but in the fully-developed syndrome due to lesions of the midbrain tectum there is often loss of the pupillary light reflexes and paralysis of convergence in addition. This may result from encephalitis, from tumours of the third ventricle, midbrain or pineal body, from Wernicke's disease or from infarction. **Paralysis of convergence** is occasionally seen in post-encephalitic Parkinsonism, as a result of head injury or midbrain infarction, and rarely results from ageing. Loss of convergence is occasionally, and spasm of convergence invariably, hysterical.

Progressive supranuclear degeneration (the Steele–Richardson–Olszewski syndrome) is a rare degenerative disorder characterised by progressive ophthalmoplegia affecting vertical and especially downward gaze with early loss of saccadic movements. The ophthalmoplegia is associated clinically with variable Parkinsonian and dystonic features, with dysarthria, pseudobulbar palsy, inconstant cerebellar and pyramidal signs and occasionally dementia; pathologically there is neurofibrillary and granulovacuolar degeneration of neurones with gliosis and demyelination in the brain stem (sometimes involving the oculomotor nuclei), basal ganglia and cerebellum. The disease is progressive and uninfluenced by treatment.

Nystagmus

Nystagmus is an oscillatory movement of the eyes which is often rhythmical and repetitive; it is sometimes present with the eyes at rest, but may only appear when they are moved conjugately, or, if present at rest, it may be accentuated by ocular movement. It can be rotary in type (occurring in more than one plane) or may occur only in a lateral or vertical direction. Occasionally both phases of the to-and-fro oscillation are of equal duration but more often there is a quick phase in one direction succeeded by a slower recoil (**phasic nystagmus**); in this case the nystagmus is said to occur in the direction of the quick phase. This phenomenon is a disorder of the posture of the eyes and can be produced by disease of the reflex pathways which influence ocular posture. Stimuli from the retina and labyrinths are important in the maintenance of posture of the eyes as of other parts of the body as is cerebellar activity, so that lesions of any of these structures can give rise to nystagmus.

Nystagmus must be distinguished from other rare spontaneous ocular movements such as **opsoclonus,** a repetitive shock-like myoclonic jerking of the eyes, seen in subacute myoclonic encephalopathy of infancy and childhood, and **ocular bobbing,** in which the eyes bob rhythmically upwards and downwards as a very rare and often transient manifestation of a pontine lesion.

Congenital nystagmus, which may be familial, is a benign disorder of unknown aetiology in which a continuous pendular movement of the eyes occurs at rest and is often accentuated by movement of the head and eyes in any direction. It is usually asymptomatic. **Optokinetic nystagmus** is a physiological phenomenon which occurs when the eyes are fixed upon a moving object such as a rotating drum or the landscape observed from a moving vehicle. The slow phase occurs in the direction in which the object moves and is followed by a quick recoil. Optokinetic nystagmus to one side may be lost as a result of lesions of the contralateral frontal or parietal cortex or of the upper brain stem and this has been used as a diagnostic test. Absent, sluggish or irregular optokinetic responses usually indicate a pontine lesion; contralateral parieto-occipital lesions impair the slow phase of optokinetic nystagmus, frontal lesions the fast. **Nystagmus of peripheral origin** may be seen in any local ocular condition (such as amblyopia or optic atrophy) which impairs visual fixation; it may then be monocular, involving only the affected eye, and is generally pendular in type.

Impairment of ocular fixation resulting from ocular muscle weakness, as in polyneuropathy or myasthenia gravis, may rarely give similar nystagmus. **Miner's nystagmus**, which was generally gross and pendular in type, was due to impaired macular vision and visual fixation resulting from prolonged work in poor illumination, but there were many associated symptoms (headaches, giddiness) and neurosis was an important complicating factor; the condition is now rare since lighting in mines has been improved.

Nystagmus of labyrinthine origin can be evoked by caloric stimulation of the semicircular canals; if only the horizontal canals are stimulated it is lateral in type, but involvement of the vertical canals gives a rotary type which is therefore more common in disease of the internal ear, and the quick phase of the nystagmus takes place in a direction away from the affected ear. This is seen in acute labyrinthine vertigo (*see below*); the amplitude of the nystagmus is increased on looking to the side away from the lesion. Sometimes nystagmus is produced only by sudden movement of the head in a particular direction (positional nystagmus); this occurs in benign positional nystagmus (*see below*), but is occasionally seen in brain stem lesions or in patients with neoplasms in the region of the fourth ventricle.

The commonest causes of nystagmus in neurological practice are **lesions of the cerebellum or of cerebellar and vestibular connexions in the brain stem**. However, phasic nystagmus on lateral gaze may be due to many drugs including alcohol, barbiturates and anticonvulsants (**toxic nystagmus**). In a unilateral cerebellar lesion the nystagmus is increased on lateral deviation of the eyes towards the side of the lesion. So profuse are the structures in the brain stem which are concerned with cerebellar, vestibular and oculomotor function (the medial longitudinal bundle is one of the most important) that virtually any lesion in this situation, whether inflammatory, neoplastic, degenerative or metabolic, gives rise to this physical sign; it is almost impossible to attribute to it any specific localising or diagnostic value under these circumstances, except in the case of the **ataxic nystagmus** previously mentioned (p. 172). Often the nystagmus due to a brain-stem lesion occurs particularly on lateral ocular movement, the quick phase occurring towards the direction of gaze, but many other varieties occur and **vertical nystagmus** is particularly common in cases of the Chiairi malformation or in other lesions at or near the foramen magnum. Statistically, multiple sclerosis is the commonest cause, but encephalitis, vascular lesions, syringobulbia, Wernicke's encephalopathy and tumours can also produce this sign. There is no convincing evidence that lesions in the cervical spinal cord, or indeed at any level lower than the medulla oblongata and cerebellar tonsils, ever produce nystagmus. **Rebound nystagmus** is an uncommon phenomenon, usually due to cerebellar degeneration, in which phasic nystagmus which appears on looking laterally quickly fatigues but recurs to the opposite side when the eyes return to the midline. In the rare **see-saw nystagmus** one eye moves up as the other moves down;

this is usually due to a third ventricular tumour or less often to a pontine lesion. **Pseudonystagmus** is sometimes seen in hysteria; crude and disorganised ocular movements superficially resembling nystagmus are seen during voluntary ocular movement but disappear during conscious ocular fixation and are often accompanied by blepharospasm.

The Auditory Nerve

Auditory impulses are received by the cells of the organ of Corti, travel along the peripheral processes of the bipolar cells of the spiral ganglion of the cochlea and thence in the central processes of these cells in the auditory nerve to the cochlear nucleus in the pons; they then cross the midline and travel upwards in the lateral field to the inferior corpora quadrigemina and medial geniculate body; from this relay station they pass to the cortical centre for hearing in the middle and superior temporal gyri. The principal symptoms of disease of the auditory system are deafness and tinnitus. **Conductive or 'middle-ear' deafness** due to inflammation or otosclerosis can generally be distinguished by tuning-fork tests, but audiometry is needed for accurate assessment (*see* Chapter 2, and p. 78).

Nerve deafness can result from damage to Corti's organ as in Ménière's disease (*see below*) or occupational deafness. Spread of inflammation from the middle ear will sometimes damage the cochlea, as may syphilis. Nerve deafness can be congenital (deaf mutism), when it is usually due to an atresia of the cochlea and labyrinth. In childhood it can also be due to head injury, perinatal anaemia, maternal rubella or kernicterus. The auditory nerve in its intracranial course may be damaged by head injury, by inflammatory lesions (meningitis, meningovascular syphilis), by drugs or toxins (streptomycin) or by tumours, of which acoustic neuroma is the commonest. Nerve deafness resulting from a lesion of Corti's organ can often be distinguished from that due to an acoustic nerve tumour by the recruitment test (*see* p. 78). Deafness due to lesions of the cochlear nucleus in the brain stem is rare (but can be seen unilaterally in pontine infarction or, less often, multiple sclerosis); it is not produced by cortical lesions unless they are bilateral and extensive.

Tinnitus, or noise in the ears, is an important symptom of disease of the auditory nerve, though it can result from wax, from Eustachian catarrh or middle-ear disease. Typically it is a hissing or machinery-like noise which may be unilateral or bilateral, continuous or intermittent. It is often severe in elderly people and can be so distressing as to interfere seriously with sleep and hearing, so that some become almost suicidal; it may be due to atherosclerotic ischaemia of the inner ear, though it can also be a manifestation of severe depression. Drugs such as quinine, salicylates and streptomycin will also produce it. When unilateral, however, it may be an important symptom of disease of the labyrinth (e.g. Ménière's disease) or of the auditory nerve (e.g. acoustic neuroma).

The Vestibular Nerve

The end-organs which subserve vestibular function are the semicircular canals, which are concerned with the appreciation of movements of the head in any direction, and the utricle and saccule which convey information concerning the position of the head in relation to gravity. In the ampullae of the semicircular canals and in the utricle and saccule, where they lie in contact with the crystalline otoliths, are hair cells which transmit impulses to the cells of the vestibular ganglion of Scarpa. Thence they are conveyed by the vestibular nerve to the vestibular nuclei of the pons which have profuse connexions with the cerebellum, with the oculomotor nuclei via the medial longitudinal bundle, and with the spinal cord via the vestibulospinal tract.

The most important symptom produced by disorders of the vestibular system is **vertigo.** This term implies a disorder of equilibrium characterised by a sensation of rotation of the self or of one's surroundings. Often it is the objects around the patient which seem to be moving, either continuously in one direction or in a to-and-fro manner, but sometimes the patient feels that it is he himself that is twisting or spinning. Commonly vertigo is accompanied by staggering or even by actual falling, with clumsiness of the limbs, vomiting, depression and pallor. Nystagmus is generally present and in severe cases the vision is blurred or momentarily lost while rarely transient fainting may occur. It is important to distinguish true vertigo from mild 'giddiness' or 'swimming in the head' which are commonly psychogenic, or else may be due to syncope or presyncope.

In considering the aetiology and diagnostic significance of vertigo one must remember the many organs and mechanisms concerned in the normal maintenance of posture, as disorders of many different nervous pathways may cause this symptom. Firstly, visual impulses from the retina and from proprioceptive receptors in the external ocular muscles convey information concerning the relationship between the individual and his surroundings. Thus we can experience transient vertigo when looking down from heights or when observing a rapidly-moving object. Secondly, the labyrinth is very important; the commonest forms of vertigo are of aural origin and will be discussed below. Thirdly, and closely related to labyrinthine function, are the proprioceptive impulses derived from neck muscles, while similar stimuli from the muscles of the trunk and limbs give information concerning the position of the body. Whereas lesions of these proprioceptive pathways do not usually cause vertigo it can, however, result from disorders of the central co-ordinating mechanisms in the brain stem and of the cerebellum; the latter is important in the efferent mechanisms controlling posture. Lesions of the cerebral cortex rarely cause vertigo, although it has been described as the aura of an epileptic fit and can occasionally result from tumours of the temporal lobe. Even though the cerebellum is so important in the control of posture, it is comparatively uncommon for cerebellar hemisphere lesions, however massive, to give rise to vertigo. An exception is primary intracerebellar haemorrhage in which intense vertigo and vomiting often occur at the outset. Brain-stem lesions involving central cerebellar connexions, however, often give severe vertigo. Whereas it may result from **encephalitis**, **pontine tumours** or **syringobulbia**, the two most common brain-stem causes are **multiple sclerosis** and **infarction** or transient ischaemia. Occasionally the first symptom of multiple sclerosis is a sudden attack of severe vertigo, often lasting for hours or days, and associated with severe nystagmus and usually with other signs of a brain-stem lesion. The lateral medullary infarct produced by posterior inferior cerebellar artery thrombosis typically produces sudden vertigo, vomiting and prostration at the outset, while less severe attacks can occur in the recurrent ischaemic episodes of vertebro-basilar insufficiency.

Lesions of the labyrinth itself are, however, the most frequent cause of vertigo. Whereas some patients with compression or irritation of the eighth nerve, say, by an acoustic neuroma, suffer from it intermittently, disease of the internal ear is more often responsible. Sudden vertigo may result from an extension of a middle-ear infection to the labyrinth, but an **'acute vestibular neuronitis'**, often erroneously called 'labyrinthitis', can occur without a preceding middle-ear infection. In such a case vertigo develops suddenly and is generally associated with severe vomiting and prostration, some ataxia of the homolateral limbs, and a rotary nystagmus to the opposite side. The patient is often pyrexial and the illness may last for hours, days or weeks. The condition can occur in epidemic form and is believed to be an acute virus infection of the brain stem, involving vestibular nuclei, rather than a labyrinthitis, as diplopia and a lymphocytic pleocytosis in the CSF may be found. Hence the title **'epidemic vertigo'** is often preferred, even for sporadic cases. A similar clinical picture, usually with a shorter time course, and generally identified by the accompanying unilateral deafness, can result from atherosclerotic **occlusion of the internal auditory artery**. The distinction between epidemic vertigo and a first episode of multiple sclerosis due to a plaque in the brain stem can be difficult and may depend solely upon the subsequent course, as acute vestibular neuronitis generally recovers completely, whereas in multiple sclerosis subsequent manifestations of neurological disease are to be expected. Furthermore, other signs of brain stem dysfunction (e.g. diplopia) may accompany the vertiginous presentation of multiple sclerosis. Even in the benign labyrinthine disorder, however, one or more relapses may occur within the first few months.

Ménière's syndrome (recurrent aural vertigo) is a condition characterised by recurrent attacks of vertigo, often with vomiting and prostration, and accompanied by unilateral tinnitus and progressive nerve deafness. The condition can occur at any age, but is rare in children; it is commonest in middle life and somewhat more frequent in males. It seems to be due to a hydrops of the membranous labyrinth, of unknown aetiology, resulting in dilatation of the endolymph system with consequent pressure atrophy of the organ of Corti. Sometimes deafness and tinnitus are present for some time before the attacks of vertigo develop but more often the latter are the presenting feature. Attacks may initially be mild and brief, increasing in severity and frequency, but the manifestations are very variable. Typically a sudden attack of vertigo occurs with unsteadiness, vomiting and prostration and can be so violent that the patient is literally thrown to the ground. Pallor, perspiration, depression and tachycardia are common accompaniments and rotary nystagmus is present. Occasionally transient loss of consciousness due to syncope occurs in a severe attack. The attack may last only a few minutes or several hours but the patient is often lethargic, unsteady and depressed for several days afterwards. The episodes can occur at intervals of a few days, weeks or even months, but tend to become less frequent and eventually to disappear completely when deafness is complete in the affected ear. Unfortunately the contralateral ear is occasionally affected, sometimes concurrently but more often subsequently. A form of self-limiting **benign paroxysmal vertigo of childhood** is recognised which gives recurrent attacks of vertigo, without deafness, in children under the age of three years; it usually resolves spontaneously after a few months and its cause is unknown.

A somewhat similar condition giving episodic attacks of vertigo is **benign positional nystagmus**, which results from a degenerative lesion, again of unknown aetiology, in the otolith of the utricle and saccule. In this condition, however, the attacks occur only on certain specific movements of the head (e.g. stooping or lying down on one side) and can be reproduced at will by carrying out this movement. Most patients learn to avoid the offending position which evokes the attacks and often the condition improves spontaneously after months or years.

Motion-sickness is also a closely related disorder, and is due to the stereotyped repetitive stimulation of the semicircular canals produced by movement of a motor car, ship, train or aeroplane. There is a wide variation in individual susceptibility. Commonly lassitude, vague depression and drowsiness are early symptoms and are followed by vomiting and vertigo, though the latter is not usually severe. Considerable adaptation usually occurs in the habitual traveller.

References

Adams, R. D. and Victor, M., *Principles of Neurology*, 2nd ed. (New York, McGraw-Hill, 1981).

Ashworth, B. and Sherwood, I. *Clinical Neuro-ophthalmology* (Oxford, Blackwell, 1981).

Baloh, R. W. and Honrubia, V., *The Clinical Neurophysiology of the Vestibular System,* in the Contemporary Neurology Series, Eds. Plum, F. and McDowell, F. H. (Philadelphia, F. A. Davis, 1979).

Cogan, D. G., *Neurology of the Visual System,* 2nd ed. (Springfield, Ill., Thomas, 1977).

Fields, W. S. and Alford, B. R. (Eds.), *Neurological Aspects of Auditory and Vestibular Disorders* (Springfield, Ill., Thomas, 1964).

Gardner, E., *Fundamentals of Neurology*, 6th ed., Chapter 12 (Philadelphia and London, Saunders, 1975).

Mayo Clinic, Section of Neurology, 'The cranial nerves, and neuro-ophthalmology', in *Clinical Examinations in Neurology*, 4th ed. (Philadelphia and London, Saunders, 1976).

Newman, P. P., *Neurophysiology* (New York, SP Medical and Scientific Books, 1980).

Patton, H. D , Sundsten, J. W., Crill, W. E. and Swanson, P. D., *Introduction to Basic Neurology* (Philadelphia, W. B. Saunders, 1976)

Walton, J. N., *Brain's Diseases of the Nervous System,* 8th ed. (London, Oxford University Press, 1977).

Walton, J. N., Section X on Neurological pathophysiology, in *International Textbook of Medicine*, Eds. Smith, J. H. and Thier, S. (Philadelphia and London, W. B. Saunders, 1981).

Wolfson, R. J. (Ed.), *The Vestibular System and its Diseases* (Philadelphia, University of Pennsylvania Press, 1966).

9 The Motor System

Disorders of movement of the parts of the body produce some of the commoner symptoms professed by patients with disease or dysfunction of the nervous system. Sometimes the ability to move a part voluntarily is impaired (weakness or paresis) and sometimes it is lost completely (paralysis). On other occasions, willed movements are clumsy, ill-directed or uncontrolled (ataxia or inco-ordination), or else the part moves spontaneously or independently of the will (involuntary movements). On examination the examiner may confirm the presence of these abnormalities and may also discover abnormalities of tone in which the normal response to passive stretching of a muscle is altered; it can be reduced (hypotonia) or increased in two ways (spasticity, rigidity). Abnormalities of this type, and particularly weakness or paralysis, are sometimes emotionally determined (hysteria); or else they can be apraxic, resulting from a cortical lesion impairing the ability to recall acquired motor skills (*see* p. 103). More often, however, they are due to a disorder of function of that motor pathway which begins in the motor area of the cerebral cortex and ends in the voluntary musculature. There are a number of important physical signs which help to localise lesions within this motor apparatus, but to appreciate their significance a working knowledge of the organisation and pathophysiology of movement is essential.

The human motor system consists first of the descending pathways derived from the cerebral cortex and brain stem (the corticospinal or pyramidal system) which are concerned with the suprasegmental control of movement, secondly of the basal ganglia and cerebellum, thirdly of the continuation of these pathways within the spinal cord, and fourthly of the neuromuscular system which is made up of the nuclei of the motor cranial nerves and the muscles which they innervate, as well as the spinal cord anterior horn cells along with the segmentally organised voluntary musculature of the trunk and limbs. Both at higher and at segmental levels major afferent pathways project to these motor structures, providing information about the relative positions of different parts of the body and about muscle length; the latter is provided through the fusimotor spindle system of the muscles, which fulfils an important role in the control of movement. The basal ganglia and cerebellum do not project directly to the segmental motor structures of the brain stem and spinal cord but process information from other parts of the nervous system and project backwards on to the cortical and brain stem structures from which the suprasegmental pathways arise. A schematic outline of the motor system is given in Fig. 10.

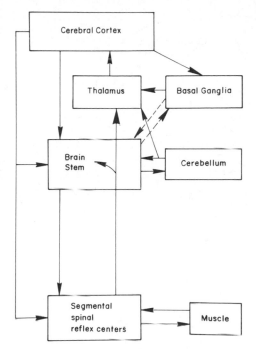

Fig. 10. A schematic 'flow' diagram of the motor system. The arrows do not necessarily represent direct monosynaptic connections.

(Reproduced from *Introduction to Basic Neurology* by Patton *et al.*, by kind permission of the authors and publisher.)

Anatomy and Physiology

The **upper motor neurones**, which constitute the pyramidal or corticospinal tracts, arise in part from nerve cells in the motor cortex of the cerebrum. This area of cortex lies anterior to the Rolandic fissure, in the precentral convolution. Whereas some of these neurones arise from the giant Betz cells which are common in this area, there are far more fibres in the pyramidal tracts than could be accounted for by the axons of all the Betz cells, so that many other upper motor neurones must arise from nerve cells in or near this area which are not structurally distinctive. Stimulation experiments have shown that activation of cells in the lower end of the precentral gyrus causes bilateral movement of the pharynx and larynx, while just above are others which, if stimulated, give movement of the contralateral half of the tongue (Figs. 11A, B, C). Facial movement can be elicited at a point slightly higher still and it is of interest that stimulation

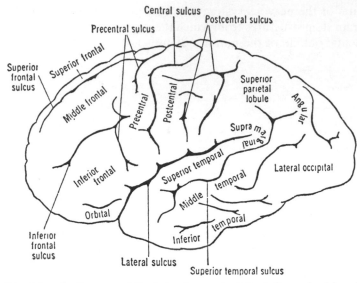

*Fig. 11*A. A diagram of the lateral aspect of the left cerebral hemisphere.
(From *Fundamentals of Neurology*, by E. Gardner, 4th edition, Saunders, Philadelphia and London, 1963)

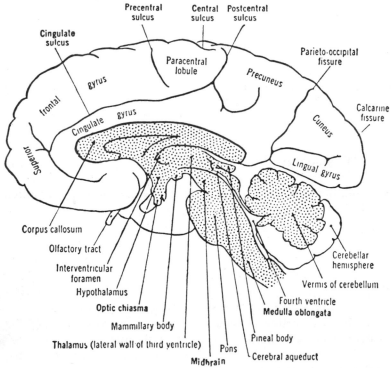

*Fig. 11*B. A diagram of the medial aspect of the right cerebral hemisphere.
(From *Fundamentals of Neurology*, by E. Gardner, 4th edition, Saunders, Philadelphia and London, 1963)

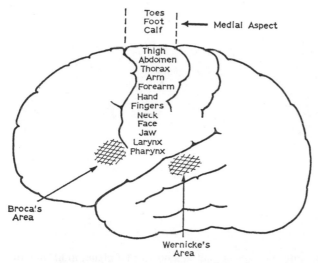

*Fig. 11*c. A diagram of the lateral aspect of the left cerebral hemisphere indicating the situation of the motor and sensory speech areas and also the 'representation' of the parts of the body in the motor area (precentral gyrus) of the cerebral hemisphere. The areas of the motor cortex concerned with movement of the lower limb lie on the medial aspect of the hemisphere in the paracentral lobule. 'Representation' in the sensory area (postcentral gyrus) is similar.

gives bilateral movement of the upper face but unilateral movement only of the lower face. Movement of the contralateral hand, arm, trunk, leg and foot is then produced in turn as one ascends the gyrus, and in each case 'representation' is strictly unilateral. The leg and foot 'area' lies partly on the medial surface of the hemisphere and partly on its superior aspect. Nerve fibres arising from the cells in this cortical area then come together in the corona radiata and converge upon the internal capsule which lies deep in the hemisphere between the thalamus and caudate nucleus medially and the lenticular nucleus laterally (Fig. 12). The pyramidal tract occupies the posterior one-third of the anterior limb, the genu, and the anterior two-thirds of the posterior limb of the capsule. Behind it lie sensory fibres travelling to the postcentral sensory cortex and others forming the optic radiation, while anteriorly are fronto-pontine fibres. From the internal capsule the tract passes down in the middle three-fifths of the cerebral peduncle to enter the mid-brain; in the pons it is broken into bundles by transverse pontine fibres, but in the medulla it is again a compact tract, the pyramid, which forms an anterior prominence. Throughout the brain stem the tract gives off fibres to the contralateral motor nuclei of the cranial nerves. In the lower medulla, most of the fibres in the pyramidal tract decussate to form the crossed pyramidal tract which travels down in the lateral column of the spinal cord on the opposite side, but a small proportion continue downwards in the anterior column of the

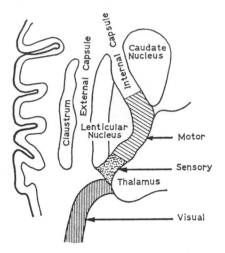

Fig. 12. A diagram of the internal capsule, cut in a horizontal plane, indicating the portions of the capsule occupied by the principal motor and sensory pathways, and the relationship of the capsule to the principal nuclei of the basal ganglia.
(Redrawn from *Introduction to Clinical Neurology*, by G. Holmes, Livingstone, Edinburgh, 1946.)

cord, forming the direct or uncrossed pyramidal tract (Fig. 13). Fibres of the pyramidal tract do not as a rule synapse directly with the anterior horn cells from which the lower motor neurones arise, but rather with internuncial neurones in the grey matter of the spinal cord, which in turn pass on to synapse in the anterior horns.

The **lower motor neurones** (alpha-neurones), which transmit impulses from the spinal cord anterior horn cells to the voluntary muscles, constitute the final common path of motor activity (Fig. 14). In other words, all nervous mechanisms which influence muscular activity produce their final effects through impulses which traverse these fibres. The axon of one anterior horn cell never innervates a single muscle fibre, but always many fibres which therefore contract simultaneously whenever the anterior horn cell discharges. It was once thought that the fibres were gathered together in bundles or fasciculi, but recent work suggests that the fibres supplied by a single neurone are widely scattered either in small groups or more often singly throughout the muscle. This basic functional unit of muscular activity, made up of one anterior horn cell, its axon, and the muscle fibres which it supplies, is known as the *motor unit*. It is now known that two types of motor unit exist in both animal and human muscle and that physical and chemical properties of their constituent muscle fibres are determined by their innervation. Thus there are slow-twitch or tonic units ('red' muscle, concerned largely with maintenance of posture and made up of type I muscle fibres which depend upon oxidative metabolism) and fast-twitch or phasic units ('white' muscle, concerned with voluntary

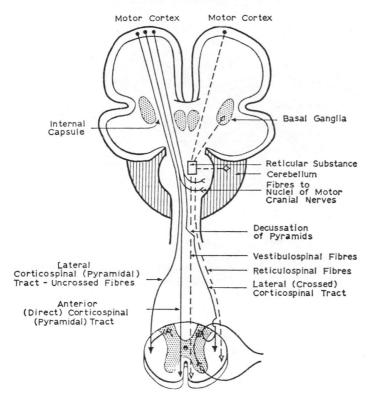

Fig. 13. A diagram of the principal pathways of the motor system. The continuous lines represent pathways of the pyramidal system, the interrupted lines those of the extrapyramidal system. The nuclear masses of the basal ganglia, the brainstem reticular substance, and the dentate nucleus of the cerebellum, which are some of the most important relay stations in the extrapyramidal system, are represented diagrammatically.

(Redrawn from *Fundamentals of Neurology*, by E. Gardner, 4th edition, Saunders, Philadelphia and London, 1963.)

activity and made up largely of type II muscle fibres which depend upon glycolytic anaerobic metabolism). During graduated voluntary contraction of a muscle, a single motor unit begins to fire with increasing frequency and gradually more and more of its fellows are recruited.

Other smaller motor neurones (gamma-neurones) innervate only the intrafusal fibres of the muscle spindle and form part of the reflex arc concerned with the control of muscle tone.

In the anatomical schema laid out above are outlined the basic functional units through which a movement is initiated and performed. However, the organisation of movement is much more complex than this simple schema would suggest. For instance, no single cell in the motor area of the cerebral cortex can be said to innervate any single muscle. Stimulation experiments

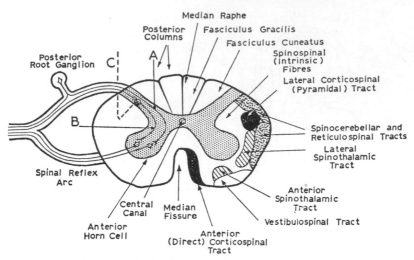

Fig. 14. Diagrammatic representation of the motor reflex arc and of the principal fibre tracts of the spinal cord. *A*, a simple two-neurone reflex arc. *B*, a three-neurone reflex arc with an internuncial neurone between the sensory and motor neurones. *C*, a corticospinal fibre influencing the activity of the reflex arc.

have shown that it is not single muscle twitches, but organised movements, which are initiated in the motor cortex. These movements involve several muscles or muscle groups, of which only some act as prime movers or agonists. Others, the antagonists, must be enabled to relax smoothly as the agonists contract, while yet others must fix a limb proximally, say, in order to allow a movement occurring distally to be efficient. Other muscles, or synergists, may also be used to counteract unwanted effects which would be produced by the unmodified action of the agonists. The many internuncial neurones in the spinal cord, which receive impulses from many pyramidal axons and may influence many anterior horn cells, are clearly important in this organisation. However, incoming sensory impulses from stretch receptors (muscle spindles) in the muscles themselves, as well as other proprioceptive impulses giving information about the position of the part which is being moved, can also modify this activity through a series of spinal reflexes. Additional modifying influences are exerted through sensory impulses from the eyes and labyrinths which enter the brain stem and initiate activity in the vestibulospinal tracts.

Not only can sensory impulses influence movement in this way, but other important effects are exerted by the **extrapyramidal motor system**. Several nuclear masses in the basal ganglia and upper brain stem, and particularly the lenticular and caudate nuclei, the thalamus, the subthalamic nuclei, the substantia nigra, the brain stem reticular formation and the olivary nuclei, exercise profound controlling influences upon movement. The basal ganglia influence movement largely through thalamic relays which project to the motor cortex, by integrating their output with cerebellar input to the ventrolateral nucleus of the thalamus and by descending impulses conveyed by the rubrospinal and reticulospinal tracts. It is now evident that the corpus striatum (consisting of the caudate nucleus, the globus pallidus and putamen, the latter two of which together form the lenticular nucleus) plays an important role in controlling posture and that the globus pallidus is the final efferent cell station; lesions of this nucleus can give akinesia (inability to initiate movement) or bradykinesia (excessively slow movement). The basal ganglia also control the balance between alpha and gamma motor neurone activity so that when disease distorts this balance, abnormalities of muscle tone or tremor result. The concerted activity of the nuclei of the basal ganglia gives smooth integration of voluntary movement; lesions of individual components of the system may allow the release, due to removal of inhibitory mechanisms, of typical involuntary movements (chorea, athetosis, dystonia, hemiballismus) which will be described below. It is now known, too, that many neurones of the substantia nigra, especially in the nigrostriatal pathway, are dopaminergic, while others in the striatonigral system employ GABA as a neurotransmitter and many neurones in the corpus striatum are cholinergic. Reserpine or phenothiazines may deplete dopamine stores giving drug-induced Parkinsonism, but may also produce troublesome facial dyskinesia; there is loss of dopamine in the substantia nigra in idiopathic Parkinsonism, but this can be restored with clinical improvement by levodopa, a dopamine precursor which, however, may cause involuntary movements like those of athetosis; and cholinergic activation can accentuate the features of Parkinsonism. It thus appears that many of the clinical features of disease or dysfunction of the basal ganglia are due to an imbalance in the relative activities of cholinergic and dopaminergic neurones and their receptors.

The **cerebellum** is made up of the archicerebellum, palaeocerebellum and neocerebellum. The archicerebellum, consisting of the flocculonodular lobe and uvula, is concerned with the control of eye movements, with postural neck and axial reflexes and thus with the maintenance of equilibrium. The palaeocerebellum, consisting of the vermis and contiguous parts of the cerebellar hemispheres, exercises a modulating influence upon muscle tone through the spindle system. Lesions of these central cerebellar structures often cause severe dysequilibrium without vertigo (truncal ataxia) with a broad-based unsteady gait and sometimes postural nystagmus. The neocerebellum, which is made up of the major part of the two cerebellar hemispheres, is especially concerned with the regulation and smooth co-ordination of limb movements, fulfilling a graduating and harmonising role.

We presume that a movement is initiated when the concept of it is first invoked in the 'association' areas of the cortex. The appropriate cells of the precentral cortex are then activated and impulses travel down the pyramidal tracts, in order to activate the appropriate anterior horn cells and their motor units. Simultaneously the movement is influenced and controlled by the activity of the cerebellum and of the extrapyramidal motor system; at the same time as agonists are being stimulated to contract, synergists to assist and fixators to fix, an inhibitory mechanism is invoked to produce controlled relaxation of antagonists. Once the movement has begun it is then subject to continued modification through sensory impulses arriving from the proprioceptors, or from the eyes and labyrinths. Clearly, therefore, movement can be disorganised by lesions of many different nervous pathways, and some principles which aid in deciding which pathway or pathways are diseased will be considered below.

Weakness and Paralysis

Weakness (paresis) of a muscle group implies that the power produced by voluntary contraction of the affected muscles is reduced, whereas paralysis indicates that the power to move the part concerned is totally lost. Weakness of one limb is called a **monoparesis**, total paralysis a **monoplegia**. **Hemiplegia** is the term used to identify paralysis afflicting one side of the body, and particularly the arm and leg, while **paraplegia** signifies a paralysis of both lower limbs. When all four limbs are paralysed, the terms **quadriplegia** or **tetraplegia** are used; a symmetrical weakness of all four limbs, affecting the lower more markedly than the upper, and occurring in children with cerebral palsy, is often called a **diplegia**. The term 'palsy' can be used interchangeably with 'paralysis', but is more often utilised in practice to identify paralysis of individual muscles or muscle groups resulting from peripheral nerve lesions.

Paralysis may be due to a lesion of the upper or lower motor neurone, and under certain circumstances it can be due to a defect in conduction at the neuromuscular junction or to a biochemical or structural abnormality of the muscle itself. Clinical methods of differentiating these causes of paralysis will be discussed below.

Disorders of Tone

The tone of a muscle is the response it shows to passive stretching. A relaxed and resting muscle is not in a state of continuous partial contraction; it has elasticity, but no tone. Tone can only therefore be assessed when the muscle is moved or when it is concerned with maintaining a posture against an applied force such as that of gravity. **Postural tone** is thus that state of partial contraction of certain muscles which is needed to maintain the posture of the parts of the body; clearly the muscles involved and the force of muscular contraction required will depend upon the position of the parts concerned at any one time.

In neurological practice, tone is usually assessed by moving a limb or some other part passively and by observing the reaction which occurs in the muscles which are being stretched. As this stretching begins, stretch receptors in the muscle concerned, and particularly the muscle spindles, give out afferent stimuli and reflex partial contraction of the muscle results. Variations in the sensitivity of this reflex, which is also responsible for the tendon reflexes, account for the alterations in tone which result from nervous disease. Forceful continued contraction of a muscle group (e.g. clenching one hand or pulling firmly with the flexed fingers of both hands opposed to one another) temporarily causes an increased flow of afferent impulses in the sensory fibres from the spindles. This in turn gives increased firing in gamma neurones throughout the body, thus causing a generalised slight increase in tone, and the tendon reflexes become more brisk as the 'set' of the spindle (the state of contraction of its intrafusal fibres) is altered, with resultant increased sensitivity to stretch. This phenomenon, often known as reinforcement, or Jendrassik's manoeuvre, is often used to bring out tendon reflexes which at first seem absent. In spasticity and extrapyramidal rigidity the 'set' of the spindles is continuously abnormal.

On stretching, the tone of the muscle may be increased (spasticity or rigidity or hypertonia) or it may be reduced (flaccidity or hypotonia) and these alterations are of great value in neurological diagnosis.

Muscle tone is normally regulated by reticulospinal fibres which accompany the pyramidal tract throughout its course and which have an inhibitory effect upon the stretch reflex. This inhibition balances the background facilitatory impulses conveyed by the pontine reticulospinal and vestibulospinal pathways; these influences are in turn modified by multisynaptic arcs traversing the cerebellum, basal ganglia and brain stem. When lesions of the pyramidal and reticulospinal tract release stretch reflexes from inhibition, the increased tone and exaggerated tendon reflexes which result are initially associated with hyperactivity in dynamic fusimotor neurones, but if such increased tone (*spasticity*) persists, increased alpha neurone discharge develops so that spasticity in man at different stages may be associated with both increased gamma (dynamic fusimotor) and alpha neurone activity. If the dorsal reticulospinal system, closely related anatomically in the spinal cord, is also damaged, afferent flexor reflex pathways are also released from inhibition giving flexor spasms in the lower limbs in response to stimulation of the legs; the 'extensor' plantar response, or Babinski reflex, one component of the flexor withdrawal reflex, is similarly released. In spasticity the affected limb or limbs show an increase in resistance to passive stretching; this resistance is particularly severe initially, but then 'gives' suddenly as the movement is continued. Hence this sign, seen particularly well in the legs of a patient with a spastic paraplegia due to bilateral pyramidal tract disease, is known as 'clasp-knife' rigidity. In individuals with spastic weakness, movement is impaired owing to defective conduction of motor impulses by the pyramidal tracts, while there is also 'clasp-knife' rigidity on passive movement.

Rigidity of extrapyramidal type, in patients with disease of the basal ganglia or substantia nigra, is different. It is seen characteristically in Parkinsonism. In such cases the rigidity is either uniform in degree throughout the entire range of passive movement, when it is known as 'plastic' or 'lead-pipe' rigidity, or else it intermittently 'gives' and returns throughout the movement, being then referred to as 'cog-wheel' in type. In extrapyramidal rigidity, unlike spasticity, alpha neurone rather than gamma neurone discharge predominates with increased activity in static as distinct from dynamic fusimotor fibres. In **dystonia** there is simultaneous contraction of agonists, antagonists and synergists, reciprocal inhibition of antagonists is seriously deranged and alpha neurone discharge is greatly increased. A particular form of muscular rigidity, known as **decerebrate rigidity**, develops as a result of severe transverse lesions of the upper mid-brain at the level of the superior colliculus or red nucleus. Excitatory mechanisms cause increased tone in extensor muscles, inhibitory mechanisms reduce tone in flexor muscles. These mechanisms are mediated by reticulospinal and vestibulospinal pathways, and tonic as distinct from phasic stretch reflexes are increased, while there is increased gamma efferent discharge to extensor muscles, involving especially static fusimotor fibres. In such a case all four limbs are rigidly extended, the back is arched and there may be neck retraction, so that the patient, if lying supine, is virtually supported by the back of the head and the heels. This posture is known as **opisthotonos**; the arching of the back is increased by any sensory stimulus and there is striking resistance to any attempt at flexing the limbs passively.

Flaccidity, or **hypotonia**, is a reduction in tone. When this is severe, as in patients with total flaccid paralysis, all resistance to passive stretch is lost and the limbs are limp and flail-like. Less severe hypotonia in the upper limbs, for instance, can be elicited by asking the patient to hold out his arms horizontally. The forearms are then tapped briskly; when tone is increased (spasticity) the recoil is sharp, immediate and exaggerated. When one limb is hypotonic the recoil is slower and the arm swings through a wider range. If the patient is asked to contract the biceps brachii against resistance, by bending the arm towards his face, and the examiner's restraining hand is suddenly removed, the patient's hand may strike his face if the limb is hypotonic, whereas if the tone is normal he will stop the movement before it does so. Furthermore, if the subject is asked to raise his arms above his head with the palms facing forwards, the palm of a hypotonic limb is externally rotated and facing more laterally than the other. In the lower limbs it is useful to place a hand beneath the knee and to lift the leg from the bed, then to allow it to fall back quickly; with experience it is soon possible to judge from the resistance of the limb to this movement, whether tone is increased or reduced.

Ataxia and Inco-ordination

Ataxia is clumsiness of motor activity, resulting from inability to control accurately the range and precision of movement. It can result from a defect in the sensory pathways carrying proprioceptive information from sensory receptors in the periphery. The appreciation of the position of the parts of the body in space is then impaired, and since controlled movement requires continuous and accurate information of this type for its continued performance, it may be seriously deranged. This phenomenon, known as **sensory ataxia**, will be considered in Chapter 10. In such a case, the cause of the unsteadiness becomes apparent on sensory examination. Similarly, sensory stimuli from the labyrinths are important in the maintenance of posture and if, as a result of disease of the labyrinths, of the vestibular nerves or of their central connexions, distorted information about the position of the head is received, the patient's gait will become grossly unsteady and the movements of his limbs clumsy and poorly controlled. Thus ataxia can also be due to **labyrinthine dysfunction**.

Most common as a cause of ataxia is **disease of the cerebellum** or of its central connexions in the brain stem. The controlling activity of the cerebellum upon the motor system is concerned particularly with the fine co-ordination of movement and with the judgement of distance; these faculties are selectively impaired as a result of cerebellar disease. Much depends upon which part of the cerebellum or its connecting pathways is diseased, and there are several general principles which help one to conclude that the function of the cerebellum or of cerebellar pathways is impaired. The archicerebellum and palaeocerebellum as defined above have important vestibular connexions and are concerned particularly with equilibration. Lesions in this situation produce an ataxia which involves central structures of the body and is thus particularly apparent when the patient walks. He is unsteady and staggers in a drunken manner, walks on a wide base and has considerable difficulty in stopping suddenly or in turning. Lesser degrees of ataxia can be brought out by asking the patient to walk 'heel-to-toe'; even in mildly ataxic individuals this is usually impossible. In such a case the tests of cerebellar function to be described below, which are concerned with demonstrating ataxia in lateral structures, such as the limbs, may be singularly uninformative. When these tests are negative it is a common pitfall to regard such patients as hysterical, particularly if the doctor fails to recognise that a central cerebellar lesion gives this particular type of so-called **truncal or central ataxia**. This sign is particularly well seen in children with medulloblastomas.

Lesions of the lateral cerebellar hemispheres, affecting the neocerebellum, give a number of physical signs which are more readily identifiable. If the lesion is predominantly unilateral, these signs are found in the limbs on the same side as the lesion. There may also be **ocular signs**; thus in an acute cerebellar lesion *skew deviation* is occasionally seen, in which the eye on the affected side is deviated downwards and inwards, while the contralateral eye is turned upwards and out; but this rare manifestation is more common in upper brain stem lesions. *Nystagmus* is commoner and usually prominent, being of greatest amplitude on looking to the side of the lesion. **Hypotonia** is often present in the ipsilateral limbs, and **ataxia** is evidenced by a striking clumsiness and inco-ordination of movement. The patient is unable to fasten buttons with the affected hand and his hand-writing may be scrawling and illegible. Judgement of distance is grossly impaired, a phenomenon known as **dysmetria**, and the hand or digit performing a movement may wildly overshoot the mark (**past-pointing**). Tremor of the limbs may be apparent at rest but is greatly accentuated by movement, being worse towards the end of an action (**intention-tremor**). The latter sign is, however, much more common in disease of central cerebellar connexions than of the cerebellar hemispheres and in fact is rarely seen in any condition other than multiple sclerosis. 'Neocerebellar' signs are particularly apparent on carrying out the 'finger–nose' and 'heel–knee' tests and there is also a gross irregularity of movement if the patient is asked to tap quickly and repetitively upon a smooth surface, or to make dots within a small circle with a pencil. Rapid alternating movements of the limbs, such as pronation and supination of the forearms, are poorly and jerkily performed (**dysdiadochokinesis**). The patient with a unilateral cerebellar lesion also tends to stagger and to deviate towards the affected side when walking. A minimal cerebellar lesion on one side is sometimes easily identified by asking the patient to walk a few paces with his eyes closed, when he will deviate to the affected side. Alternatively, if asked to walk in a circle around the examiner, first clockwise then anticlockwise, the deviation away from the examiner in one direction and towards him in the other will be apparent.

The Reflexes

The simplest reflex arc consists of an afferent or sensory neurone and an efferent or motor neurone with whose parent cell the terminal fibres of the afferent neurone synapse (Fig. 14). Stimulation of the sensory neurone then produces a motor response mediated by the motor neurone. Few reflexes are as simple as this, though the spinal reflex arc through which withdrawal of a limb follows a painful stimulus cannot be much more complex. In many pathways concerned with reflex activity, however, the sensory and motor neurones are separated by connecting or internuncial neurones, most of which lie in the spinal grey matter; they receive impulses from ascending and descending fibre pathways which exercise important controlling influences upon reflex activity. Unquestionably some long reflex pathways run a course involving brain stem as well as spinal structures, while some may even traverse the cerebral cortex. There are many reflexes concerned with autonomic and visceromotor activity, and even endocrine secretion, but in clinical neurology we are largely concerned with the simpler reflexes which, when activated, result in somatic motor activity.

Clearly reflex activity is lost or impaired if a lesion is present at any point in the reflex arc. Thus a break in the afferent or efferent pathway will mean that a particular reflex can no longer be obtained. For instance, the **corneal reflex** (the contraction of the orbicularis oculi which follows stimulation of the cornea) is lost if the cornea is anaesthetic due to a lesion of the trigeminal nerve or if the face is paralysed due to a lesion of the seventh nerve. Similarly, the **palatal and pharyngeal reflexes** which give contraction of muscles of the soft palate or pharynx on tactile stimulation may be impaired unilaterally. This occurs if one trigeminal (palate) or glossopharyngeal (pharyngeal) nerve is diseased (the afferent pathway), or if there is a lesion of the vagus (the efferent pathway).

The most informative reflexes in the physical examination of patients with nervous disease are the stretch and cutaneous reflexes.

The first of the **stretch reflexes** is the *jaw jerk,* elicited by means of a sharp downward tap on the chin with the mouth held partly open. A positive response consists in contraction of the masseters with elevation of the lower jaw; if this reflex is exaggerated it usually indicates a bilateral pyramidal tract lesion in or above the upper brain stem. The **'snout' reflex** (*see* p. 24) occurs under similar circumstances, while if there is bilateral frontal lobe destruction or degeneration as in certain varieties of dementia, a **'sucking'** reflex, like the normal sucking response of the young infant, may be present.

The stretch reflexes normally utilised on examining the limbs are the **tendon reflexes**. These consist in a reflex contraction of the muscle concerned, produced in practice by a sharp blow upon the tendon of the muscle near its point of insertion. Those commonly elicited have been described in Chapter 2. In the upper limb they are the biceps and radial jerks which obtain their motor innervation from the fifth and sixth cervical roots, the triceps jerk which is mainly innervated by the seventh, and the finger jerk which receives its supply from the seventh and eighth roots. In the lower limbs, the knee jerk is innervated by the second, third and fourth lumbar roots, the ankle jerk by the first and second sacral. Any tendon reflex can be diminished or lost if there is a lesion of the sensory pathway which carries afferent impulses from the muscle to the spinal cord, if there is a lesion at any point in the lower motor neurones supplying the muscle concerned, or even if a primary disorder of the muscle itself, a myopathy, has impaired its ability to contract. These reflexes are also lost temporarily during the stage of so-called 'shock' which follows an acute and severe lesion of the brain or spinal cord, even if there is no break in the reflex arc. All the tendon reflexes may be symmetrically exaggerated by tension and anxiety or by increased neuromuscular excitability due to metabolic or other causes, but they are most strikingly increased when there is a lesion of the pyramidal tract. A unilateral lesion is easier to identify, as the reflexes are exaggerated on one side of the body and not on the other. The finger jerk, for instance, is normally present in some patients and not in others; it is only of real significance if present unilaterally. The phenomenon of *clonus* often accompanies exaggeration of the stretch reflexes. It consists of an intermittent muscular contraction and relaxation evoked by sustained stretching of a muscle; it can occur apparently spontaneously in spastic limbs, but is best elicited as a physical sign in the lower limbs by sudden pressure applied in a distal direction to the upper margin of the patella (*patellar clonus*), or by a sharp dorsiflexion of the foot carried out with the leg extended (*ankle clonus*).

Inversion of upper-limb reflexes may be an important physical sign of spinal cord disease. Thus if there is a lesion of the C5 or C6 segments of the spinal cord, this will break the reflex arc for reflexes innervated by these segments, namely the biceps and radial jerks, which are therefore lost or diminished. If, however, the same lesion is compressing the spinal cord and giving pyramidal tract dysfunction, reflexes innervated by lower segments (triceps, finger jerks) are exaggerated and are obtained by stimuli applied over a wide field. Thus tapping the biceps tendon may produce contraction of triceps, while on attempting to elicit the radial jerk, finger flexion, but no radial jerk, is obtained. This so-called inversion of either reflex is diagnostic of a cervical cord lesion.

The **cutaneous or superficial reflexes** commonly utilised in neurological diagnosis are the abdominal reflexes, the cremasteric, anal and plantar reflexes. The *abdominal reflexes* are elicited by stroking the skin of the abdomen (the point of a pin is a suitable instrument), when movement of the umbilicus towards the stimulus should follow. The level of a segmental lesion in the dorsal spinal cord can sometimes be identified by loss of the lower abdominal reflexes and preservation of the upper. Even more useful is the fact that the abdominal reflexes are unilaterally diminished in amplitude or lost, or may simply fatigue rapidly on repetitive stimulation, when there is a lesion of the pyramidal tract on the same side of the body. There are some conditions (e.g. multiple sclerosis) in which the abdominal reflexes are lost at a comparatively early stage of the disease, whereas in others (e.g. motor neurone disease), in which there is also evidence of pyramidal tract disease, they often survive much longer. Total absence of the abdominal reflexes is usually a finding of pathological significance, except in the very obese, in multipara with lax abdominal muscles, and in the elderly. The *cremasteric reflex* (contraction of the cremaster on stroking the medial side of the thigh) is also impaired or lost in pyramidal tract lesions. The *anal reflex* (contraction of the external sphincter on scratching the perianal skin) is particularly likely to be lost when there is a lesion of the cauda equina involving the fourth and fifth sacral roots.

A most important reflex in clinical neurology is the **plantar response**. On stroking the lateral aspect of the sole of the foot from the heel towards the fifth toe, there is normally plantar-flexion of all five toes (the flexor response). The abnormal response which consists of dorsiflexion of the great toe and a simultaneous downward and 'fanning-out' movement of the remaining toes, is known as an extensor response or the Babinski response. The Babinski response refers only to the abnormal extensor reflex and it is semantically inaccurate to say that 'the Babinski was negative or positive'. It is better to avoid the eponymous term and to refer to the plantar response as being 'flexor' or 'extensor'. An extensor plantar reflex is virtually diagnostic of a lesion of the pyramidal tract at any point in its course from the contralateral motor cortex down through the brain stem and the ipsilateral lateral column of the spinal cord. It is part of a primitive withdrawal response 'uncovered' or 'released' by a pyramidal tract lesion; often it is accompanied by contraction of the hamstrings. Indeed, if the spinal cord lesion is severe and complete, stroking the sole will also evoke flexion at the hip and knee and even evacuation of the bladder and bowels (a 'mass' reflex). In such a case the extensor plantar response is readily elicited by a variety of stimuli applied over a wide area (e.g. pressure upon the shin, pricking the leg with a pin, etc.).

Among the many other reflexes which are altered by nervous disease there are few which are of sufficient practical importance to be mentioned here. However, in decerebrate patients, as in neonates, the **tonic neck reflexes** may be greatly exaggerated so that on forcibly turning the head to one side the limbs on that side extend while the contralateral limbs flex (Magnus–de Klejn reflex). Persistence of this reflex after the first three months of life, and of the Moro reflex (flexion of all four limbs on sharply tapping the bed upon which the baby lies) indicates a serious disorder of cerebral development. Similarly, the activity of the frontal lobes in man is sufficient after the first year or two of life to inhibit the reflex grasping and groping which results from stroking the palm of the hand. This **grasp reflex** may, however, return unilaterally due to a lesion of the contralateral frontal lobe.

The Clinical Features of Upper and Lower Motor Neurone Lesions

Let us take as an example of the effects of an **upper motor neurone lesion** the hemiplegia which is produced by an extensive lesion of the contralateral motor area of the cerebral cortex, or of the internal capsule. If the lesion is acute, say, a massive haemorrhage, the paralysed limbs are at first flaccid, immobile and without tone, owing to the phenomenon of 'shock', through which a sudden and extensive lesion causes an abrupt depression of reflexes subserved by relatively remote areas of the nervous system, even though the reflex arcs concerned remain intact. All reflexes are absent at this stage on the affected side. Gradually over the course of days or weeks this flaccidity lessens and the affected limbs become spastic, though there are a few cases in which, particularly if there is also an extensive parietal lobe lesion, the hemiplegia remains permanently flaccid. Whereas the affected arm and leg are completely paralysed, those parts of the body which are bilaterally 'represented' in the cerebral cortex can still be moved voluntarily, even on the paralysed side. Thus facial weakness affects mainly the lower part of the face and the upper part slightly or not at all, while there will be no defect of palatal movement. Furthermore, since emotional movement of the face, as in smiling, seems to be controlled not by the cerebral cortex but by thalamic mechanisms, a patient who cannot move the lower half of one side of the face at will may yet smile symmetrically.

As flaccidity passes off in the paralysed limbs and spasticity appears, so the tendon reflexes return, become greatly exaggerated and may be accompanied by clonus. The abdominal and cremasteric reflexes on the affected side remain absent and the plantar response extensor. Spasticity is often greatest in the flexor muscles of the upper limbs and in the extensor muscles of the lower, so that in a patient with a long-standing hemiplegia, the arm is flexed at the elbow and at the wrist and fingers, while the leg remains extended.

When the lesion of the pyramidal tract is not sufficiently severe to cause total paralysis, but only relatively slight weakness, it is the finer and more skilful movements, those most recently acquired by man in the process of evolution, which are most severely impaired (Hughlings Jackson's law). Thus independent finger and toe movements are poor, though the strength of movement at proximal joints such as the elbow and knee remains good. A useful sign of early pyramidal tract dysfunction is to observe the hands and arms outstretched in front of the patient when the eyes are closed; a downward 'drift' is an early sign of upper motor neurone weakness. Furthermore, while difficulty in opposing the thumb and individual fingers may be an early sign, objective testing of muscle power often shows that 'pyramidal' weakness is first apparent on abduction of the shoulder and in hand-grip in the upper limbs and in hip flexion and foot dorsiflexion in the lower. And during the process of recovery from a pyramidal tract lesion, movement usually returns first at the proximal joints; the cruder movements are first regained, while the more delicate and precise activity of the fingers and toes is the last to return. A patient recovering from a hemiplegia resulting from, say, cerebral thrombosis, may be able to use his hand to grip or to lift objects, but is often unable to write or to fasten buttons or shoelaces. He walks with his arm flexed across his chest and with stiffness, dragging and circumduction of the affected leg.

Similar physical signs are found in patients with bilateral pyramidal tract lesions causing spastic paraplegia. If the lesion responsible is an acute transverse lesion of the cord, say, from infection or injury, there is total flaccid paralysis of the limbs below the affected segment during the initial stage of spinal shock; subsequently spasticity, increased tendon reflexes and extensor plantar responses appear. As the lower motor neurone and the spinal reflex arc are intact, severe wasting of muscles does not occur, although when paralysis has been present for some time, disuse atrophy, affecting all muscles of the limb or limbs, appears. When the spinal cord lesion is incomplete, the tone of the spastic lower limbs may be particularly increased in the extensor muscles (paraplegia-in-extension) but when both pyramidal tracts are severely diseased and there are lesions of reticulospinal and vestibulospinal pathways, the legs become progressively flexed at the knees and hips and stimulation will provoke painful flexor spasms (paraplegia-in-flexion).

It is important to realise that much depends, in an individual case, upon the rate of evolution of any upper motor neurone lesion. Whereas an acute lesion, e.g. cerebral haemorrhage or cord transection, gives a total flaccid paralysis initially with spasticity evolving slowly over subsequent days or weeks, a chronic or slowly progressive lesion such as a tumour may give little more initially than a slight impairment of fine finger movement in one hand, or else a minimal increase in tendon reflexes in the affected arm; subsequently, however, a spastic monoparesis or hemiparesis slowly develops.

The pathological causes of upper motor neurone lesions are many and varied—too many for their differential diagnosis to be considered in detail here. Once the lesion has been localised by means of the physical signs, the clinical history should again be analysed to see if any clue can be obtained as to the nature of the pathological process. The scheme of pathological classification given in Chapter 2 is often useful. Thus if we take the cerebral causes of spastic weakness, these may include traumatic (cerebral contusion, extradural haematoma), developmental (cerebral palsy), inflammatory (cerebral abscess, encephalomyelitis), neoplastic (meningioma, glioma, metastases), and degenerative (cerebral infarction or haemorrhage) causes.

The natural history of these and of the many other conditions which may affect the pyramidal tract differ considerably, and associated signs indicating involvement of other nervous structures or other systems may be invaluable. Similarly, there are many possible causes of spinal cord disease giving rise to spastic paraplegia. These include developmental causes (basilar impression, Chiari malformation), trauma (fracture dislocation of spine, haematomyelia), inflammation, either extradural (abscess) or intramedullary (transverse myelitis), neoplasia (meningioma, neurofibroma, glioma, metastases, reticulosis) and a group of common degenerative, demyelinating and metabolic disorders. Of these, multiple sclerosis is characterised by a remittent course and often by involvement of brain-stem structures; it sometimes gives temporal pallor of the optic disks, nystagmus or diplopia and cerebellar signs as well as signs of a spastic paraplegia with impaired appreciation of 'posterior column' type sensation in the lower limbs. Some few cases, however, run a progressive course with only a spastic paraplegia and no signs of involvement of brain-stem structures, although even in these, visual evoked potential measurement may demonstrate unsuspected lesions of the optic nerves or pathways. In these cases the condition may be difficult to distinguish from amyotrophic lateral sclerosis or cervical cord compression due to tumour or cervical spondylosis. In the latter disorder, however, particularly if the long-standing disk protrusions extend laterally, spinal roots are often compressed as well as the cord, and there may be muscle wasting and weakness in the arms or inversion of upper limb reflexes as well as a spastic paraplegia. Patients with motor neurone disease usually demonstrate some wasting, weakness and fasciculation of muscles in the limbs, as well as signs of a spastic paraparesis, and in this condition there is no sensory impairment, but in early cases presenting with the clinical syndrome of amyotrophic lateral sclerosis, as distinct from progressive muscular atrophy, the signs may simply be those of spastic paraparesis. In syringomyelia, on the other hand, dissociated anaesthesia to pain and temperature sensation with retention of touch is often found in one upper limb, combined with some wasting and weakness of muscles due to lower motor neurone involvement, while in the lower limbs there are usually signs of a spastic paraparesis. Spastic weakness of the legs is also present in some cases of subacute combined degeneration of the cord, but here sensory symptoms and signs indicating dysfunction of the posterior columns of the cord usually predominate; there may be tenderness of the calves and absent ankle jerks owing to a neuropathy interrupting the sensory side of the reflex arc, while signs of pyramidal tract disease, though present, are often relatively unobtrusive. In spinal cord infarction, if the cord is infarcted over several segments, due to occlusion of the anterior spinal artery resulting from thrombosis, embolism or compression, the paraplegia may be permanently flaccid, but the plantars, if not absent, are extensor.

The features of a **lower motor neurone lesion** are different. As the final common path of all forms of motor activity is interrupted, the muscle or muscle groups involved become totally paralysed and flaccid, and remain so. Any reflex movement for which the paralysed muscles are necessary is lost. Another invariable feature is that all muscles deprived of their motor nerve supply undergo rapid atrophy; they may shrink to half normal size within about six weeks and eventually disappear almost completely, being virtually replaced by fibrous connective tissue. Before this stage of total atrophy is reached, and particularly if the lesion responsible lies in the anterior horn cells of the spinal cord (e.g. motor neurone disease), **fasciculation** is common. The latter is a phenomenon, visible through the intact skin unless the subject is very obese, in which individual muscle fasciculi contract spontaneously, and random, repetitive flickering of these fibre bundles is seen to be occurring in a muscle which is apparently at rest. Fasciculation, though most often seen in motor neurone disease, is not diagnostic of that condition, as it may occur after old poliomyelitis, and is also seen occasionally in polyneuropathy and in other conditions involving anterior horn cells and peripheral nerves. Furthermore, it may be benign and of no pathological significance; it is often noticed by doctors in their calf and small hand muscles. A benign condition in which widespread and coarse fasciculation occurs along with profuse sweating and muscular cramps is known as one variety of **myokymia**. Benign myokymia of the lower eyelid is a flickering in that lid often experienced by normal individuals when fatigued. Another rare and obscure form of myokymia is characterised by fasciculation, myotonia, distal muscular wasting and contracture and by continuous muscle fibre activity in the EMG (Isaacs' syndrome or neuromyotonia).

Fibrillation, or spontaneous contraction of single muscle fibres, also follows a lesion of the lower motor neurone, but cannot be seen through the skin, though it can be recorded in the EMG. Hence the clinical features of an acute lower motor neurone lesion are flaccid paralysis, absent reflexes, and rapid atrophy of the affected muscle or group of muscles. In a slowly progressive lesion weakness and atrophy increase gradually, and eventually the reflexes are lost. In such a case it can be difficult to decide whether the lesion involves a single peripheral nerve, multiple peripheral nerves, spinal anterior roots, or the anterior horn cells of the cord. All-important in making this distinction is a knowledge of the anatomy and innervation of muscles. If more muscles are affected than could be supplied by one peripheral nerve, it must then be asked whether lesions of one or several spinal roots could be responsible, in which case there may be other evidence of spinal cord dysfunction. If the muscular weakness and wasting is more widespread still, and particularly if it occurs symmetrically in the periphery of the limbs, the two most likely diagnoses are polyneuropathy and motor neurone disease (progressive muscular atrophy). The presence of sensory loss, particularly if present symmetrically and distally, will support the former diagnosis, while if there is widespread fasciculation, no sensory loss, and some evidence of pyramidal tract disease, motor neurone disease can be diagnosed with reasonable confidence.

Muscular weakness and wasting which can mimic that due to a lower motor neurone lesion may result from disease of the muscles themselves, a myopathy. Here too there is flaccid weakness with atrophy and absence of tendon reflexes. Even in disorders of conduction at the motor end-plate, such as myasthenia gravis, the muscles may be weak and hypotonic, though atrophy is uncommon. In general, however, myopathic as distinct from neuropathic disorders (*see* Chapter 18) tend to affect the proximal rather than the distal muscles of the limbs; fasciculation is rare. Considerable help in differential diagnosis is obtained from electromyography, since in polyneuropathy and motor neurone disease the motor unit potentials, though reduced in number, are often normal or larger than normal, whereas in myopathy, owing to patchy degeneration of individual muscle fibres, they are broken-up and polyphasic or of short duration.

Involuntary Movements

Movements which do not occur in response to the will and are thus involuntary can be of great importance in neurological diagnosis.

The first type of movement commonly classified in this group, though not strictly involuntary, is the so-called **tic** or **habit spasm**. This term embraces many twitching or jerking movements which occur irregularly and involve particularly the muscles around the eyes, the remainder of the face and the shoulders. The subject is aware of the movement, and on close questioning it is evident that it is performed voluntarily as from it the patient obtains relief of tension which would otherwise become intolerable. This affliction is clearly related to anxiety. Though initially under the control of the will the movements become so habitual as to be almost involuntary.

The epileptic fit or convulsion, whether focal or general, clearly involves involuntary movement, but has been considered (*see* Chapter 6). A closely related phenomenon is **myoclonus**, a sudden shock-like muscular contraction which can involve a small group of muscles, several muscle groups or even the greater part of the voluntary musculature, either simultaneously or successively. Myoclonic jerks may occur while falling asleep and are not then pathological, though when they occur repeatedly throughout the night they become in all probability an epileptic manifestation and many affected individuals have occasional major seizures. A brief myoclonic jerk of the limbs is a common accompaniment of an attack of petit mal. Myoclonus in response to startle (say, by noise) is a feature of cerebral lipidosis, but in some individuals it is a benign but troublesome disorder unaccompanied by other evidence of disease (hyperekplexia, or the 'essential startle disease'), while myoclonic jerks also occur in several cerebral degenerative diseases such as subacute sclerosing panencephalitis and Creutzfeldt–Jakob disease (*see* pp. 289 and 241). When myoclonus involves many parts of the body and occurs repetitively or at times almost rhythmically, this clinical syndrome has been called paramyoclonus multiplex; sometimes the condition is familial and the patients show no other features of epilepsy (hereditary essential myoclonus). However there are some patients developing severe myoclonus in childhood who go on to develop major epilepsy and dementia with progressive degenerative changes in the cerebrum and cerebellum. This fatal condition is known as **progressive myoclonic epilepsy** (or Lafora body disease, since the affected nerves, especially in the dentate nuclei of the cerebellum, show cytoplasmic acidophilic inclusions consisting of abnormal polysaccharides, known as Lafora bodies). Occasionally in elderly persons a repetitive myoclonus of palate and throat muscles develops. This condition, **palatal myoclonus**, also interferes with respiration and speech which then occur in a series of staccato jerks. Though distressing, the condition, which is due to degenerative changes in the olivary nuclei and the central tegmental tract of the mid-brain, is not progressive.

Repetitive irregular twitching of one half of the face must not be confused with either habit spasm or myoclonus, as this condition, **hemifacial spasm** (*see* p. 366) is probably due to an irritative lesion of the facial nerve.

Tremor is a rapid, rhythmically repetitive movement which tends to be consistent in pattern, amplitude and frequency, and usually consists of intermittent contraction of a muscle group and then of its antagonists. It may be *static* (present at rest), *action* (present throughout the range of movement), or *intention* (accentuated towards the end of movement) in type. A *static tremor* of the head and hands, rapid in frequency and small in range, and not generally abolished by movement, constitutes the so-called *senile tremor* which is seen in some elderly persons. A more coarse rhythmical nodding of the head is seen in some patients with cerebellar disease. Senile tremor is closely related to, if not identical with, benign familial tremor (*see* below), but comes on later. The most typical form of static tremor, however, is the 'pill-rolling' movement of the fingers and hands, often with associated tremor of the arms and legs and sometimes the lips and tongue, which is seen in Parkinson's disease. Though accentuated by embarrassment and attention, this tremor is generally abolished by movement, though occasionally in Parkinsonism an action tremor is present as well. The principal lesion responsible for this tremor appears to be in the substantia nigra. Rarely, a similar tremor (often called, perhaps erroneously, 'striatal' tremor) is seen in other degenerative diseases of the nervous system (e.g. olivo-ponto-cerebellar degeneration).

Many different diseases can cause an *action tremor* which is readily observed in the actions of writing, of taking hold of an object, or in holding the arms outstretched. The fine tremor of the outstretched hands in thyrotoxic patients is usually easy to recognise, while much coarser movements occur in individuals with many toxic and metabolic disorders including delirium tremens (alcoholism), mercury poisoning and chronic liver disease; in the latter condition there is 'flapping' movement of the outstretched hands, like the beating of wings ('asterixis'). In Wilson's disease (hepatolenticular degeneration), this movement of the hands is seen if the liver disease is severe, but facial grimacing, rigidity and tremor of the limbs are also present as a result of the pathological changes which occur in the lenticular nuclei. In general paresis, tremor not only affects the hands but often also lips and tongue. So-called *benign familial* or *essential tremor* is also accentuated by movement. It is remarkable that this tremor, though sometimes gross, does not often interfere with fine movements such as threading a needle which would at first sight seem impossible. Curiously, this condition, which often develops first in early adult life but occasionally not until middle life, is often relieved considerably by alcohol. Some patients also develop tremor of the head, as in senile tremor. The most bizarre and gross form of tremor is often that of hysteria, and is produced for histrionic effect; it is coarse, irregular and variable and diminishes when the patient's attention is distracted.

Intention tremor is diagnostic of disease of the cerebellum or more often of its brain-stem connections. When unilateral it indicates a lesion on the affected side. Whereas the lesion, if severe, may also give rise to static tremor, this invariably becomes much worse towards the end of movement, which cannot therefore be accurately controlled, and activities such as writing and feeding are grossly disorganised. The patient may spill a cup whenever he brings it towards his mouth.

Many types of involuntary movement result from lesions of the extra-pyramidal system, in addition to the Parkinsonian tremor already described. The movements of **chorea**, for instance, though involuntary, may seem at first sight to be semipurposive and to show a high degree of organisation. Facial grimacing, raising of the eyebrows and rolling of the eyes, curling of the lips and protrusion and withdrawal of the tongue are common. In the limbs the movements are largely peripheral with intermittent 'wriggling' or 'squirming' of the fingers and toes. Often, too, there is striking limb hypotonia, and the reflexes may be 'pendular' in type in that a single blow on the quadriceps tendon causes the dependent leg to swing forwards and backwards several times like a pendulum. The limb movements cease during sleep. The exact situation of the causal pathological change is not known, though the caudate and lenticular nuclei have been implicated. The condition occurs in two main forms, namely rheumatic or Sydenham's chorea, and Huntington's chorea, a degenerative disease of late adult life, which is inherited as an autosomal dominant trait, and in which progressive dementia also occurs. A choreiform syndrome can also occur in chronic liver disease. Chorea, particularly the rheumatic form, is often accompanied by emotional lability and movement is often uncontrolled and ill-directed with undue expenditure of effort in performing simple actions. In other words, 'associated' movements are increased in chorea, in contrast to Parkinsonism in which they are diminished.

Athetosis involves the more proximal limb muscles to give movements which are writhing in character, slower in their execution and of greater amplitude than those of chorea. Often choreiform and athetotic movements occur together in the same patient, when the condition is called choreo-athetosis. Athetosis can be bilateral and congenital due to degenerative changes (*état marbré*) in the corpus striatum. It is sometimes a sequel of birth injury, occurring particularly in those children with cerebral palsy who initially have a flaccid diplegia, and it rarely follows kernicterus due to Rh-factor incompatibility. It may also occur unilaterally in children with infantile hemiplegia in whom the lesion responsible has extended to involve the basal ganglia.

Another type of involuntary movement with an ill-defined pathological basis in which the trunk muscles are predominantly involved, is **dystonia musculorum deformans** or **torsion spasm**. In this condition there is a striking increase in tone with irregular spasmodic contraction of the muscles of the neck, back and abdomen, and also of the limbs, giving bizarre alterations in posture. These postural changes are often constant over long periods with superimposed painful spasms and the affected muscles often show marked hypertrophy. The condition often begins in childhood with an abnormal posture of a limb (e.g. inversion of one foot) resulting in a gait which is so remarkable that it may at first be thought hysterical. It is unfortunately progressive, depending upon degenerative changes of unknown aetiology which occur in the basal ganglia and is sometimes inherited as a dominant trait. Many believe that **spasmodic torticollis**, a condition of frequent spasm of the sternomastoid and of other neck muscles, which results in a spasmodic turning of the head and neck to one side, is a fractional variety of dystonia; there is often a constant increase in the tone of neck and shoulder muscles, and in some cases the condition progresses to involve other parts of the body, although in others it remains localised. Spasmodic retrocollis (backward movement of the head) is similar. The inadequacy of present histopathological methods is revealed by the fact that the situation and nature of the lesion responsible for this condition too, are not yet clearly defined.

That biochemical rather than structural abnormalities often account for involuntary movements is evident from recent work in neuropharmacology. Drugs of the phenothiazine group, given over long periods, can cause irreversible **facial** or **'tardive' dyskinesias** (involuntary grimacing and protrusion of the tongue), while athetosis, foot-tapping and paddling movements are among the many side-effects of treatment of Parkinsonism with levodopa.

One final but characteristic form of involuntary movement which can result from extrapyramidal disease is **hemiballismus**, a wild, purposeless, 'flinging' movement of one arm and leg which may occur in elderly patients as a result of a lesion, generally an infarct, which involves particularly the subthalamic nucleus of Luys on the opposite side. The movements can be so violent and distressing that if untreated they result in death from exhaustion. The condition resembles in many respects a very violent form of unilateral chorea and similar but less severe movements occurring in the elderly, often unilaterally but occasionally bilaterally, are often called **senile chorea**.

Conclusions

Although the organisation of voluntary movement is complex and still holds many mysteries, a careful analysis, based upon anatomical and physiological knowledge, of the ways in which it is disorganised in any single case, whether through weakness or paralysis, ataxia or involuntary movements, can be of the greatest value in localising the situation of the lesion responsible; observed changes in muscle tone and in the reflexes may give invaluable aid. Once localised, reconsideration of the mode of evolution of the lesion will often indicate its nature.

References

Adams, R. D., 'Motor paralysis' and 'Tremor, chorea, athetosis, ataxia and other abnormalities of movement and posture', in *Harrison's Principles of Internal Medicine,* Ed. Isselbacher, K. J., *et al.,* 9th ed., Chapters 15 and 16 (New York, McGraw-Hill, 1980).

Adams, R. D. and Victor, M., *Principles of Neurology,* 2nd ed. (New York, McGraw-Hill, 1981).

Denny-Brown, D., *The Basal Ganglia and their Relation to Disorders of Movement* (London, Oxford University Press, 1962).

Ford, F. R., *Diseases of the Nervous System in Infancy, Childhood and Adolescence,* 6th ed. (Springfield, Ill., Thomas, 1973).

Gardner, E., *Fundamentals of Neurology,* 6th ed. (Philadelphia and London, Saunders, 1975).

Gordon, N., *Paediatric Neurology for the Clinician* (London, Spastics International Medical Publications. Heinemann, 1976).

Holmes, G., *An Introduction to Clinical Neurology,* revised by Matthews, W. B., 3rd ed. (Edinburgh, Livingstone, 1968).

Martin, J. P., *The Basal Ganglia and Posture* (London, Pitman Books, 1967).

Matthews, W. B., *Practical Neurology,* 3rd ed. (Oxford, Blackwell, 1975).

Patton, H. D., Sundsten, J. W., Crill, W. E. and Swanson, P. D., *Introduction to Basic Neurology* (Philadelphia, W. B. Saunders, 1976).

Schadé, J. P. and Ford, D. H., *Basic Neurology,* 2nd ed. (Amsterdam, Elsevier, 1973).

Spillane, J. D., *An Atlas of Clinical Neurology,* 2nd ed. (London, Oxford University Press, 1975).

Walton, J. N., *Brain's Diseases of the Nervous System,* 8th ed. (London, Oxford University Press, 1977).

Wartenberg, R., *The Examination of the Reflexes* (Chicago, Year Book Publishers, 1945).

10 The Sensory System

The examination of sensory function and the interpretation of abnormalities in sensory perception present considerable difficulties, as in no part of the neurological examination is the patient's co-operation more important. Objective assessment of the degree and extent of sensory impairment can thus be difficult and it is often necessary to make considerable allowance for the patient's state of co-operation and intellectual capacity. Areas of cutaneous sensory impairment, particularly to light touch and pinprick, subsequently shown to be spurious, are not uncommonly elicited even by the most skilled observers. Few parts of the clinical examination are as liable to error. In fact, sensory examination is sometimes easier in children and in adults of comparatively low intellect, as it is virtually impossible to achieve uniformity of sensory stimulation in clinical practice. Intelligent patients often perceive and remark upon relatively slight variations which prove in the end to be of no pathological significance, but which nevertheless give some confusion during the course of the examination. Furthermore, individuals vary considerably in their reaction to sensory stimuli, a sensation which appears acutely painful to one being well tolerated by another. And whereas it is conventional to examine sensory function and to record the results of this examination independently of those obtained on examining the motor system, motor and sensory functions are intimately connected, the one being largely dependent upon the other. Thus motor activity is grossly impaired if there is a defect in proprioception: a limb from which no afferent stimuli are received (deafferentation) is virtually immobile even though its motor pathways are intact. A serious disorder of movement can therefore be due entirely to a defect of sensation in the affected part.

The Anatomical and Physiological Organisation of Sensation

The sensory apparatus consists first of a series of sensory receptors in the skin and other organs, secondly of the first sensory neurone, whose cells lie in the posterior root ganglia, and thirdly of secondary sensory neurones which conduct impulses through the spinal cord and brain stem to the thalamus and thence, sometimes, to the cerebral cortex. Cells in the substantia gelatinosa of the spinal cord, and the internuncial neurones which arise from them, probably play a major rôle in modulating sensory input. Visceral sensation, which is conveyed initially alongside fibres of the autonomic nervous system, enters the spinal cord along with somatic sensory impulses and is conveyed centrally in a similar manner.

Sensory receptors can be divided into **exteroceptors** which are largely situated in the skin and which record information about the external environment of the body, and **proprioceptors** which are situated in muscles, tendons, joints and viscera and which inform us of the position and condition of these deeper structures. Many **exteroceptors** consist of no more than a network of fine nerve endings terminating in the skin, but there are also more specialised receptors such as the basket-like nerve endings which surround hair follicles, as well as Merkel's disks and Meissner's corpuscles which are thought to record touch sensation, and Krause's bulbs and Ruffini's corpuscles which appear to respond to thermal stimuli. Indeed it was once believed that specific sensory receptors were necessary to record each form of sensation, but recent work on the cornea has shown that touch, pain and thermal sensations can all be appreciated through undifferentiated nerve endings. Each so-called 'sensory spot' on the skin may receive filaments from several branches of a nerve and it is probably the pattern of stimulation and the frequency of discharge in these fibres which determines the nature of the sensation perceived, rather than any specificity of the nerve endings themselves. It is, however, true that certain cutaneous 'spots' are particularly sensitive to pain, and others to cold or warmth. This is why there is considerable variation in the sensation evoked by uniform stimuli in contiguous skin areas. Thus a touch on a cold spot will feel cold, or a pin-prick on a pain spot may be more painful than one applied with similar force nearby. Fortunately these fine distinctions are of little significance in clinical neurology, since sensory abnormalities, to be of practical importance, must generally be relatively crude.

The **proprioceptive receptors** are the muscle spindles and the Golgi–Mazzoni tendon organs which respond to muscle tension or stretch, and the Pacinian corpuscles which are probably responsive to pressure. Comparatively few proprioceptive stimuli reach consciousness; many are concerned with reflex activity mediated through the spinal cord or cerebellum, through which posture and movement are controlled.

The Simpler Sensory Modalities

While all forms of sensory experience are interrelated, several clearly definable forms of somatic sensation can be recognised whose integrity is customarily assessed during a neurological examination. The first of these is **touch**, commonly tested with a light application to the skin of a pledget of cotton wool. Touch may be assessed quantitatively by using von Frey hairs, so graduated that differing pressures are needed to bend them. The threshold for touch appreciation varies considerably on different parts of the body surface, depending upon such variables as the thickness of the epidermis and the number of hair follicles present. **Pain** sensation is generally assessed by pin-prick, which can also be of graduated severity if an algesiometer is used. The patient must be asked to assess the painful quality of this stimulus and not the sensations of pressure or touch which may be simultaneously evoked. Squeezing of the tendo Achilles or of other deep tendons will determine whether appreciation of **deep pressure** is intact, but this sensation can also be painful. **Thermal sensation** is generally tested by applying metal test-tubes to the skin, one filled with ice, the other with water at 45°C. Again the patient is told that it is the feeling of heat or cold he is being asked to note and not the sensation of touch or pressure. The assessment of **position and joint sense** is generally carried out by moving the terminal phalanx of the forefinger or the great toe in a vertical plane and by asking the patient, whose eyes are closed, to describe the direction of movement each time the digit is moved. After making initial movements of considerable amplitude it must then be decided whether the patient can appreciate movements through a very small range (about 1 mm). Another test of position and joint sense is to ask the patient, with his eyes closed, to point towards a part of his body (such as the other forefinger), when the position of the part in space has been altered by the examiner. **Vibration sense**, as tested with a tuning fork of 128-frequency applied to bony prominences, is not a physiological sensation, being compounded of both touch and pressure, but nevertheless the ability to perceive this form of somatic sensibility, more complex in nature, is commonly tested in the neurological examination. And **tactile discrimination** is assessed by recording the threshold distance at which the two blunt points of a compass, simultaneously applied, are independently perceived. The normal threshold for two-point discrimination on the tip of the tongue is 1 mm, on the tips of the fingers 2–3 mm, on the palm of the hand or sole of the foot 1.5–3 cm, and in the centre of the back 6–7 cm. The appreciation of **texture**, **weight**, **size** and **shape** of objects can also be assessed crudely by asking the patient, with his eyes closed, to identify objects placed in the hand, while tactile localisation is tested by asking him to identify on a diagram or model, or on the examiner, the point or points on his body which had been stimulated. He may also be asked to identify figures or letters traced with a blunt point on his skin. There is considerable individual variation in the ability to perceive and interpret these more complex sensations, but retention of them on one side of the body and their absence on the other is always of pathological significance.

The Sensory Pathways

The cells of the first sensory neurone are situated in the posterior root ganglia and are bipolar in type, having peripheral axons which convey afferent impulses from the sensory receptors, and central axons which enter the spinal cord in the posterior nerve roots. Sensory fibres in the **peripheral nerves** vary in diameter and in their rate of conduction; the large, heavily-myelinated, rapidly-conducting *A* fibres are primarily concerned with the conduction of impulses subserving touch, pressure and proprioceptive sensation, but some undoubtedly transmit painful and thermal sensations. The most slowly-conducting unmyelinated *C* fibres seem capable of carrying touch, temperature, and pain sensation so that there is no exact relationship between the size and myelination of sensory axons on the one hand and their function on the other. Since some peripheral nerve disorders, and especially peripheral neuropathy, may have a selective effect upon fibres of one particular size or degree of myelination, there are certain cases in which the appreciation of painful stimulation is more severely affected than that of touch or vice versa. And whereas cutaneous and pressure sensations travel in pure sensory (cutaneous) and later in mixed sensory and motor nerves, proprioceptive stimuli, particularly from the muscle spindles, travel centrally first of all in motor nerves.

As the central axons of the first sensory neurone enter the spinal cord, some regrouping of these fibres occurs, according to their function. Initially most enter the posterior column, lying just medially to the posterior horn of grey matter. At this point internuncial neurones arising from cells in the substantia gelatinosa exert a modifying or 'gating' influence (*see* p. 81), especially upon painful sensations. Fibres concerned with proprioception, position and joint sense, vibration sense and tactile discrimination, and some conveying touch, turn immediately upwards in the **posterior columns** and travel to the nuclei of Goll and Burdach in the medulla. Since entering fibres continually displace medially those which entered the cord at a lower level, it follows that fibres from the lower limbs lie medially in the posterior column (the fasciculus gracilis or column of Goll), while those from the upper limbs lie more laterally (the fasciculus cuneatus or column of Burdach) (Fig. 15 (*a*)).

A second group of entering fibres, concerned with the appreciation of touch, also enters the lateral part of the posterior column where they ascend for several segments, then entering the posterior horn of grey matter to synapse with cells in this area. The axons of these cells then cross the midline close to the central canal to join the **ventral spinothalamic tract**. Fibres subserving pain and temperature sensation run a similar course, but only ascend in the posterior column for a few segments before crossing the midline to end in the more **lateral portion of the spinothalamic tract** in the opposite lateral column of the cord (Fig. 15(*b*)). As in the posterior columns, there is some lamination of fibres in the spinothalamic tracts, those from the lower limbs lying nearest the cord surface and those from the upper limbs being situated more centrally. This probably explains why a lesion causing spinal cord compression may impair pain sensation first in the lower limbs; the sensory 'level' then ascends steadily but finally

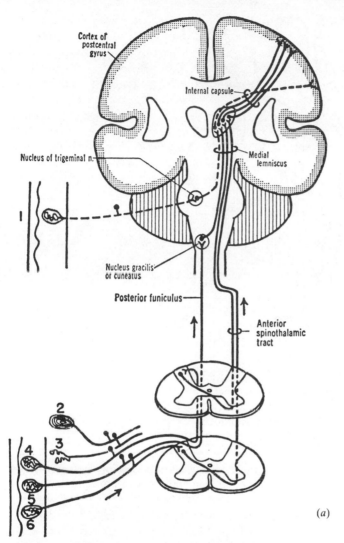

Fig. 15. A diagram of the principal pathways of the sensory system. (*a*) The pathways followed by impulses subserving touch, tactile discrimination, position and joint sense and related sensations. 1, 4, 5 and 6 represent Meissner's corpuscles; the pathways from 2 (Pacinian corpuscle) and 3 (joint receptor) are similar to those followed by impulses from 5.

(From *The Fundamentals of Neurology*, by E. Gardner, 5th edition, Saunders, Philadelphia and London, 1968.)

becomes arrested on the trunk at the level of a dermatome corresponding to a cord segment several segments below the actual point of compression; presumably fibres situated nearest to the surface of the cord are the first to be affected by pressure.

When the sensory fibres of the spinal cord reach the medulla oblongata,

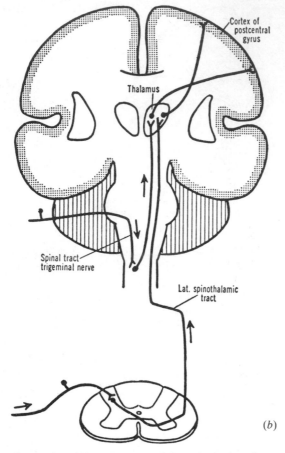

Fig. 15 (contd.) A diagram of the principal pathways of the sensory system. (*b*) The pathways followed by impulses subserving pain and temperature sensation.
(From *The Fundamentals of Neurology* by E. Gardner, 5th edition, Saunders, Philadelphia and London, 1968.)

the spinothalamic fibres enter it laterally and pass upwards through the pons and mid-brain to the thalamus. The fibres of the posterior columns, however, end in synapses in the nuclei of Goll (nucleus gracilis) and Burdach (nucleus cuneatus). From the cells of these nuclei new axons arise which immediately cross the midline and then travel upwards as the **medial fillet** or **lemniscus,** again to enter the thalamus.

The pathway followed by sensory impulses from the face deserves special mention. The fibres of the trigeminal nerve which carry touch and tactile discrimination enter the main trigeminal nucleus and then, in the **quintothalamic tract**, cross the midline to join the medial fillet. Those subserving pain and thermal sensation enter the pons but then travel downwards in the **descending root of the trigeminal nerve** to end in a nuclear mass which extends downwards as far as the second cervical segment of the cord; then they, too, forming another part of the quintothalamic tract, cross the midline and travel upwards in the spinothalamic tract. 'Representation' of the parts of the face in the descending root is inverted; thus a lesion of its lower end in the upper cervical cord gives loss of pain and temperature sensation only, but not of touch, over the area supplied by the ophthalmic division on the same side of the face. It should also be noted that proprioceptive stimuli from the face travel centrally in the facial nerve, so that sense of position in the facial muscles (a difficult faculty to test) is not abolished by a lesion of the trigeminus.

Thus all sensory pathways which ascend as far as the brain stem terminate in the thalamus. Throughout their course in the spinal cord and brain stem many of these fibres give off collaterals or synapse with internuncial neurones. These connexions complete the sensory side of the arcs concerned with those spinal and brain-stem reflexes which are necessary for the maintenance of posture and other functions. There are, for instance, many sensory fibres, some of which synapse in Clarke's columns of the posterior horn of grey matter, which ascend the spinal cord in the dorsal and vertral spinocerebellar tracts and which are concerned with supplying information through which the cerebellum exerts control over posture and movement. The **thalamus** is, however, the first important sensory relay station. The sensory relay nuclei which are concerned with somatic and visceral sensation are the nucleus ventralis posterolateralis (VPL), which receives afferent stimuli from the trunk and limbs, and the ventralis posteromedialis (VPM), which is similarly concerned with input from the face. Both nuclei send thalamocortical neuronal projections to the somatosensory and parietal association areas of the cortex and receive corticothalamic projections from the same areas. The dorsomedial nucleus (DM), which projects to the prefrontal cortex, appears to have a rôle relating to the affective response to sensory input, especially of pain. The lateral and medial geniculate bodies are concerned respectively with vision and audition, the ventralis lateralis (VL) with cerebellar and extrapyramidal function, the ventralis anterior (VA) with activity of the basal ganglia, and the nucleus anterior (A) with hypothalamic function.

The **primary somatosensory area of the cerebral cortex** is concerned with the appreciation of most of those stimuli which enter consciousness. The integrity of the sensory cortex is particularly important if we are to recognise form, texture, size, weight and consistency of objects, or changes in position of parts of the body. It is also essential for the accurate localisation and recognition of the nature of stimuli applied to the body, for discrimination between two simultaneously applied stimuli, and even more for the ability to relate sensory experiences to others experienced previously, or to sense data perceived through the special senses. Clearly, numerous association pathways are concerned in the interpretation and recognition of these more complex sensory experiences, which may nevertheless be grossly deranged if there is a lesion of the primary sensory cortex, an important cell-station in all sensory association mechanisms. As with the motor cortex, stimulation experiments have revealed that specific portions of the postcentral gyrus are concerned with the appreciation of sensations from particular areas of the opposite side of the body. 'Representation' in the sensory cortex corresponds topographically with that in the motor area; thus a lesion of the lower end of the postcentral gyrus will impair sensory perception in the contralateral face and hand, while a lesion on the superior and medial aspects of the hemisphere will result in a failure to appreciate 'cortical' forms of sensation in the opposite leg.

However, cortical or subcortical lesions, even if they divide all thalamocortical fibres, do not destroy completely the ability to perceive sensory experiences in the opposite half of the body. In the presence of such a lesion, sensitivity to pain and temperature is affected comparatively little, while crude touch is still felt, though finer forms of sensory experience are greatly impaired. Hence it is that the cruder varieties of sensation can be recorded in consciousness at a thalamic level.

Some Common Abnormalities of Sensation

In considering the disorders of sensation commonly noted in clinical neurology, it is first essential to understand clearly the meaning of several terms often utilised to describe disorders of sensation. The word **numbness** can have many meanings; when a patient says that a part of the body is numb he may mean that sensation in the part is abnormal, but sometimes the term is used to denote weakness or clumsiness. Hence careful enquiry is needed in order to determine the significance of this symptom. Many other sensory abnormalities, occurring apparently spontaneously, can be found in patients with neurological disease. Of these, one of the commonest is **pain**, which has been discussed fully in Chapter 4. Pain may result from disease of any pain-sensitive structure; if, for instance, it is due to irritation of a sensory nerve or root, the distribution of the pain will be in the cutaneous area supplied by the nerve or root concerned. Pain can alternatively be felt in the organ or organs which are diseased, while if arising in a viscus or in a muscle, it can be referred to an area of skin which sometimes overlies the viscus but may be anatomically remote. Referred pain seems to be due to a spread of impulses to contiguous sensory neurones within the cord (*see* p. 82). Spontaneous pain in the limbs or trunk can result from thalamic lesions, when it has a peculiarly unpleasant burning character, often with additional 'grinding' or 'tearing' qualities. This so-called **thalamic pain** is most often felt in the face, around one angle of the mouth and in the hand and foot on the affected side. A closely-related sensation of continuous burning, of pricking, of warmth or even cold, may result from a spinothalamic tract lesion, but tends to be more diffusely felt in the area of altered cutaneous sensation. Disordered sensations of this type, occurring spontaneously, are called **dysaesthesiae**. In addition, patients who have lesions of the spinothalamic tract often observe that they cannot feel pain or temperature in the affected part. They have perhaps injured or burned a limb without discomfort or may admit that they are unable to assess the temperature of bath water.

Other abnormal sensations which the patient may feel are called **paraesthesiae**. These include feelings of tingling, pins and needles, of swelling of a limb, sensations suggesting that tight strings or bands are tied around a part of the body, or as if water were trickling over the skin. These sensory experiences result from disordered function in the pathways conducting the finer and discriminative aspects of sensibility. Thus tingling or pins and needles can result from ischaemia of peripheral nerves, from polyneuropathy, from transient ischaemia of the sensory cortex, or from sensory Jacksonian epilepsy due to a cortical lesion. Similar symptoms are described by patients with lesions of the posterior columns of the cord and it is usually in such individuals that the 'tight, constricting band' or the 'trickling' type of sensation is felt. Often the affected part feels swollen, although inspection shows that this is not the case, or the patient may feel, for instance, as if the limb is encased in a firm glove or plaster cast. If there is a lesion of the posterior columns in the cervical region, sudden flexion or extension of the neck may give an 'electric shock' sensation which travels rapidly down the trunk and sometimes into the hands and feet; this sign (Lhermitte's sign) is most often due to multiple sclerosis or cervical spondylotic myelopathy. Similarly, tapping over the trunk of an ischaemic nerve (as in patients with median nerve compression in the carpal tunnel) or over a sensory nerve which has been injured in some other way, often gives paraesthesiae which shoot along the cutaneous distribution of the nerve concerned. A comparable sign produced by tapping a nerve in which regeneration is occuring is known as Tinel's sign.

As well as experiencing paraesthesiae, patients with dysfunction of the spinal posterior columns or of the sensory cortex often find that the affected part has become clumsy or even useless. If a hand is affected, they may be unable to use it except under direct vision and cannot recognise objects felt in a pocket or handbag, unless they can be taken out and examined visually. Fine movements such as fastening buttons or threading needles are grossly impaired. If both lower limbs are affected the patient is unsteady; he feels as if he were walking on cotton wool, and is worse in the dark. When the eyes are covered while washing the face, he tends to fall forwards into the washbasin.

Turning to the sensory abnormalities discovered on physical examination, **anaesthesia** is generally used to describe a cutaneous area in which the sensation of touch is totally lost, while **hypaesthesia** implies impaired touch appreciation. Similarly, **analgesia** is absence of and **hypalgesia** diminution of the appreciation of painful sensations. When thermal sensations cannot be appreciated the term **thermoanaesthesia** is sometimes utilised, but this is rarely found unless hypalgesia is also present. **Hyperalgesia** is allegedly an increased sensitivity to painful stimuli and **hyperaesthesia** a heightened perception of touch. In fact, however, careful examination will usually show that in the one case the pain threshold, and in the other that for touch, is actually raised above normal, owing to a disorder of the pain or touch pathways. The apparent over-reaction is due to an abnormal and often unpleasant additional quality added to the primary sensation which is in itself impaired; for this reason the term **hyperpathia** (Head's protopathic pain) is preferred to hyperalgesia which is semantically incorrect.

Romberg's sign is an important sign of impaired position and joint sense in the lower limbs. The preservation of the upright position depends upon labyrinthine, cerebellar and visual postural reflexes as well as upon those reflexes whose afferent pathway is from the lower limb proprioceptors. So long as the eyes are open, even if the conduction of proprioceptive stimuli from the lower limbs is grossly impaired, the patient can maintain his position, but once the eyes are closed he will sway or fall. Cerebellar or labyrinthine disease can also cause excessive swaying, but severe instability and a tendency to fall results only from severe impairment of position and joint sense in the lower limbs. The same patient will show **sensory ataxia** when he walks; being unsure of the position of his feet in relation to the ground, he lifts them unusually high and then bangs them down heavily (the steppage gait). Owing to loss of visual control of posture, he is much more unsteady in the dark.

Ataxia of sensory type is also found in the upper limbs if affected by similar lesions. The hands are clumsy, and fine movements are impossible, particularly when the hands are out of sight (e.g. tying a necktie). If the affected arm is held outstretched with the eyes closed, it 'wanders' in space, upwards or sideways or indeed in any direction, unlike the downward drift of the limb showing motor weakness from pyramidal tract disease. There are also purposeless movements of the outstretched fingers, of which the patient is unaware, and these may have a 'writhing' character **(pseudoathetosis).**

Abnormalities of the finer and discriminative aspects of sensibility are more difficult to assess, although in a patient with a lesion of the sensory cortex, the threshold for two-point discrimination is much greater on the abnormal than on the normal side, and there may be total inability to recognise figures or letters drawn on the skin. Sensory stimuli are also incorrectly localised. Lesions of the parietal lobe of less severity may be demonstrated by the phenomenon of **sensory inattention**. The patient is well able to appreciate stimuli applied independently to the two sides of the body, but when two similar stimuli are applied simultaneously to homologous points on the skin of the two sides, one is ignored, a finding which implies dysfunction of a centralateral sensory association area of the cerebral cortex. It is well-known that after amputation of a limb or of another member, it takes time, in a sense, for the brain to realise that the limb is no longer there, and there is often a clear-cut 'phantom' sensation as if the amputated part were still present and were able to move; sometimes the phantom is painful. A phantom limb can be abolished by a lesion of the contralateral sensory cortex.

Another defect observed in some patients with lesions of the arm area of the opposite sensory cortex is an inability to appreciate the form and texture of objects placed in the hand. Correctly this abnormality is entitled **stereoanaesthesia,** but the term **astereognosis** is more often used. Strictly speaking the latter term should be reserved for a failure to recognise the nature of objects when the primary sensory modalities are intact. This is an agnosic defect, due to a disorder of sensory association and akin to the other more complex disorders of parietal lobe function which were described in Chapter 5 (p. 103).

The Clinical Significance of Sensory Abnormalities

In localising the lesion causing an abnormality of sensation, it must be asked whether the sensory changes found could be due to a lesion of one or several peripheral nerves, to one of sensory roots, of the spinal cord, of the brain stem, of the thalamus, or of the sensory cortex.

Identification of the sensory abnormalities which result from **peripheral nerve lesions** or from lesions of the brachial and lumbosacral plexuses can only stem from a knowledge of the cutaneous distribution of the various peripheral nerves and of the components of the plexuses (Fig. 16). If a nerve is divided, and it is one with an extensive cutaneous distribution, there is a central area of sensory loss to all forms of sensation and a surrounding zone in which tactile loss is more extensive than that for pain and temperature sensation. There is considerable overlap in the cutaneous supply of individual peripheral nerves so that section of a small cutaneous nerve may produce no definable sensory abnormality. This fact is even more true of the dermatomes innervated by the individual **sensory roots**; these have a strictly segmental distribution (Fig. 17) but if a single root is divided it may be impossible to distinguish any area of sensory loss, in view of the overlap in the supply of neighbouring roots. When more than one root is interrupted, however, there is generally some cutaneous sensory loss and its distribution clearly indicates the roots involved. A working knowledge of the dermatome distribution of the individual sensory roots is essential in clinical neurology. With this information it is relatively easy to distinguish on clinical grounds the sensory loss resulting from a root lesion from that due to a peripheral nerve lesion. Associated signs of a lower motor neurone lesion can be of great value in confirming the distinction.

In clinical practice, for instance, the sensory loss due to an ulnar nerve lesion affects mainly the little finger and the ulnar half of the ring finger,

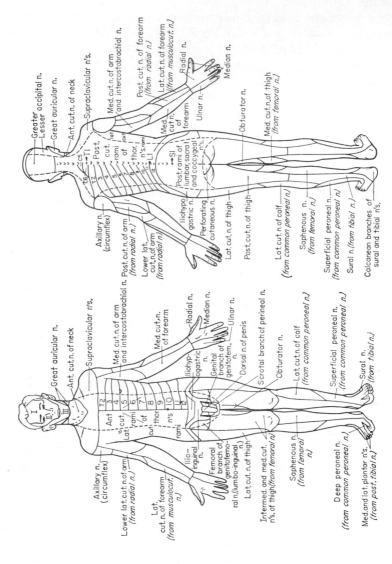

Fig. 16. The cutaneous fields of peripheral nerves.

(From *Peripheral Nerve Injuries,* by W. Haymaker and B. Woodhall. Saunders, Philadelphia and London, 1945.)

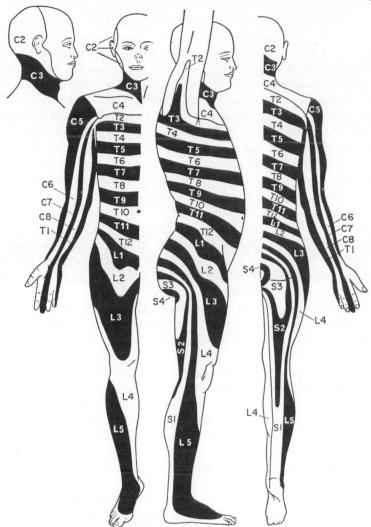

Fig. 17. A diagram of the distribution of the sensory spinal roots on the surface of the body.

(From *Introduction to Clinical Neurology*, by G Holmes, Livingstone, Edinburgh, 1946.)

while that due to a disorder of the median nerve involves chiefly the thumb, the first two fingers and the radial half of the ring finger. An ulnar nerve lesion also gives wasting of most of the small hand muscles, while median nerve damage affects only those in the lateral part of the thenar eminence. In contradistinction, compression of the inner cord of the brachial plexus, which can also give wasting and weakness of small hand muscles, gives sensory impairment in the medial aspect of the arm and forearm and only occasionally in the little finger.

When multiple peripheral nerves are symmetrically involved, as in **polyneuropathy**, it is the longest sensory fibres which tend to be most severely affected. Hence sensory impairment, which usually involves all forms of sensation, but may affect one more severely than the others, is most severe in the periphery of the limbs. Although this type of sensory loss is often described as of 'glove and stocking' distribution, the borderline between normal and abnormal areas of sensory perception is not usually abrupt, but there is a gradual transition between the two. When there is widespread disease of posterior spinal roots (as in the Guillain–Barré syndrome) there is occasionally ascending sensory loss which eventually involves the entire trunk and all four limbs, but the disease can cease to progress at any stage. The condition may mimic a transverse lesion of the spinal cord, as motor paralysis is often severe. Indeed in many cases motor weakness predominates and sensory impairment is slight or absent. A rare variety of hereditary sensory neuropathy exists in which pain fibres are affected almost exclusively and there is peripheral insensitivity to pain, often giving perforating ulcers of the feet and extensive destruction of bones and joints (Morvan's syndrome).

Sensory abnormalities resulting from **spinal cord disease** depend upon which sensory pathways are principally affected. Total transection of the cord gives total loss of all forms of sensation below the dermatome level on the trunk corresponding to the segment at which the cord transection took place. Often there is a zone of 'hyperaesthesia' (*see* p. 214) in the skin area supplied by the segment immediately above the lesion. In hemisection of the spinal cord **(the Brown–Séquard syndrome)** there is loss of tactile discrimination, impaired touch perception and loss of position and joint sense on the same side of the body as that on which the cord has been divided, and these sensory faculties are impaired on the trunk up to the dermatome of the cord segment at which the lesion is present. There are also signs of pyramidal tract dysfunction on the same side. On the opposite side of the body there is loss of pain and temperature sensation, but the sensory level for these modalities is a few segments lower, since pain fibres ascend in the posterior horn for a few segments before crossing to join the contralateral spinothalamic tract. A Brown–Séquard syndrome can result from trauma or from asymmetrical cord compression and is occasionally the initial manifestation of multiple sclerosis.

The principal lesion of **tabes dorsalis** is in the root entry zone of the posterior roots; there is ascending degeneration of the posterior columns and to a lesser extent of the spinothalamic tracts. Hence patients with this disease have severe sensory ataxia and there is often pain loss, and impairment of deep pressure sensation, over the bridge of the nose, centre of sternum, perineum and Achilles tendons, while position and joint sense and vibration sense are greatly impaired in the lower limbs. The tendon reflexes are lost owing to a break on the sensory side of the reflex arc. Similar impairment of lower limb tendon reflexes may be seen in **subacute**

combined degeneration of the cord, in which disease sensory ataxia is also usual and vibration and position sense are commonly lost in the lower limbs; signs of pyramidal tract disease are also present as a rule. The cavity of **syringomyelia** usually damages the central grey matter of the cervical spinal cord; hence decussating pain and temperature fibres are interrupted, resulting in dissociated anaesthesia, i.e. loss of pain and temperature sensation but preservation of touch and of position and joint sense. Commonly, but not invariably, this sensory loss is unilateral, affecting the whole of one upper limb and shoulder and ending on the trunk at the mid-line and with a sharp lower level like the edge of a cape. As the cavity generally extends into the anterior horns, there is loss of tendon reflexes and muscular atrophy in the affected upper limb or limbs, while compression of the pyramidal tracts gives spastic weakness of the legs. The sensory changes of **multiple sclerosis** are usually due to lesions of the posterior columns, giving impaired tactile discrimination, vibration sense and sense of position, sometimes in one arm, in both lower limbs, or even in all four limbs. Occasionally, however, a plaque of demyelination affects one trigeminal nucleus to give facial hemianaesthesia and sometimes, though rarely, a unilateral lesion of the cord involves the spinothalamic tract and gives loss of pain and temperature sensation in one lower limb.

Lesions of the brain stem give sensory abnormalities which can easily be interpreted anatomically. Dissociated sensory loss in the face can result from syringobulbia, due to involvement of the descending root of the trigeminus, while lesions of the pons and medulla can give unilateral facial sensory loss (due to a lesion of the trigeminal nucleus) with hemianaesthesia and/or hemianalgesia of the trunk and limbs on the opposite side due to involvement of ascending sensory tracts. A lesion of the upper pons or mid-brain, however, can give a complete contralateral hemianaesthesia. More often such unilateral sensory loss is dissociated, involving only pain and temperature sensation, owing to selective involvement of the spinothalamic tract.

Patchy contralateral hemianaesthesia and hemianalgesia can also be due to a **thalamic lesion** and there is often in addition spontaneous pain of a peculiarly unpleasant and disturbing nature on the partially anaesthetic side. Fortunately this **thalamic syndrome**, which usually results from cerebral infarction, is rare. The pain usually affects the face, arm and foot.

Lesions of the **sensory cortex**, if irritative in type, give sensory Jacksonian epilepsy, often in the form of spreading paraesthesiae whose 'march' corresponds closely to the anatomical 'representation' of the parts of the body in the postcentral gyrus. This symptom is easy to confuse with the paraesthesiae which often occur during the aura of migraine, or during transient cerebral ischaemic attacks. When there is destruction of a part of the gyrus, then in the corresponding part of the opposite half of the body there is no impairment of pain sensibility and comparatively little of touch, but the appreciation of position, of tactile discrimination and localisation and of form and texture is profoundly impaired. Figures written upon the skin cannot be recognised, and the threshold for two-point discrimination is raised. In a less severe cortical lesion, there may simply be tactile inattention on the affected side. Defects of recognition and interpretation of sense data found in parietal lobe lesions were discussed in Chapter 5.

One final diagnosis which must be considered as a possible cause of sensory abnormalities found on clinical examination is **hysteria**. In a suggestible patient it is only too easy to discover areas of spurious sensory loss. A total hemianaesthesia affecting all modalities of sensation, even including vibration sense over one half of the skull or sternum, is a common hysterical manifestation, as is anaesthesia of the palate or of the limbs in 'glove and stocking' distribution. Alternatively such sensory loss may be found in one limb only, particularly after minor injury in a compensation setting, when there is usually associated hysterical weakness and the sensory impairment ends at the level of a joint (e.g. the elbow, shoulder, knee or hip). In such cases in contradistinction to polyneuropathy, there is an abrupt line of demarcation between the area of complete sensory loss and that where all sensation is normal. In a patient with hysterical sensory loss it may be possible to 'find' (with suggestion) an area within the anaesthetic region (impossible to explain on an anatomical basis) where pin-prick is felt acutely. Another useful pointer is that the patient, though claiming that all forms of sensation are impaired in the affected part, is yet able to localise accurately in space one finger or toe, say, with his eyes closed, indicating that the sense of position is in fact well preserved.

Sensory examination is a technique which can only be learned by experience and which even so is full of pitfalls, particularly with an anxious and suggestible patient. Nevertheless consistent and clear-cut sensory abnormalities are of great value in localising accurately a lesion within the nervous system, while the precise nature of the changes may give invaluable aid in determining its character.

References

Adams, R. D. and Victor, M., *Principles of Neurology*, 2nd ed. (New York, McGraw-Hill, 1981).

Bickerstaff, E. R., *Neurological Examination in Clinical Practice*, 4th ed. (Oxford, Blackwell, 1980).

Gardner, E., *Fundamentals of Neurology*, 6th ed. (Philadelphia and London, Saunders, 1975).

Haymaker, W. and Woodhall, B., *Peripheral Nerve Injuries*, 2nd ed. (Philadelphia and London, Saunders, 1953).

Head, H., *Studies in Neurology* (London, Oxford University Press, 1920).

Holmes, G., *Introduction to Clinical Neurology*, 3rd ed., revised by W. B. Matthews (Edinburgh, Livingstone, 1968).

Lance, J. W. and McLeod, J. G., *A Physiological Approach to Clinical Neurology*, 3rd ed. (London, Butterworths, 1981).

Matthews, W. B., *Practical Neurology*, 3rd ed. (Oxford, Blackwell, 1975).

Mayo Clinic, Section of Neurology, *Clinical Examinations in Neurology*, 5th ed. (New York, Saunders, 1981).

Medical Research Council, *Aids to the Examination of the Peripheral Nervous System* (London, HMSO, 1976).

Patton, H. D., Sundsten, J. W., Crill, W. E. and Swanson, P. D. *Introduction to Basic Neurology* (Philadelphia, W. B. Saunders, 1976).

Sunderland, S., *Nerves and Nerve Injuries* (Edinburgh, Livingstone, 1968).

11 The Autonomic Nervous System

The autonomic nervous system is largely concerned with the control of visceral activity; its influences are widespread, affecting the cardiac rhythm and output, respiration, blood-vessel tone and the behaviour of the hollow viscera of the alimentary and urogenital systems, as well as the secretion of the ducted and ductless glands. It is probably as well that these activities are in a sense automatic and reflexly controlled, and that they are but little influenced by the will, for many of them are too vital to allow of any interference from the capricious behaviour of the mind. The combined activities of the autonomic nerves and of the endocrine glands are concerned in maintaining the constant internal thermal and biochemical environment of the body, a function which Cannon entitled homeostasis. Although many of the visceral functions of the autonomic nervous system and particularly its control of the heart, lungs and abdominal viscera are beyond the scope of this volume, there are many ways in which disease of the central or peripheral nervous system can affect autonomic activity, and accurate interpretation of the abnormalities so produced may be invaluable in diagnosis. Owing to the complex arrangement of the autonomic pathways it is easy to overlook some of the general principles upon which interpretation of autonomic disorders depends. However, a basic knowledge of the anatomy and pathophysiology of these nerves is necessary for these principles to be rationally applied.

Anatomy and Physiology

The autonomic nervous system can be divided into two principal components, namely the **sympathetic** and the **parasympathetic** systems (Fig. 18). These two systems are in a sense antagonistic in their effects for where one excites the other inhibits. Thus activity of the sympathetic system produces dilatation of the pupil and slight protrusion of the eye, increased cardiac output with tachycardia, dilatation of the bronchioles, vasoconstriction of skin vessels but dilatation of the coronary and intramuscular arteries, sweating, inhibition of intestinal movement, and probably closure of vesical and rectal sphincters, and erection of hairs (the pilomotor effect) on the skin. In other words the animal is prepared for action in response to an

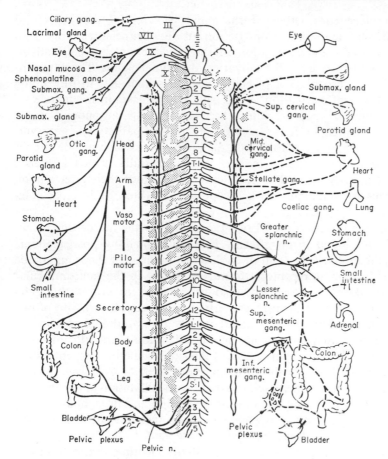

Fig. 18. A diagram of the spinal cord and brain stem showing thoracolumbar or sympathetic nerves and ganglia on the right, and craniosacral or parasympathetic nerves and ganglia on the left. The dual autonomic supply of the viscera is demonstrated.

(By courtesy of the late Dr Eaton and W. B. Saunders Co.)

emergency. Most sympathetic fibres are adrenergic, i.e. they produce their effects upon smooth muscle or other tissues by secreting noradrenaline at their nerve-endings, and their effects can be reproduced by an increase in the amount of circulating adrenaline or noradrenaline in the blood. Some few sympathetic fibres, however, and particularly those which innervate the sweat glands (sudomotor fibres) are cholinergic, i.e. they produce their effects by secreting acetylcholine at the effector organ. In skeletal muscle, there are adrenergic fibres which cause constriction of intramuscular blood vessels and cholinergic fibres which cause dilatation. Parasympathetic fibres are, on the contrary, mainly cholinergic, secreting acetylcholine which then combines with specific receptors. Activity of the parasympathetic system gives constriction of the pupil, slowing of the heart and diminished cardiac output, constriction of the bronchioles, increased intestinal peristalis and evacuation of the bladder and bowels, and increased secretory activity of the salivary and lacrimal glands. The parasympathetic system also plays a principal role in sexual activity, including penile erection and ejaculation in the male, and orgasm in the female.

Acetylcholine or noradrenaline are released at autonomic nerve endings; all preganglionic fibres (*see below*), both sympathetic and parasympathetic, are cholinergic. Circulating biogenic amines such as noradrenaline and adrenaline, secreted by the adrenal medulla, which influence sympathetic activity, as well as acetylcholine, produce their effects upon target organs by combining with receptor sites which lie in close relationship to the nerve endings.

Acetylcholine receptors are of two types, namely the muscarinic receptors which are found in all effector cells stimulated by postganglionic parasympathetic neurones (and in cholinergic endings of the sympathetic system), and nicotinic receptors, found especially in the neuromuscular junctions of skeletal muscle but also at synapses in sympathetic and parasympathetic ganglia themselves. Adrenergic receptors are also of two types; alpha receptors are stimulated mainly by noradrenaline and are concerned especially with vasoconstriction, dilatation of the iris, intestinal relaxation and pilomotor contraction in the skin, while beta receptors are stimulated mainly by adrenaline and to a lesser extent by noradrenaline; the latter account for an increased heart rate, vasodilatation of intramuscular blood vessels, intestinal and uterine relaxation and bronchodilatation. The rational use of many drugs depends upon receptor specificity. Thus parasympathomimetic drugs like pilocarpine and methacholine have a muscarinic effect and neostigmine is essentially nicotinic; atropine blocks the muscarinic but not the nicotinic effect of such drugs. Similarly the activities of sympathomimetic drugs depend upon their relative affinities for alpha and beta receptors. Guanethidine appears to block noradrenaline release, phenoxybenzamine and phentolamine block alpha receptors and propanolol beta receptors.

Unquestionably there are areas of the **cerebral cortex** which exercise a controlling influence upon autonomic activity, but the exact areas of the cerebrum concerned and the mechanisms by which they produce their influence are not yet fully defined. However, certain areas of the prefrontal cortex, and particularly the cingulate gyrus, are clearly important, as lesions of the cingulate area may dull the emotions, a fact sometimes made use of in the operation of cingulectomy. Stimulation of the prefrontal cortex may also provoke sweating in the opposite arm and leg. Furthermore, the voluntary act of evacuation of the bladder and bowels seems to be initiated in the paracentral lobule; probably motor impulses from this area, destined to activate the appropriate parasympathetic nerves, travel downwards with the pyramidal tract. It is also evident that certain areas of cortex in the temporal lobe and insula, and particularly the hippocampal gyrus, may, with the amygdaloid nucleus, exercise important control over visceral as well as emotional activity.

Although the cerebrum influences autonomic activity, it is now clear that the most important cell stations from which visceral and other autonomic activity are finally controlled lie in the **hypothalamus**. Nuclei in this area receive fibres from the 'visceral' areas of cerebral cortex mentioned above and in turn they give rise to descending pathways which enter the brain stem and spinal cord. The hypothalamic nuclei not only exert important controlling influences upon all autonomic activity but some nuclei also control secretion from the posterior pituitary, to which, through the infundibulum and tuber cinereum, they are closely related anatomically. Thus the cells of the supraoptic nuclei form antidiuretic hormone (ADH) and vasopressin which then travel down axons into the posterior lobe of the pituitary, being stored there in the form of neurosecretory granules. Similarly oxytocin, which stimulates contraction of the lactating mammary gland and of the pregnant uterus, is found in the paraventricular nucleus and is then conveyed to the posterior pituitary. Although the anterior lobe is not under direct nervous control, humoral substances (mainly polypeptides) secreted by hypothalamic neurones are conveyed to the anterior pituitary through the vessels of the hypophysial venous system, thus exciting gonadotrophic, adrenocorticotrophic, somatotrophic, lactogenic and thyrotrophic secretion. In general, the anterior hypothalamic nuclei are particularly concerned with parasympathetic activity and with controlling the pituitary gland, while posterior nuclei, by contrast, influence sympathetic activity. Lesions of this area give rise to emotional disturbances such as 'sham rage' in animals or to lethargy and hypersomnia. Temperature regulation, control of the emotions and of sleep are also mediated through hypothalamic nuclei. The corpora mammillaria, too, which form a part of the hypothalamic system, are clearly important in memory regulation, as lesions in this area may prevent the patient from recording new impressions, a feature seen typically in the Korsakoff syndrome (*see* Chapter 6, p. 120).

Descending pathways from the hypothalamus control both sympathetic and parasympathetic activity. These travel downwards, in the case of the sympathetic fibres, to the dorsal portion of the spinal cord to end in relation to the cells in the lateral horn of grey matter, while the parasympathetic fibres end in the nuclei of the oculomotor, facial, glossopharyngeal and vagus nerves, or in the sacral region of the spinal cord. No central autonomic fibres travel directly to any viscus, but in each case a ganglion lying outside the central nervous system is interposed, so that there are always preganglionic fibres arising within the central nervous system and postganglionic fibres arising in the ganglia. The sympathetic ganglia lie lateral to the vertebral bodies and with connecting fibres form the sympathetic chain; the postganglionic fibres to the effector organs are therefore long. Many of the parasympathetic ganglia are situated close to the effector organ so that in this case the preganglionic fibres are long.

The Sympathetic Nervous System

Preganglionic medullated sympathetic fibres (white rami) arise from the lateral horn of grey matter in each segment of the spinal cord from the first thoracic to the second lumbar. They then pass laterally to the sympathetic chain in which there are ganglia corresponding to each of those segments of the cord from which sympathetic fibres arise; from these ganglia non-medullated postganglionic fibres (grey rami) join the corresponding somatic spinal nerve, to be distributed to the blood vessels and skin of the appropriate dermatome. However, fibres also run up and down in the chain to three cervical ganglia (superior, middle and inferior or stellate) and to four lumbar ganglia; these are necessary since there is no sympathetic outflow from the spinal cord in these regions. The thoracic and abdominal viscera receive a sympathetic supply through postganglionic fibres of the thoracic ganglia; these fibres form the splanchnic nerves and the coeliac, mesenteric and hypogastric plexuses. The sympathetic innervation of the cranium and of the upper limbs comes from the cervical ganglia and that of the lower limbs from the lumbar ganglia. Fibres travelling to the cranium traverse the inferior and middle cervical ganglia to synapse with nerve cells in the superior cervical ganglion, whence postganglionic fibres arise which enter or overlie the cranium in the coats of the internal and external carotid arteries and are then distributed to the blood vessels, smooth muscle, sweat glands, lacrimal and salivary glands.

Whether there are afferent sympathetic fibres concerned with the transmission of visceral sensation is controversial. Some regard the autonomic nervous system as entirely motor and suggest that afferent fibres accompanying sympathetic efferents are not themselves sympathetic. Whatever their nature, these fibres enter the posterior nerve roots, and visceral sensation is thereafter conveyed centrally along with somatic sensation.

The Parasympathetic Nervous System

This part of the autonomic system is often called the craniosacral outflow as its function is motor and its fibres only leave the central nervous system in the cranial nerves and in the sacral region. Fibres arising in the oculomotor nucleus (its parasympathetic portion, the Edinger–Westphal nucleus) travel with the oculomotor nerve to enter the ciliary ganglion in the orbit, whence long and short ciliary nerves to the ciliary and pupillary muscles arise. The superior salivary nucleus in the brain stem gives origin to fibres which travel with the facial nerve; in the geniculate ganglion some of these leave to form the greater superficial petrosal nerve. This nerve enters the sphenopalatine ganglion from which arise secretomotor fibres to the lacrimal gland. Other fibres from the superior salivary nucleus are conveyed by the chorda tympani to the submaxillary ganglion from which come fibres which innervate the submaxillary and sublingual glands. The axons of the inferior salivary nucleus, on the other hand, travel with the glossopharyngeal nerve; they form the lesser superficial petrosal nerve, enter the otic ganglion, and its postganglionic fibres promote secretion by the parotid gland. Finally, so far as the cranial outflow is concerned, the preganglionic fibres which arise in the dorsal nucleus of the vagus nerve end in many ganglia which lie in the walls of the numerous viscera innervated by this nerve.

The sacral outflow of the parasympathetic system leaves the spinal cord in the second, third and fourth sacral nerves, the so-called nervi erigentes. These preganglionic fibres pass to the vesical plexus and to numerous ganglia in the walls of the bladder, rectum and other pelvic organs, and from these ganglia postganglionic fibres arise.

The Bladder and Bowel

The wall of the bladder consists of unstriped muscle, which forms the detrusor; it and the internal sphincter are both supplied by parasympathetic nerves arising from the nervi erigentes. Stimulation of these fibres gives contraction of the detrusor and relaxation of the internal sphincter. Evacuation of the bladder cannot, however, occur until the external sphincter relaxes; this consists of striped muscle, being supplied by the pudendal nerve and being thus under voluntary control. Normally the tone of the detrusor keeps the bladder contracted upon its contents, but when the intravesical pressure rises to a certain level rhythmical contractions of the bladder wall develop and after a time there is reflex relaxation of the internal sphincter; evacuation is then resisted only by voluntary contraction of the external sphincter. When the latter is relaxed and micturition occurs, the abdominal muscles also contract.

Sympathetic fibres from the hypogastric nerves also supply the bladder wall and, if stimulated, may inhibit contraction. In fact, however, section of these nerves has little practical effect upon bladder function. Some of the afferent fibres concerned in the vesical reflexes travel with these fibres but others travel with the pelvic nerves.

The physiological stimulus for bladder evacuation is an increase in the intravesical pressure which gives the desire to micturate. If this desire is unfulfilled, repeated contractions eventually follow. As previously mentioned there are also higher centres in the paracentral lobule of the cerebral cortex and probably also in the mid-brain which exercise control over micturition; these produce their influence through fibres which descend with the pyramidal tracts. Hence disease of the spinal cord, as will be seen below, can profoundly influence bladder function. Disordered function is often assessed by measuring with a manometer the changes in intravesical pressure which follow the introduction of a standard volume of fluid into the bladder via a catheter. Normally this **cystometrogram** reveals a sudden rise in pressure as the fluid is introduced, followed by a gradual fall and thereafter by rhythmical contractions of the bladder wall. But if the bladder is hypotonic as a result of nervous disease these reflex contractions fail to occur.

In many respects the innervation of the rectum resembles that of the bladder. Stimulation of the parasympathetic nerves gives contraction of the rectal musculature but relaxation of the internal sphincter, as both consist of smooth muscle. The striated external sphincter of the anus, however, is supplied by the pudendal nerve and enables evacuation to be resisted voluntarily. As with the bladder, distension with faeces give reflex rectal contraction and the desire to defaecate.

Sexual Activity

Sexual function in the male can be divided into first, desire or libido which is essentially an emotional function; secondly, erection of the penis due to tumescence of the corpora cavernosa, and thirdly, ejaculation of semen. The second and third functions are mediated through the activity of parasympathetic nerves, while closure of the internal sphincter through sympathetic action is also necessary during ejaculation. Loss of libido may be due to disease of the mind or of the endocrine glands, while impotence (retention of desire but inability to achieve an effective penile erection) can also be psychologically determined. However, impotence can also result from disease of the sacral cord or cauda equina, and is then due to a lesion of the parasympathetic motor pathway or of the afferent sensory pathways; in such a case the ability to ejaculate is also absent. However, since the sexual act is a function which, once initiated, is largely controlled reflexly, erection and ejaculation can occur despite a severe transverse lesion of the cord above the sacral segments. Indeed in some cases of spinal cord injury persistent erection of the penis (priapism) is seen. Disorders of sexual function in the female are less well understood. Lack of desire (frigidity) is relatively common in otherwise normal females and is usually psychogenic. Disease of the cauda equina or of the lower spinal cord may abolish the ability to achieve orgasm, but the effects of nervous disease upon female sexuality are much less apparent than in the male.

Precocious sexual development is generally due to overactivity of the adrenals or ovaries but is occasionally seen in patients with hypothalamic or mid-brain neoplasms or in male patients with pinealomas. Excessive sexuality is generally a constitutional disorder, of psychic rather than physical origin, and often shows some affinities with psychopathy.

Some Autonomic and Related Sensory Reflexes

In addition to the visceral reflexes mentioned above, certain cutaneous reflexes dependent upon autonomic pathways assist in neurological diagnosis. Thus local warming of a limb initially gives vasodilatation and flushing of the skin, followed by sweating in the part that is warmed. Subsequently general vasodilatation and sweating occur in other parts of the body; this occurs even when all nervous connexions between the stimulated limb and the remainder of the body have been divided and must therefore depend upon stimulation of the hypothalamus by the warmed blood. Converse effects (vasoconstriction, pilomotor responses) follow cooling of a limb. Sweating and pilomotor activity are, however, lost in a part of the body which has lost its sympathetic nerve supply, whether the postganglionic or preganglionic fibres have been divided. Absence of cutaneous sweating can be demonstrated by dusting the skin with either quinizarin powder or a starch and iodine mixture; sweat turns quinizarin purple and starch and iodine blue.

The 'flare' reaction is another important reflex. It is an axon reflex; in other words the afferent stimulus travels centrally along a fibre, but then spreads to other branches of the same fibre, in which stimuli travelling peripherally are evoked; these produce a peripheral effect. If the skin is scratched firmly there is temporary blanching along the scratch-line due to local capillary injury, but this is soon followed by a spreading vasodilatation or 'flare', resulting from the axon reflex. A central weal also occurs due to local histamine release, but the 'flare', and the pilomotor response which may also occur in the same area, are reflexly determined. Since this axon reflex does not traverse the spinal cord it remains intact in spinal cord lesions and in lesions lying central to the posterior root ganglia; it is only impaired when the afferent sensory fibres or the ganglia themselves are diseased. Hence absence of the 'flare' can be a valuable physical sign of a lesion of somatic sensory nerves. Another useful test is the cold vasodilatation response; if normal fingers are immersed in water at 5°C they cool rapidly but 5 or 10 minutes later there is vasodilatation. This does not happen if the finger is denervated; like the flare, this is not strictly an autonomic reflex as it depends upon the integrity of sensory axons. Thus in disease of the efferent sympathetic pathways, whether preganglionic or postganglionic, reflex vasodilatation (flushing of the skin) and sweating are abolished but a 'flare' will develop. When the sensory nerves from an area of skin are diseased, sweating may occur, but the 'flare' and cold vasodilatation are abolished.

Some Common Disorders of the Autonomic Nervous System

Horner's Syndrome

A lesion of the cervical sympathetic chain or ganglia causes constriction of the pupil on the same side due to unopposed action of the parasympathetic; drooping of the eyelid, due to paralysis of that part of the levator palpebrae superioris which is composed of smooth muscle and is innervated by sympathetic nerves; slight retraction of the globe of the eye into the orbit because of paralysis of smooth orbital muscle which is similarly innervated; and loss of sweating on the affected side of the head and neck. Hence the features of Horner's syndrome are myosis, ptosis, enophthalmos and anhidrosis of head and neck, all on the same side as the lesion. This condition can result from a lesion of sympathetic ganglia in the neck, whether due to disease or operation; it is rarely congenital or may result from a lesion of the cervical and upper dorsal spinal cord (such as syringomyelia), which destroys the lateral horn of grey matter. It can also be due to a lesion of the lateral part of the medulla, as in infarction due to thrombosis of the posterior inferior cerebellar artery, causing division of sympathetic fibres descending from the hypothalamus. Rarely, a lesion destroying sympathetic fibres which ascend into the cranium in the coat of the internal carotid artery (e.g. aneurysm or carotid thrombosis) gives all the ocular features of Horner's syndrome, but facial sweating is normal as fibres responsible for the latter sign travel in the unaffected external carotid and its branches. This combination of signs is called Raeder's paratrigeminal syndrome. Finally, in a few patients a Horner's syndrome appears for which no cause is ever determined.

Cranial Nerve Syndromes

A lesion of one oculomotor nerve usually gives a fixed dilated pupil on the affected side, owing to paralysis of parasympathetic fibres and unopposed action of the sympathetic. Diseases of the glossopharyngeal and vagus nerves rarely produce any clinical evidence of autonomic disturbance, but after a facial palsy misdirection of regenerating parasympathetic fibres can result in fibres intended for the salivary glands reaching the lacrimal gland so that lacrimation occurs when the patient eats (the syndrome of crocodile tears). Facial sweating during meals (gustatory sweating) is another reflex phenomenon which is occasionally seen in apparently normal individuals and can often be controlled by atropine and related drugs. The myotonic pupil (Adie's syndrome), due to a lesion of the ciliary ganglion of undetermined cause, is described on p. 162.

Lesions of the Cauda Equina and Spinal Cord

A severe lesion of the cauda equina can have profound effects upon bladder and bowel function because of damage to the sacral parasympathetic outflow. The bladder becomes toneless and reflex contraction can no longer occur as it distends, so that urinary retention develops. As distension increases so the elasticity of the bladder wall forces urine into the urethra, and as the external sphincter is usually paralysed as well, dribbling incontinence or retention with overflow occurs. If the cauda equina lesion is permanent, reflex bladder activity cannot be re-established and owing to enforced catheterisation and urinary stasis, severe urinary infection often supervenes. In some such cases permanent suprapubic drainage of the bladder is necessary but eventually in many cases evacuation by manual compression is achieved. Similarly, faecal retention often occurs, with incontinence, and regular enemas may be required to empty the bowel.

The initial effects of an acute transverse lesion of the spinal cord are similar; there is retention of urine with overflow and also faecal retention. As spinal shock wears off, reflex bladder and bowel evacuation are gradually established, occurring solely in response to increasing intravesical and intrarectal pressure and independently of the will. Thus automatic bladder and bowel activity develop; micturition and defaecation can be evoked by anything which increases intravesical pressure, including pressure upon the abdomen, or straining. They can also occur as a result of stimuli applied to the lower limbs, as part of the 'mass reflex' which includes flexor withdrawal of the limbs. The patient with a total transverse cord lesion may become aware that his bladder is full through sensations of headache, sweating or abdominal fullness and may then be able to initiate micturition by pressure upon the abdomen.

Retention of urine can also result from parasagittal lesions affecting both cerebral paracentral lobules, while incomplete lesions of the spinal cord affecting the pyramidal tracts, in relation to which descending fibres controlling micturition are believed to travel, can also affect bladder function. Sometimes, in such a case, there is delay in the initiation of micturition and even incomplete retention with overflow. More often, in a patient with spastic paraplegia, say, as a result of multiple sclerosis, there is heightened reflex activity of the bladder and precipitancy or urgency of micturition results. The patient cannot resist the desire to micturate and precipitate bladder evacuation occurs. Incontinence of urine also occurs in some patients with bilateral lesions of the medial aspect of the frontal lobes, as in some elderly atherosclerotic or demented individuals or occasionally as a result of aneurysms of the anterior communicating or anterior cerebral arteries.

Apart from their effect upon bladder and bowel function, lesions of the spinal cord influence other autonomic activities. Thus after an acute transverse lesion, and during the stage of spinal shock (diaschisis) the skin of the body below the level of the lesion is dry, pale and cool, but subsequently when reflex activity is established, profuse sweating in the affected area is common and can be provoked by many cutaneous or other stimuli. It should also be remembered that local disease of the dorsal spinal cord may damage the lateral horn of grey matter and will give sympathetic denervation of the affected segments with signs corresponding to those produced by division of preganglionic fibres.

Referred Pain

The afferent pathway for visceral sensation is initially along afferent fibres which accompany autonomic nerves, and particularly the sympathetic. These fibres enter posterior nerve roots and travel centrally with somatic afferents. Visceral pain is often felt in skin areas which are not at first sight anatomically related to the viscus concerned; thus cardiac pain may be preferred to the substernal region, but also to the left arm, to both arms or to the jaw. The mechanism of referred pain is discussed on p. 82.

Degenerative Disorders of the Autonomic Nervous System

In **familial orthostatic hypotension** (the Shy–Drager syndrome) (*see* p. 133) attacks of fainting occur whenever the patient assumes the upright posture. The condition is due to degeneration of unknown aetiology in the cells of the intermediolateral column of the spinal cord and the patients often show features of dementia, Parkinsonism or cerebellar ataxia. The latter combination is often called progressive multi-system degeneration.

Familial dysautonomia (the Riley–Day syndrome) is a rare disorder of autosomal recessive inheritance, usually seen in Jews, in which defective lacrimation, hyperhidrosis, epilepsy, and episodic hyperpyrexia generally occur. Most patients have no sense of taste and are relatively insensitive to pain, and they usually die in childhood from respiratory infection. There is evidence of an inborn error of catecholamine metabolism in such cases and of a marked reduction in the numbers of unmyelinated nerve fibres in peripheral nerves.

Acute autonomic neuropathy is a rare disorder of unknown cause presenting in childhood or adult life with the rapid onset of postural hypotension, paralysis of ocular accommodation, anhidrosis and urinary and faecal retention. Spontaneous recovery usually occurs within a few months, so that the condition is also known as 'pure pan-dysautonomia with recovery'.

Peripheral Nerve Lesions

Whereas section of a sensory nerve peripheral to its posterior root ganglion usually abolishes the 'flare' response in the cutaneous anaesthetic area, a lesion of the lower motor neurone usually produces no recognisable autonomic effects. However, as a result of disuse the skin of the affected part may become smooth, shiny and inelastic, while subcutaneous tissue and even bone, as well as denervated muscle, will atrophy. Owing to loss of the 'pumping' action of muscles upon the veins, the affected part, especially a hand or foot, is often cyanosed and oedematous. These so-called trophic changes are due to disuse and not to a lesion of autonomic nerves; the autonomic reflexes are intact. The sequelae of a sensory nerve lesion are often more serious, particularly if pain fibres are involved as, if the part is analgesic, injury to the insensitive skin and joints readily occurs, giving indolent or perforating ulcers and gross disorganisation of joints (Charcot's arthropathy). Other trophic changes, such as loss of sweating and of the pilomotor response, only follow a lesion of preganglionic or postganglionic sympathetic efferents and hence do not always result from lesions of somatic peripheral nerves, unless these contain sympathetic fibres.

After an incomplete lesion of a peripheral nerve, particularly in the region of the forearm and wrist, a curiously unpleasant type of pain may develop in the affected hand, with excessive sweating and excessive sensitivity to touch and pain. This syndrome is called **causalgia**; it seems that stimuli responsible for the pain travel with autonomic nerves and not along somatic afferents, as block or division of somatic sensory nerves fails to relieve the pain, while sympathectomy does so. The pathogenesis of causalgia is poorly understood (p. 91). Similarly, the mechanism by which painful swelling of the hand, often giving eventually atrophy of muscles and even of bone (Sudeck's atrophy), develops in some cases of pericapsulitis of the shoulder joint or 'frozen' shoulder (**the 'shoulder-hand' syndrome**) is obscure, but this condition, too, is often relieved by cervical sympathectomy.

Hyperhidrosis

Though excessive sweating, particularly of the hands and feet, can be due to emotional disturbances or to endocrine disorders such as thyrotoxicosis, it may also be congenital and, if intolerable, can be alleviated by sympathectomy. It is also seen sometimes in Parkinson's disease. Localised cutaneous areas of increased sweating can occur following peripheral nerve lesions, as in causalgia, while excessive perspiration in response to any peripheral stimulus is seen below the level of a transverse lesion of the spinal cord.

Hypothalamic Syndromes

That **disorders of sleep**, taking the form of either hypersomnia or wakefulness with reversal of the sleep rhythm, may result from hypothalamic lesions has been mentioned in Chapter 6. **Excessive appetite** can also occur, and in the so-called Kleine–Levin syndrome, which usually occurs in adolescent males, hypersomnia and megaphagia occur, but may resolve spontaneously after some weeks in which the patient does little but sleep and eat. Conversely, some hypothalamic lesions produce **anorexia** leading to extreme **cachexia**; a syndrome of this nature may also result from a hypothalamic lesion in infancy and early childhood. The affected children show rapid longitudinal growth with almost total loss of subcutaneous fat despite an adequate food intake; they are alert and often hyperactive. Usually a hypothalamic or optic nerve glioma is eventually found, but rarely no cause is demonstrable.

Disorders of memory, and Korsakoff's syndrome in particular, result from lesions of the corpora mammillaria. Actual **visual hallucinations** (so-called peduncular hallucinations) can also be produced by lesions in this area, while many **emotional** and **personality disorders**, including excessive anger and irritability on the one hand, and apathy leading to akinetic stupor on the other, have been attributed to hypothalame lesions. The region plays a major rôle in regulating **body temperature**, and irritation of hypothalamic nuclei, say as a result of sudden distension of the third ventricle by haemorrhage, can give rise to hyperpyrexia. A similar mechanism probably accounts for the **hyperglycaemia** and **glycosuria**, **albuminuria**, and acute **gastric ulceration** with haemorrhage, which sometimes occur in patients with brain disease; basal neoplasms and subarachnoid haemorrhage are particularly liable to produce these effects.

Diabetes insipidus, a condition in which the patient passes very large quantities of dilute urine and consequently has polydipsia or excessive thirst, may also be the result of an anterior hypothalamic lesion. A reduced output of ADH, resulting in diabetes insipidus, may follow a lesion of the hypothalamus or of the posterior pituitary, or even of the pathways joining the two in the tuber cinereum.

Obesity and sexual underdevelopment are other signs which are sometimes due to disease of the hypothalamus or pituitary or both. Diabetes insipidus and obesity may both be seen as a result of pituitary or para-pituitary neoplasms (e.g. chromophobe adenoma, prolactinoma, craniopharyngioma), following head injury, as a result of hydrocephalus with third ventricular distension, and in patients with granulomatous processes involving the base of the brain (e.g. sarcoidosis). There are also several hypothalamic disorders of early life whose cause is unknown. In idiopathic adiposogenital dystrophy (Frohlich's syndrome) the obesity is present from birth, is greatest around the shoulders and hips, and there is genital hypoplasia and immaturity. The condition is more common in males, but when females are affected sexual function is more often normal.

The Laurence–Moon–Biedl syndrome is another congenital disorder of the hypothalamic–pituitary axis and is almost certainly genetically determined. Like Frohlich's syndrome it is characterised by obesity and hypogonadism but in addition there is mental retardation, polydactyly (usually there are six fingers and toes) and retinitis pigmentosa, giving rise to progressive visual impairment.

Conclusions

Disease or dysfunction of the hypothalamus, which is the control centre from which autonomic activities are regulated, can produce many variable clinical manifestations, but through an understanding of some simple principles governing the behaviour of this part of the nervous system, it is possible to interpret the significance of many important symptoms and physical signs. Similarly, a knowledge of the structure and function of the peripheral components of the autonomic nervous system is necessary in order to interpret those symptoms and signs of autonomic dysfunction, and particularly those of abnormal bladder and bowel activity, which occur in patients with nervous disease.

References

Appenzeller, O., *The Autonomic Nervous System,* 2nd ed. (Amsterdam, North-Holland, 1976).

Holmes, G., *Introduction to Clinical Neurology,* 3rd ed., revised by Matthews, W. B., Chapters 16 and 17 (Edinburgh, Livingstone, 1968).

Johnson, R. H. and Spalding, J. M. K., *Disorders of the Autonomic Nervous System* (Oxford, Blackwell, 1974).

Patton, H. D., Sundsten, J. W., Crill, W. E. and Swanson, P. D., *Introduction to Basic Neurology,* (Philadelphia, W. B. Saunders, 1976).

Walton, J. N., *Brain's Diseases of the Nervous System,* 8th ed. (London, Oxford University Press, 1977).

Walton, J. N., Section X on Neurological pathophysiology, in *International Textbook of Medicine,* Ed. Smith, J. H. and Thier, S. (Philadelphia and London, W. B. Saunders, 1981).

12 Developmental, Hereditary and Degenerative Disorders

Among the many disorders of the nervous system which are considered in this volume there exist a group of syndromes or diseases which are difficult to classify according to rational criteria. Some are clearly inherited but we do not know how the gene or genes responsible for them produce their effects upon the nervous system. Nor do we know in the case of many of them whether they constitute separate diseases or are merely variants of a single disease process. Others are clearly due to an abnormality of unknown cause which has afflicted the developing nervous system of the affected individual *in utero*, while others which are normally grouped together for convenience on account of clinical similarities are probably due to a variety of causes, some well-recognised and others obscure. And in yet another group of conditions there is evidence of a pathological process involving part of the central or peripheral nervous system, a process so inexplicable in our present state of knowledge that we can only classify it as being degenerative in type. In this chapter an outline of some of the commoner nervous disorders which fall into these categories will be given and their interrelationship will be considered. Many uncommon developmental defects, such as the microcephalies, macrocephalies and ageneses of portions of the brain will not be considered, in view of their rarity. These are described in some of the larger textbooks to which reference is made at the end of the chapter.

Cerebral Palsy — $\frac{1-2}{1000}$ children

The term cerebral palsy is used to identify a group of nervous disorders which are apparent from birth, which are very variable in their clinical manifestations and severity, and probably also in their aetiology. Although abnormalities of movement are generally the most prominent clinical features in such cases there are often associated defects of intellect, of emotional development, of speech in the broadest sense, and of sensation. Between one and two in every thousand children are victims of some form of cerebral palsy. In most of the affected children the limbs are stiff and spastic and this is why these cases are often referred to, particularly by the lay public, as spastic children. In fact, in as many as 10 per cent of cases it is involuntary movements of athetoid type and not spasticity which constitute the principal disability, while in about 5 per cent, the limbs are actually hypotonic and the child is ataxic rather than spastic.

The aetiology of cerebral palsy has been a fertile source of dispute. Some claimed that virtually all cases are due to **birth injury** with meningeal haemorrhage, a view now clearly untenable, while others suggested that an encephalitis, or some degenerative cerebral process of known aetiology, occurring *in utero*, is the cause. The truth appears to be that the pathological changes seen in such cases are so diverse that no single cause can be implicated. A **genetic factor** may be responsible for the condition in up to 10 per cent of cases, as other members of the family, particularly sibs, are afflicted, either with cerebral palsy or with mental defect or epilepsy. Probably in some cases, **intra-uterine cerebral anoxia** due to placental insufficiency is responsible, and there is certainly a high incidence of threatened abortion or accidental haemorrhage in pregnancies resulting in the birth of spastic children. Possibly, too, the anoxia resulting from a prolonged convulsion in early infancy can give rise to similar changes, as may anoxia or direct trauma to the brain during a breech or forceps delivery or any prolonged labour. Certainly 50 per cent of spastic children have abnormal deliveries and many are born prematurely. There is increasing evidence that prenatal or perinatal anoxia is the predominant aetiological factor, but complex neonatal metabolic abnormalities, including hypoglycaemia, as well as disorders of cerebral perfusion resulting from cerebral oedema and hypotension all play a part. Pathologically the principal changes are those of periventricular encephalomalacia, but multiple areas of cortical scarring are found in some cases, porencephalic cysts communicating with the ventricles in others and spongiform changes in the basal ganglia in yet others. **Kernicterus**, the degeneration and bilirubin-staining of the basal ganglia which frequently resulted from Rh-incompatibility (icterus gravis neonatorum) often caused a variety of cerebral palsy in which mental defect, deafness and athetosis were prominent features.

Although all forms of cerebral palsy usually reveal themselves through delay in development, and failure to pass intellectual and physical milestones at a normal age, most cases fall into one of several distinctive clinical syndromes. The age at which the parents realise that their child is abnormal varies depending upon severity, but it is usually within the first 12 to 18 months of life; in some, delay and difficulty in walking are not apparent until late in the second year.

The condition can simply cause **mental retardation**, but more often there is clumsiness and spasticity of the limbs as well. The diagnosis of mental defect in early life, depending as it does upon failure to achieve new milestones of intellectual development (smiling, following lights, groping for objects, forming syllables and words, etc.) at the normal age, is a matter which requires great skill and experience in assessing the infant's behaviour against a background of known developmental variations. Certain children with cerebral palsy have specific defects of motor function (**apraxia**), of sensory function (**agnosia**), of the special senses (**nerve deafness**) or of speech (**aphasia, articulatory apraxia, dyslexia**) which can give a false impression of mental defect if the clinical appraisal is too superficial. In some cases developmental disorders of execution and cognition (learning defects) occur in isolation without accompanying manifestations of spasticity or ataxia. Congenital reading defect (developmental dyslexia) is a good example, but apraxic and agnosic disorders ('clumsy children') also occur (p. 105) and are difficult to recognise in the early stages, though a discrepancy between high verbal and low performance scores in an I.Q. test may be a useful pointer. These and other forms of so-called minimal cerebral dysfunction are often overlooked.

The commonest form of cerebral palsy is **spastic diplegia** (Little's disease) which may or may not be associated with mental defect. In its mildest form it presents with little more than a delay of a few months in learning to walk, with some clumsiness and unsteadiness of gait, symmetrical exaggeration of the lower limb reflexes and extensor plantar responses. In a severe case, walking is never possible, all four limbs are spastic and there is also severe spastic dysarthria and/or dysphagia. More often the patient cannot walk until the fifth or sixth year and then does so with the characteristic 'scissors gait', and contractures develop in the Achilles tendons and hamstrings.

In patients with **athetosis** (p. 202) which is usually bilateral and symmetrical, there may also be facial grimacing and an intermittently explosive dysarthria. Voluntary movements of the limbs sometimes override the abnormal movements but are slowly and clumsily performed. Often the athetotic movements are not seen until the second year of life or later, and at an earlier stage the limbs are hypotonic and movement is inco-ordinate while the plantar responses are flexor. Some cases, however, show associated spasticity. More rarely patients with a hypotonic or flaccid variety of diplegia do not develop involuntary movements but have nystagmus and asymmetrical **ataxia** of all four limbs, usually due to cerebellar dysfunction (**cerebellar diplegia**).

The prognosis of cerebral palsy varies, depending upon the severity of the intellectual and motor deficit. When mental retardation is severe, little can be done and this is unfortunately true of some cases in which the motor abnormality is gross. Sometimes abnormal movements can be alleviated surgically (*see* p. 459), while many patients, with appropriate training, can be helped to lead useful lives. Children with specific disorders of language and reading, though requiring patient individual training, are particularly profitable subjects.

Infantile hemiplegia is another condition commonly classified as a form of cerebral palsy, although it clearly differs considerably from the diffuse and symmetrical cerebral disorders mentioned above. It can occur bilaterally (double hemiplegia) and is then distinguished from cerebral diplegia through the fact that the upper limbs are more severely affected than the lower. The condition can be present from birth (congenital hemiplegia), when it may be due to a congenital cystic deformity of one cerebral hemisphere (porencephaly), to the Sturge–Weber syndrome (*see* p. 356), or possibly to infarction occurring *in utero*. More commonly it develops acutely in infancy or early childhood, often during an acute illness such as whooping cough or an exanthem, or after a so-called 'febrile convulsion'. Probably the commonest pathological cause is infarction due to either arterial or venous occlusion, resulting in scarring and atrophy of the hemisphere and localised dilatation of the lateral ventricle (secondary porencephaly). It may in some cases be due to an inflammatory process of unknown cause involving the wall of the internal carotid artery. Characteristically the arm on the affected side is severely paralysed, finger and hand movement being virtually abolished, and the hand and forearm assume a typically flexed posture, lying across the front of the chest. The leg, though spastic with exaggerated deep reflexes and an extensor plantar response, is less severely affected, and all patients eventually walk, often with surprisingly little difficulty. If the dominant hemisphere is involved, aphasia occurs; the earlier the age at which the hemiplegia develops, the more complete and rapid is the recovery of speech function. Indeed if the patient is a young infant, the development of speech is not perceptibly delayed and this function becomes established in the contralateral hemisphere. The residual neurological deficit can be of all grades of severity and occasionally the resulting disability is trivial. In more severe cases, however, epilepsy is a common complication, as the scar in the affected hemisphere acts as a focus of epileptic discharge. Particularly in those cases in which epileptic seizures are frequent and severe, intellectual impairment and behaviour disorders are common.

Hydrocephalus

Hydrocephalus can be defined as an increase in the volume of CSF within the cranial cavity. This may occur as a compensatory phenomenon when the brain or any part of it is atrophic through disease (hydrocephalus *ex vacuo*), but no symptoms then result from the presence of excess fluid. It is when the increase in fluid is accompanied by a rise in the intracranial pressure that clinical effects become apparent. This variety of hydrocephalus results from increased formation of CSF (possibly due to hyperaemia of the choroid plexuses as in meningitis), from obstruction to the circulation of the fluid, or from impaired absorption (as in thrombosis of the superior longitudinal sinus).

When hydrocephalus is due to an obstruction to the flow of fluid through a part of the ventricular system (lateral ventricle, third ventricle, aqueduct, fourth ventricle), it is known as **obstructive hydrocephalus** and there is enlargement of those ventricles which lie between the choroid plexuses and the block. An obstruction to the flow of fluid through the subarachnoid space gives **communicating hydrocephalus** and there is then dilatation of all the cerebral ventricles.

Obstructive hydrocephalus may be **congenital** or acquired. The commonest congenital cause is stenosis or malformation of the aqueduct of Sylvius (aqueduct stenosis, in which the third and lateral ventricles are dilated but the posterior fossa is small), but less often there is membranous occlusion of the foramina of Magendie and Luschka (the so-called Dandy–Walker syndrome, in which the fourth ventricle is also dilated and the posterior fossa is large). Another cause is the Arnold–Chiari malformation which is often, but not always, associated with a spinal meningomyelocele. The medulla oblongata is elongated and the cerebellar tonsils protrude downwards through the foramen magnum; in this condition, and in basilar impression (*see below*) there may be an obstruction to the outflow of fluid from the fourth ventricle into the basal cisterns and syringomyelia may develop. In most cases of congenital hydrocephalus there is conspicuous enlargement of the head, present sometimes at birth, but usually developing subsequently. The head is excessively translucent, it yields a typical 'cracked-pot' note on percussion, there is separation of the sutures and the eyes tend to be pushed forwards and downwards (the rising-sun sign). Convulsions, mental impairment, optic atrophy and spastic weakness of the limbs often develop, and many patients die within the first four years of life, but the condition becomes arrested in many patients, who then survive with a variable degree of disability. **Acquired** obstructive hydrocephalus can result from any lesion, whether inflammatory or neoplastic, which distorts intracranial hydrodynamics in such a way as to cause an obstruction to CSF flow in a cerebral ventricle or in the aqueduct. This is why a cerebral tumour often presents with the clinical features (headache, vomiting, papilloedema) which are the typical symptoms of hydrocephalus occurring in adult life.

The clinical effects of **communicating hydrocephalus** are similar to those of the obstructive variety, but except in severe cases this is frequently a self-limiting disorder. It generally follows conditions such as meningitis (or rarely subarachnoid haemorrhage) which lead to the formation of inflammatory adhesions in the subarachnoid space; sometimes these absorb with time. In some such cases the condition develops insidiously and although the lateral ventricles are enlarged the pressure of the fluid within them, measured at ventriculography, is found to be unexpectedly low so that the condition may be erroneously attributed to cerebral atrophy. Such cases of **low-pressure hydrocephalus**, in which a history of antecedent head injury or cerebral illness is often lacking, frequently present with fluctuating confusion, ataxia and eventually with progressive dementia in middle or late life. As in some cases ventricular drainage produces prompt clinical improvement, these cases must be distinguished by the CAT scan and sometimes by air encephalography and isotope ventriculography (*see* p. 54), from those suffering from presenile or senile dementia (*see below*). The principal distinguishing characteristic is that in low-pressure hydrocephalus the ventricles are dilated but the cortical sulci are not, whereas the latter are enlarged due to gyral atrophy in the presenile dementias.

The syndrome of **otitic hydrocephalus** is one of headache and severe papilloedema which may complicate middle-ear disease and is generally due to aseptic thrombosis of the lateral and/or superior longitudinal sinuses, giving impaired absorption of CSF. This condition is self-limiting, and complete recovery usually occurs provided vision is preserved; a similar disorder may follow trauma; it can complicate pregnancy or cachexia, or can occur apparently spontaneously, especially in plump young women, when it has been variously entitled 'toxic hydrocephalus', 'pseudotumour cerebri', or **'benign intracranial hypertension'**. Although in some such cases venous sinus thrombosis is the cause, many are unexplained and the fact that the lateral ventricles are often shown by the CAT scan to be small or normal in size suggests that swelling of the brain tissue itself causes the increased intracranial pressure and that there is no true hydrocephalus.

Presenile and Senile Dementia

This condition has been considered in Chapter 7 (p. 139). Whereas a syndrome of progressive intellectual deterioration in late middle-life (the presenium) can be due to many causes (general paresis, frontal neoplasm, cerebral atherosclerosis, liver disease, vitamin B_{12} deficiency, myxoedema), some of which are remediable, there is a group of progressive degenerative cerebral diseases which give dementia as their principal presenting feature. The pathological changes (atrophy of gyri with senile plaques of argyrophilic glial fibres in the cortex) are identical with those of senile dementia and the separate recognition of a presenile group of cases is no longer thought to be valid. **Alzheimer's disease**, in addition to progressive dementia, often gives aphasic and apraxic defects and convulsions; it occurs sporadically, while **Pick's disease** may affect more than one member of a sibship and gives focal cortical atrophy, particularly in the frontal lobes, so that euphoria and volubility often precede florid dementia. A form of degenerative cerebral disease of undetermined aetiology in which a progressive dementia is associated with Parkinsonian features, signs of pyramidal tract disease, and muscular wasting in the periphery of the limbs due to degeneration of anterior horn cells in the spinal cord, is sometimes referred to as **Creutzfeldt–Jakob disease**. This condition, which is sometimes familial, is probably a form of cortico-striato-nigro-spinal degeneration. Pathological observations suggest that a rare form of rapidly progressive presenile dementia, often associated with intermittent myoclonic jerks which are accompanied by an irregular spike-and-wave pattern in the EEG and which results from a spongiform degenerative change in the brain with marked astrocytic hyperplasia (subacute spongiform encephalopathy), comes closer to the original description of Creutzfeldt and Jakob. This condition, unlike the degenerative disorders referred to above, has been transmitted to the chimpanzee by intracerebral inoculation and is believed to be due to a slow virus infection.

Huntington's Chorea

This genetically-determined degenerative disorder, in which pathological changes are most striking in the frontal and temporal cortex and caudate nuclei, is inherited as an autosomal dominant trait and is usually apparent first in late middle-life. The characteristic features are progressive dementia, facial grimacing and uncontrollable choreiform movements of the limbs. Rarely, dementia develops before the choreiform movements; more often the latter are evident for some years before intellect declines. Very occasionally the condition presents in childhood or early adult life, with generalised rigidity of the limbs (the 'rigid' form of the disease). The CAT scan or air encephalography in such cases often demonstrate atrophy of the caudate nuclei. Neuropharmacologists are attempting, so far without success, to define the fundamental biochemical defect in such cases. A specific diagnostic test, applicable in the preclinical phase of the illness, is urgently required since each child of an affected individual has a 50:50 chance of developing the disease and most sufferers have passed through their active reproductive phase before manifestations of the condition are first recognisable.

Tuberous Sclerosis (Epiloia)

This degenerative disorder, which occasionally affects more than one member of a sibship, is characterised pathologically by the development of sclerotic masses of glial overgrowth in the cerebral cortex and by a hyperplasia of sebaceous glands upon the face, affecting the cheeks and lower lip, but often sparing the upper lip (adenoma sebaceum). Most sufferers are mentally retarded and all are epileptic. Convulsions usually begin early in life and are intractable. In some cases the condition presents in early infancy with infantile spasms (*see* p. 127). The disorder is sometimes recognised in infancy or early childhood if the typical yellowish plaques or phakomata are seen in the retina. The CAT scan or air encephalography usually demonstrates glial masses protruding into the cerebral ventricles. Cerebral gliomas commonly develop in such cases and few patients survive beyond the third decade.

Cerebral Lipidosis

Many inherited diseases exist which result in the accumulation of abnormal lipids within cells, often including those of the central nervous system. In **Niemann–Pick's disease** the cortical nerve cells contain sphingomyelin, as do reticuloendothelial cells in many other parts of the body, but nervous symptoms are usually unobtrusive, while splenomegaly and hepatomegaly are striking. Neurological involvement may also be seen in **Gaucher's** disease in which kerasin accumulates, particularly in the cells of the spleen and liver; occasionally neurological symptoms and signs (paresis of the limbs, fits, and intellectual deterioration) occur. In **Hand–Schuller–Christian** disease the accumulation of cholesterol gives xanthomatous deposits, particularly in the bones of the skull and pelvis. The disease is commonest in childhood and usually causes diabetes insipidus and exophthalmos. The commonest lipidosis to affect the central nervous system, however, is **cerebromacular degeneration** in which gangliosides are deposited in central nervous system neuronal perikarya which become enormously ballooned. The infantile variety of this disorder, which often affects more than one member of a family, is usually called **Tay–Sachs disease** or **amaurotic family idiocy** and is confined to the Jewish race. Other varieties of the disorder, to which many eponymous titles have been given, may develop in later childhood and even in early adult life. The characteristic features of all varieties of the disease are progressive dementia and paralysis and epilepsy of myoclonic type; the myoclonic jerks are frequently evoked by startle, while major convulsions also occur. In infancy and early childhood, blindness frequently develops and there is a typical cherry-red spot at the macula. The EEG often reveals almost continuous irregular spike-and-wave discharges. The condition in all its forms is invariably progressive to a fatal termination, usually in from one to ten years, the course being shorter in younger patients.

Another variety of lipidosis, inherited as an autosomal recessive trait, is **metachromatic leukodystrophy** (sulphatide lipidosis). Difficulty in walking usually occurs in the second or third year of life and spastic paralysis and dementia usually supervene. Convulsions occur in some cases and death is usual in one to two years. Rarely the condition presents in adult life with manifestations of polyneuropathy and progressive dementia. Material staining metachromatically (brown instead of blue) is seen in the brain and peripheral nerves stained with toluidine blue; the deep tendon reflexes are lost early and motor nerve conduction is slowed. Diagnosis is made by finding metachromatic material in the urine or in a peripheral nerve or brain biopsy or by finding that the urinary or leucocyte aryl-sulphatase is low.

Krabbe's disease (globoid cell leucodystrophy) is another rare autosomal recessive disorder in which galactocerebroside accumulates in the brain and peripheral nerves and causes convulsions, rigidity and ultimately bulbar paralysis beginning in infancy and leading to death within a few months or years.

Refsum's disease (heredopathia atactica polyneuritiformis) is another recessive disorder which begins in childhood or early adult life and gives rise to retinitis pigmentosa, nerve deafness, cerebellar ataxia and a polyneuropathy with hypertrophy of peripheral nerves. The disorder has been shown to be due to an accumulation of phytanic acid in the tissues and the isolation of phytanic acid (which is a derivative of chlorophyll) from the urine is a valuable diagnostic test. Some patients have improved on a chlorophyll-free diet.

Progressive Myoclonic Epilepsy

In this familial disorder, first described by Unverricht, repeated myoclonic jerking of the face, trunk and limbs of increasing and uncontrollable severity is associated with progressive dementia; this disease, too, is eventually fatal. Pathologically there is degeneration of the dentate nuclei of the cerebellum. In many such cases abnormal mucopolysaccharides can be found in the serum and inclusion bodies (Lafora bodies) may be found in affected cells in the cerebellum and even in voluntary muscle.

Neurofibromatosis

This disorder, which is inherited as an autosomal dominant trait, is characterised by the development of widespread benign tumours which grow from the neurolemmal sheaths of nerves. **Cutaneous pigmentation** in the form of *café-au-lait* spots and/or larger areas of diffuse pigmentation with an irregular edge, is an almost invariable association. Cutaneous fibromata are often widespread throughout the body as sessile or pedunculated soft pink swellings, while firmer beady nodules may be found attached to peripheral nerves. Sometimes plexiform neuromatous enlargement of nerves occurs and is associated with an overgrowth of skin and subcutaneous tissue to give an appearance resembling localised elephantiasis. Bone involvement can produce hyperostosis of the facial or long bones while small plaques or phakomata may be seen in the retina. Even in the absence of intrathecal neurofibromas, a characteristic concave 'scalloping' of the posterior borders of the vertebral bodies may be seen in spinal radiographs. Neurofibromas sometimes cause painful compression of peripheral nerves; they may grow on spinal roots, giving root pain and spinal cord compression; and they can develop intracranially on cranial nerve sheaths (e.g. acoustic neuroma, trigeminal neuroma) to give clinical features indicating intracranial neoplasia. A neurofibroma on a spinal root often causes enlargement of the appropriate intervertebral foramen, and a soft-tissue shadow of the extraspinal portion of the growth (a dumb-bell tumour) may be seen in radiographs. Intracranial meningiomas and gliomas also occur in these patients more often than can be accounted for by chance, and an optic nerve glioma is particularly common. Sarcomatous change in a fibroma is a rare complication. In severe cases multiple neurosurgical operations may be required to relieve symptoms as neurofibromas in different situations produce their effects, but many cases run a relatively benign course and the patients survive to a normal age. Remarkably in some patients in whom radiographs clearly demonstrate several large intraspinal neurofibromas, signs and symptoms of spinal cord compression remain slight for many years and pain is the most prominent symptom. Surgery is best avoided in such cases unless increasing limb weakness or severe sphincter dysfunction appear.

The Hereditary Ataxias and Related Disorders

Among the degenerative disorders of the nervous system there exists a group of comparatively rare progressive disorders or syndromes, many of which are identified by eponymous titles, and which have in common the fact that they are all genetically determined. In some families these diseases, if distinctive diseases they be, appear to be inherited as autosomal dominant traits, in others, despite similar clinical features, as autosomal recessives. Only in one condition which is provisionally included in this group, namely **Leber's optic atrophy,** does an X-linked recessive mechanism hold. This inherited disorder is characterised by sudden bilateral visual impairment developing, usually in males, in early adult life, and bilateral central scotomas are found in the visual fields. It can be regarded as an inherited form of retrobulbar neuritis; it may be due to a disorder of cyanide metabolism (*see* p. 160).

The remaining clinical features which can appear alone or in combination in the diseases of the hereditary ataxia group include progressive dementia, insidiously progressive optic atrophy, pigmentary retinal degeneration, agenesis or degeneration of cranial nerve nuclei, including those of the oculomotor, facial and auditory nerves, cerebellar ataxia, sensory ataxia and/or peripheral loss of pain sensation, due either to lesions in the posterior root ganglia or in the posterior columns of the spinal cord, spastic paraplegia or quadriplegia, wasting and weakness of peripheral limb muscles, hypertrophy of peripheral nerves, and skeletal deformities. A bewildering variety of individual syndromes has been described within the confines of this group. Whereas there are some disorders which appear repeatedly in different families with reasonably stereotyped clinical manifestations, many different combinations of the clinical features outlined above have been reported occasionally in individual families, and many of these rare combinations have received distinctive names.

Retinitis Pigmentosa

This condition is characterised in the beginning by night blindness but later by progressive visual deterioration and constriction of the visual fields. Epilepsy and nerve deafness are commonly associated. The optic disk is pale, the retinal vessels are attenuated and there is a typical arborisation of dark pigment in the retina, particularly towards the periphery.

Agenesis or Degeneration of Cranial Nerve Nuclei

A condition which gives progressive bilateral ptosis and impairment of ocular movement in all directions was once called progressive nuclear ophthalmoplegia, but it is now apparent that in some such cases the condition is one of muscular dystrophy of the external ocular muscles. However, a similar syndrome is sometimes seen in association with cerebellar ataxia and retinal pigmentation and with abnormal mitochondria in muscle and in the cerebellum (the Kearns–Sayre syndrome). Bilateral facial paralysis present from birth (facial diplegia–Möbius' syndrome), is probably due to an agenesis of the facial nerve nuclei. Progressive nerve deafness can also be an inherited disorder, occurring either alone or in combination with other neurological manifestations.

Hereditary Spastic Paraplegia

This is a genetically determined disorder (usually dominant) in which spastic weakness of the lower limbs generally develops in early adult life and progresses slowly over many years, eventually involving the upper limbs and even the bulbar muscles. Pes cavus is usually present.

Friedreich's Ataxia

This is the most common and stereotyped of the hereditary ataxias. In addition to a spastic paraparesis, there are usually signs of cerebellar ataxia in all four limbs and also of impairment of sensation mediated through the posterior columns of the cord (absent vibration sense, impaired position and joint sense). Scoliosis and pes cavus are usual and occasionally there is amyotrophy in the legs, while there is often associated myocardial degeneration. Diabetes mellitus is seen more often in association with this condition than can be coincidental. Owing to an associated polyneuropathy the deep tendon reflexes are usually absent, even when the plantar responses are clearly extensor. There is often dysarthria of 'cerebellar' type and nystagmus is common. The condition is slowly progressive, beginning usually in childhood—the patient may be able to walk for several years but death is usual, often from heart failure, in middle-life. Frequently, apparently unaffected relatives of patients with Friedreich's disease show mild stigmata of the disease (pes cavus, scoliosis) without neurological signs, and benign varieties (formes frustes) of the syndrome are also seen occasionally, in which signs of spinal cord disease are few and the pathological process appears to become arrested.

Hereditary Cerebellar Ataxia

This is a term applied to a group of inherited disorders which are mainly characterised by a progressive and symmetrical cerebellar ataxia. In most families symptoms first appear in early adult life but sometimes the condition develops in late middle-age (late-life cerebellar ataxia). When the neurological signs indicate that the disease process is virtually limited to the cerebellum and its connexions, the condition is often referred to as delayed cortical cerebellar atrophy (*Holmes type*), but when there is associated optic atrophy, external ophthalmoplegia and spastic parapare-sis, without skeletal deformity, a diagnosis of the *Sanger–Brown variety* is often made. *Marie's cerebellar ataxia* is characterised by a combination of signs of ataxia and pyramidal tract dysfunction. If, in addition to cerebellar ataxia, there are also dementia, a titubating tremor of the head, static tremor of the limbs and a spastic paraplegia, then this clinical picture is typical of *olivo-pontocerebellar atrophy*. The *Roussy–Levy* syndrome is a name given to a syndrome of hereditary areflexia which is sometimes accompanied by cerebellar ataxia and pes cavus and by peripheral amyotrophy. Recent evidence suggests that most cases of the Roussy–Levy syndrome are closely related to, if not identical with, the hypertrophic form of peroneal muscular atrophy. It seems likely that many of these disorders of cerebellar function are interrelated. These disorders develop-ing in middle or late life must be distinguished from the variety of cerebellar degeneration which may complicate malignant disease in the lung or elsewhere (*see* p. 338). Yet another variety of familial cerebellar ataxia may be associated with consistent amino-aciduria, and may well be due to some specific but as yet unidentified metabolic disorder (*Hartnup disease*). A rare disorder, entitled *ataxia telangiectasia* (the Louis–Bar syndrome) is characterised by ataxia developing in childhood and by telangiectasia in the conjunctiva and skin. The patients show a deficiency of serum γ-globulin and usually die from respiratory infection in adolescence.

Hereditary Sensory Neuropathy

While symptoms and signs of dysfunction of the posterior columns of the spinal cord and a mild neuropathy are common in Friedreich's ataxia, there is a more severe inherited disorder of sensory pathways in which the principal pathological change is one of degeneration in posterior root ganglia. The appreciation of pain and temperature sense and of touch and position are greatly impaired, particularly in the lower limbs, so that perforating ulcers of the feet, disorganisation of joints (Charcot-type arthropathy) and eventual destruction of terminal phalanges (Morvan's syndrome) are common. The condition bears a superficial resemblance to syringomyelia, in which, however, sensory loss of dissociated type (*see below*) is generally confined to the upper limbs.

Peroneal Muscular Atrophy (Charcot–Marie–Tooth Disease)
This is in many ways the most benign of the hereditary degenerative nervous diseases, for despite the gross muscular atrophy and weakness which affect particularly the muscles of the foot and leg below the knee, and later, as a rule, the small muscles of the hands, sufferers generally remain active for many years and even into late adult life. The condition is due to changes in motor neurones, nerve roots or peripheral nerves, so that it is properly regarded as a neuropathy. Yet the involvement is curiously localised, for in the upper limb the muscular atrophy rarely advances beyond the forearm, while in the lower limbs it affects the legs and distal one-third of the thighs but spreads no further (the inverted champagne-bottle leg). Bilateral foot drop and claw hands are characteristic and the appreciation of vibration is absent at the ankles in some cases, but there is little else to find, as a rule, on sensory examination. The condition appears to occur in three forms which are probably distinct, both clinically and genetically. In most families the condition is inherited as an autosomal recessive trait, but it is occasionally dominant, and rarely X-linked. The commonest and most benign variety is due to a hypertrophic demyelinating neuropathy in which nerve conduction is greatly slowed. There is also an axonal variety which is often more severe and less strictly confined to distal muscles, while in occasional families this clinical syndrome seems to be due to distal spinal muscular atrophy, the primary pathological change being one of the anterior horn cells. Dyck and Lambert have identified these three sub-varieties as hereditary motor and sensory neuropathy, types I, II and III.

Progressive Hypertrophic Interstitial Polyneuropathy (Dejerine–Sottas)
This is another hereditary disease of early onset in which the distribution of the muscular involvement is similar to that seen in peroneal muscular atrophy, though there is often more extensive peripheral sensory impairment. Furthermore, the peripheral nerves (the ulnar and the common peroneal are easiest to feel) are often greatly enlarged, due to proliferation of the Schwann cells, which form concentric layers around the nerve fibres in an 'onion-skin' manner. The condition is similar to peroneal muscular atrophy but usually runs a more rapid course.

In this short account of the so-called hereditary ataxias, no attempt has been made to cover the ground comprehensively, but it is important to realise that although some such conditions breed true, many atypical and transitional forms appear; there are also sporadic cases which do not at first sight seem to fit into any single category of neurological disease. Prognosis and management become more straightforward once it is found that such a case belongs to the hereditary ataxia group.

Parkinsonism

Parkinsonism, or 'the shaking palsy', as first described by James Parkinson in 1817, is a common degenerative nervous disorder. It occurs in two principal forms, namely **paralysis agitans** ('idiopathic' Parkinsonism), and **post-encephalitic** Parkinsonism which develops as a sequel of encephalitis lethargica. Similar clinical manifestations can result from cerebral atherosclerosis, from head injury (as in the punch-drunk boxer), from neurosyphilis and from poisoning with carbon monoxide or manganese, but in such cases the resemblance to typical Parkinson's disease is generally superficial. The syndrome of so-called **atherosclerotic Parkinsonism** usually occurs in elderly hypertensive patients; facial masking and progressive stiffness of the limbs and a shuffling gait may develop but tremor is not seen, the plantar responses often become extensor, dementia commonly supervenes and many patients eventually develop signs of 'pseudobulbar palsy' due to progressive cerebral and brain-stem softening. In both paralysis agitans and the post-encephalitic variety, the maximal site of pathological change is in the substantia nigra of the mid-brain.

The clinical features of the two varieties of the disease are broadly similar, differing only in detail, but the post-encephalitic variety is now rare as most survivors of the epidemic of encephalitis lethargica which occurred in the 1920's have died. For instance, the age of onset was generally earlier and the rate of progress of the disorder more rapid in postencephalitic Parkinsonism; in this variety, too, rigidity was often more striking than tremor, while in paralysis agitans the reverse is usually the case. Limb contractures and deformity and dystonic features (*see* p. 203) were seen in some post-encephalitic but not in idiopathic cases. Oculogyric crises (*see below*) occurred only in the post-encephalitic variety, while in this type mental symptoms such as emotional lability, dementia, or even psychotic features including paranoia and delusions, were more common. Paralysis agitans is commoner in men than women, and usually develops after the age of 50, while in postencephalitic cases an onset in early adult life and even in childhood was once frequent, following almost immediately upon the acute encephalitic illness. New post-encephalitic cases are now very rare since the virtual disappearance of encephalitis lethargica, but it is possible that a few cases of Parkinsonism which have developed in recent years may nevertheless be the sequel of a mild encephalitis occurring many years ago, or of an unrecognised, more recent, sporadic outbreak of the disease, different in its clinical presentation from the classical variety.

The typical clinical features of Parkinsonism include disorders of facial expression, posture, gait, attitude and movement, and also rigidity and tremor. The recognition of early paralysis agitans can be very difficult, even for the most skilled clinician. It has been said that in some cases the diagnosis will easily be missed despite meticulous examination unless it is made as the patient enters the room. And sometimes the condition begins unilaterally with clumsiness of one hand and slight dragging of one leg. When tremor is inconspicuous it is easy to overlook the correct diagnosis in such a case, unless one recalls that Parkinsonism often gives a slowly progressive hemiparetic syndrome in late middle-age.

The immobile, unblinking **facial expression** of the established case is characteristic; if the disorder is more severe there may be a trickle of saliva from the mouth. Tapping above the bridge of the nose often gives rhythmical blinking which continues indefinitely in time with the taps (glabellar tap sign). The speech may be slow, quiet and monotonous. Usually, too, the patient is slightly stooped; he walks with quick, shuffling steps as if constantly about to fall forwards while chasing his own centre of gravity **(the festinant gait)**. Typically there is a deficiency of associated movements; swinging of the arms when walking, is notably impaired. Characteristically the patient will say that he has become greatly slowed in all his activities and that fine movements carried out with the affected hand or hands have become more clumsy; usually the handwriting has become much smaller **(micrographia)**. Also characteristic is **akinesia** (difficulty in initiating movement). Thus the patient may be unable to begin walking for several seconds as his feet seem frozen to the floor; or he might be incapable of rising from a chair or of getting out of bed or out of the bath unaided. **Bradykinesia** is a term often used to indicate slowness of movement. One of the earliest signs in the limbs may be a reduced range and amplitude of movement, well shown by asking the patient to carry out repeated opposition of the thumb and individual fingers of an affected hand. Less typically, occasional patients show intolerable restlessness **(akathisia)**.

The **muscular rigidity** of Parkinson's disease varies greatly in distribution and severity. In one case it may be mild and localised, affecting only one arm and leg, in another profound and generalised, rendering the patient mute and virtually immobile. Typically it affects flexor and extensor muscles equally, unlike spasticity, and it can be of the plastic or 'lead-pipe' variety or else 'cog-wheel' in type. Often the tendon reflexes are increased in moderately rigid limbs; contractures of the fingers and feet may occur in advanced post-encephalitic cases.

Tremor, of the static type, is the typical involuntary movement of Parkinsonism. It is most evident in one or both hands and/or feet but may involve the head, lips and other mid-line structures. Usually it is abolished by voluntary movement, but may persist while the movement is performed (action tremor). It is typically rhythmical and sometimes of pill-rolling type, occurring four to eight times a second and generally being accentuated by stress and excitement.

The **oculogyric crises** of the post-encephalitic form consist of attacks of involuntary conjugate upward movement of the eyes, with retraction of the upper lids; sometimes the head tilts backwards (retrocollis) and the patient may fall. The attacks are distressing and difficult to control.

Sensory disorders are not seen in the Parkinsonian syndrome, but **autonomic disturbances** (excess salivation and sweating, retention of urine) occasionally occur. The disease is progressive but varies greatly in its clinical course. The more severely affected post-encephalitic patient can be totally disabled and bed-ridden within a few years from the onset, but, with few exceptions, paralysis agitans is much more benign and patients may live reasonably active lives, but with increasing restrictions, for many years. The prognosis is less good in paralysis agitans when akinesia and severe rigidity develop early; the course of the disease in cases presenting first with tremor is usually less rapid. The lot of the patient with this disease, has, however, been greatly alleviated by the many new drugs and surgical procedures which have been introduced recently (*see* Chapter 20, p. 446).

Syringomyelia

Syringomyelia is a slowly progressive disorder in which cavitation develops within the central grey matter of the spinal cord, sometimes extending into the lower brain stem **(syringobulbia)**. This cavitation usually occurs in the cervical cord and may extend over many segments from the lower medulla into the upper dorsal region. Similar changes in the lumbar region rarely occur; they may develop above a complete or incomplete transection of the cord (post-traumatic syringomyelia) or in relation to an intra-medullary tumour. The disorder is usually sporadic, though rare familial cases have been described; it is commoner in males than in females and is generally first apparent clinically between the ages of 20 and 40 years.

Maldevelopment or incomplete closure of the central canal of the cord was once thought to be responsible for this condition. Sometimes the syringomyelic cavity is separate from the central canal; it is occupied by clear gelatinous material, is not lined by ependyma, and is surrounded by an area of gliosis. However, it has long been known that a true dilatation of the central canal or hydromyelia, with similar clinical effects, may develop in a patient with a cervical cord tumour, basilar impression, or other congenital abnormalities in this region. Indeed, recent evidence, based largely upon supine myelographic studies, indicates that in most cases syringomyelia is associated with a Chiari anomaly with descent of the cerebellar tonsils into the upper cervical canal. Occasionally the mechanism responsible is an arachnoiditis around the foramen magnum. In either event the exit foramina of the fourth ventricle are blocked so that the pressure wave of CSF passing downwards in the fourth ventricle enters the central canal of the cord and dilates it instead of spreading laterally into the subarachnoid space. Diverticula from the central canal may form and dissect downwards in the central grey matter; this is why the syringomyelic cavity sometimes seems to lie alongside a normal central canal in the lower cervical region.

Since the centrally-situated cavity interrupts the decussating sensory fibres carrying pain and temperature sensation which are destined to ascend in the spinothalamic tract, the most prominent clinical feature of syringomyelia is dissociated anaesthesia (loss or impairment of pain and temperature sensation with preservation of light touch, position and joint sense and tactile discrimination). The cavity may also extend anteriorly to destroy anterior horn cells and laterally to compress the pyramidal and spinothalamic tracts. The posterior columns are usually affected late in the course of the disease if at all. In the brain stem the motor nuclei of the lower cranial nerves and the spinal tract and nucleus of the trigeminal nerve are commonly involved.

The onset of the disease is typically insidious. The first symptoms are usually sensory; the patient may notice numbness of a part of one hand or becomes aware that injuries to the hand are no longer painful. Sometimes aching or burning pain is felt in the limb. Less commonly the earliest manifestations are those of progressive weakness of a hand, with inability to extend the fingers, and flexion contracture soon develops. Often the symptoms and signs are unilateral for some time.

Dissociated anaesthesia is often found initially in a part of the hand or forearm, or else it may form a 'half-cape' over the shoulder and upper arm with a sharp line of demarcation at the midline and horizontally across the upper chest wall. Eventually the whole of one arm and a 'cape' area is affected and later still the sensory loss may become bilateral. Not infrequently the upper cervical segments are also involved to give hypalgesia and thermoanaesthesia over the neck and scalp; the forehead may then become analgesic or else the sensory loss shows a 'balaclava helmet' distribution, with only the more central portions of the face being sensitive. Similar sensory impairment is uncommon in the lower trunk and in the lower limbs; when it does occur it is generally more patchy in distribution, resulting from compression of the spinothalamic tract in the cervical region. Only rarely is it due to a lumbar syrinx. Destruction of anterior horn cells causes **wasting and weakness of upper limb muscles**, often with some fasciculation. Usually the small muscles of the hands are first involved, but later the upper arm and shoulder girdle are affected. Extension of the disease process to the brain stem results in nystagmus, atrophy of the tongue and/or the sternomastoids, weakness of palatal, pharyngeal and laryngeal muscles, and occasionally a Horner's syndrome develops. Compression of the pyramidal tracts in the cervical region eventually leads to **spastic weakness of the lower limbs** with increased deep reflexes and extensor plantar responses; impaired vibration sense and position and joint sense in the lower limbs are less common, but sometimes appear in advanced cases.

Trophic changes, resulting in the main from impaired pain sensation, are often striking. The affected hand is brawny and swollen with multiple scars resulting from previous trauma; indolent ulcers frequently follow minor injury. Disorganisation of joints (Charcot's arthropathy) often occurs, particularly in the shoulder or elbow and swelling of the joint with gross but painless crepitus on movement will then be apparent. In severe cases, actual necrosis of terminal phalanges is rarely seen (Morvan's syndrome). Straight radiographs of the cervical spine and myelography often demonstrate widening of the spinal cord and cervical bony canal in such cases, as well as cerebellar tonsillar descent. Sometimes there are associated congenital abnormalities (e.g. fusion of the bodies of several cervical vertebrae).

In general, syringomyelia is a relatively benign disorder. Progression is usually slow and the disease process often seems to become arrested for many years, although occasional cases deteriorate more quickly. Death usually results in the end from an unrelated disease, though bulbar paralysis may be responsible for fatal bronchopneumonia. Treatment in the past was largely symptomatic. Recent work has clearly indicated that when a Chiari anomaly is demonstrated myelographically, surgical decompression of the upper cervical cord and at the foramen magnum, if carried out sufficiently early in the course of the disease, can produce striking improvement; in some cases all the symptoms and signs have resolved completely.

Spina Bifida

Incomplete closure of the vertebral canal can be associated with many abnormalities in the underlying spinal cord and in the roots of the cauda equina. In severe cases there is a protruding sac containing the meninges and the termination of the spinal cord and cauda equina (meningo-myelocele). In such cases there is a soft swelling over the lumbosacral area, the legs are generally paralysed from birth, there may be associated cerebral abnormalities (hydrocephalus, the Arnold–Chiari malformation) and the condition often proved in the past to be incompatible with prolonged survival. However, it has been shown that the survival rate is greatly increased and subsequent disability may be markedly reduced by operative closure of the sac within the first 48 hours of life. Subsequently, hydrocephalus and limb deformities may require surgical treatment and bladder and bowel training can present serious difficulties; nervertheless the quality of life achieved by many such children is better than was ever anticipated in the past.

The criteria for the selection of cases for early surgery are still, however, a matter of dispute. There is some hope that estimation of alpha-fetoprotein in the amniotic fluid, or less certainly, in the blood, may help in the antenatal diagnosis of neural tube defects, thus allowing therapeutic abortion before the affected fetus is viable.

In spina bifida occulta there is generally no palpable swelling and the bony defect is only apparent on X-ray. Many individuals with such a congenital defect are symptom-free throughout life, but others are late in walking. Subsequently a variety of neurological abnormalities may develop, varying from mild pes cavus and some precipitancy of micturition on the one hand to severe disorders of urinary, faecal and sexual function with muscular weakness, wasting and sensory loss in the legs and perineal area of variable degree on the other. These symptoms are due to disordered function of the nerve roots of the cauda equina; in many such cases of **spinal dysraphism** treatment can only be symptomatic, but in some it is possible to divide surgically a fibrocartilaginous band constricting roots within the spinal canal or to remove an associated intraspinal cyst or lipoma of congenital origin. Hence in such a case, clinical deterioration is generally an indication for investigation, including myelography. It is now evident that in some children with atrophy or deformity of one foot, with or without localised reflex changes and/or sensory loss, minor forms of dysraphism may be found and are always associated with some degree of occult spina bifida. Occasionally this mild form of the condition first produces symptoms in adolescence or adult life and in these patients, too, surgery may be helpful.

Myelodysplasia (Diastematomyelia)

This developmental anomaly of the lower spinal cord, which is probably due to an incomplete closure of the neural tube in the embryo, gives symptoms which are similar to those of spina bifida occulta, with which it is usually associated. The clinical picture is in some respects like that of lumbar syringomyelia, but the condition is non-progressive. Pes cavus, muscular weakness and wasting and sensory loss in the lower limbs of variable extent are generally combined with sphincter disturbances (intermittent urinary and faecal incontinence).

Basilar Impression of the Skull

A congenital malformation of the occipital condyles of the skull can lead to the partial invagination of the first cervical vertebra into the foramen magnum. This generally results in an upward movement of the odontoid process of the axis with consequent compression of the lower cranial nerves, cerebellar tonsils, upper cervical nerve roots and the upper part of the spinal cord. In such individuals the neck is unusually short and there are typical radiological appearances. Thus the body of the atlas vertebra is tilted in relation to the skull and in lateral skull radiographs the tip of the odontoid process extends above a line drawn from the posterior margin of the hard palate to the posterior border of the foramen magnum (Chamberlain's line). The clinical features are variable in degree and severity, but include hydrocephalus (due to partial obstruction of CSF circulation through exit foramina of the fourth ventricle and basal cisterns), cerebellar ataxia in the limbs, and a spastic quadriparesis with posterior column involvement often giving severe loss of position and joint sense in both hands. Sometimes syringomyelia also develops. The clinical features of the condition can be mimicked by separation of the odontoid process from the axis vertebra, an occasional complication of rheumatoid arthritis. Once symptoms and signs have appeared they tend to progress, but the condition may be alleviated by surgical decompression, involving removal of the posterior border of the foramen magnum. The syndrome is often called platybasia, as the skull base is flattened, but there are other causes of radiological platybasia (e.g. Paget's disease—*see below*). Basilar impression may be associated with congenital anomalies of the cervical spine (e.g. fusion of multiple cervical vertebrae—the Klippel–Feil syndrome), while such anomalies in turn can be associated with features suggesting a lesion in the neighbourhood of the foramen magnum, even when no significant degree of basilar impression is present. Mirror movements (a voluntary movement in one hand is copied involuntarily by the other) are common in cases of the latter type.

Paget's Disease and Other Skeletal Abnormalities

The progressive thickening and distortion of bone which occurs in Paget's disease of the skull can produce neurological manifestations. Thus optic atrophy may result from compression of the optic nerves in their exit foramina and other cranial nerves can be similarly involved. As a result of the platybasia caused by the disease, a clinical picture resembling basilar impression may develop. Other rare bony disorders which may give rise to overgrowth of skull and facial bones with consequent cranial nerve palsies include **leontiasis ossea** and **polyostotic fibrous dysplasia**. Paget's disease of the vertebral column is occasionally responsible for a progressive paraplegia due to spinal cord compression and a similar syndrome occurs infrequently in **achondroplasia**.

Craniostenosis

This is an uncommon congenital abnormality due to premature fusion of the cranial bony sutures. It is characterised by an abnormal shape of the skull, optic atrophy, exophthalmos, and signs of increased intracranial pressure. Neurosurgical treatment (separation of the fused cranial bones) is often required early in life.

Facial Hemiatrophy

This uncommon disorder of unknown aetiology (often called the Parry–Romberg syndrome) gives rise to a progressive atrophy of subcutaneous tissue, muscle, bone, and cartilage on one half of the face. Occasionally there is associated atrophy of the ipsilateral cerebral hemisphere.

Vascular Malformations

Many developmental vascular anomalies of the nervous system have been described. The intracranial **arteriovenous angioma**, which is one of the commonest, will be considered in Chapter 17. A similar anomaly is occasionally found in the spinal cord; here too, malformations and dilatations of the smaller blood vessels (**telangiectases**) sometimes occur, and may give rise to intramedullary haemorrhage with consequent clinical symptoms.

One unusual but stereotyped cerebral vascular malformation is the **Sturge–Weber syndrome**. In this condition a subcortical angiomatosis of precapillaries, a lesion which eventually becomes calcified after a few years of life to give a characteristic radiological pattern outlining the gyri of the posterior part of one cerebral hemisphere, is associated with a port-wine naevus of the face on the same side. Often the eye on this side is also enlarged (buphthalmos or ox-eye). Usually these patients show a contralateral infantile hemiplegia and suffer from recurrent epileptiform convulsions. Some cases can be helped by removal of most of the affected cerebral hemisphere (hemispherectomy).

Neuromuscular and Muscular Disorders

In addition to the conditions considered in this chapter, there are many neuromuscular and muscular disorders which are clearly genetically-determined. These conditions, including the muscular dystrophies, will be considered in Chapter 18.

References

Barnett, H. J. M., Foster, J. B. and Hudgson, P., *Syringomyelia and Other Cord Cavities*, Major Problems in Neurology, No. 1 (London and Philadelphia, Saunders, 1973).

Calne, D. B., *Parkinsonism* (London, Arnold, 1970).

Ford, F. R., *Diseases of the Nervous System in Infancy, Childhood and Adolescence*, 6th ed., Chapters 1 and 2 (Springfield, Ill., Thomas, 1973).

Gamstorp, I., *Paediatric Neurology* (London, Butterworth, 1970).

Gordon, N. *Paediatric Neurology for the Clinician* (Spastics International Medical Publications, London, Heinemann, 1976).

Holt, K. S., *Assessment of Cerebral Palsy* (London, Lloyd-Luke, 1965).

Ingram, T. T. S., *Paediatric Aspects of Cerebral Palsy* (Edinburgh, Livingstone, 1964).

James, C. C. M. and Lassman, L. P., *Spinal Dysraphism* (London, Butterworths, 1972).

Menkes, J. H., *Child Neurology*, 2nd ed. (Philadelphia, Lea and Febiger, 1980).

Tyler, H. R. and Dawson, D. M. (Ed.), *Current Neurology*, Volume 2 (Boston, Houghton Mifflin, 1979).

Walton, J. N., *Brain's Diseases of the Nervous System*, 8th ed. (London, Oxford University Press, 1977).

13 Trauma and the Nervous System

The function of the various parts of the central and peripheral nervous system can be gravely disturbed by physical injury. Although penetrating wounds of the brain, spinal cord and peripheral nerves are often seen in war-time, they are relatively uncommon in civil practice. Nevertheless, closed head injuries (in which the skull is not penetrated), resulting in the main from road and industrial accidents, are a major problem. Although the finer points of diagnosis and management in cases of severe craniocerebral injury are largely a matter for the specialist neuro-surgeon, every physician, accident surgeon and general practitioner re-quires a working knowledge of the nosology of the different types of head injury, of their clinical course and of their sequelae. To refer all patients with minor head injuries for neurosurgical advice would impose an impossible load upon these special units and it is essential that the physician or surgeon who may care for these cases initially should be able to recognise major complications. It may also be difficult to decide in an individual case whether neurological symptoms and signs have resulted from a head injury or whether the initial event had been a cerebral vascular accident, say, due to which the patient had fallen and injured the head. The clinical syndromes produced by injury to or compression of the spinal cord and peripheral nerves can also present difficult problems in diagnosis and management. This chapter will therefore deal first with head injuries, their effects, complications and sequelae, secondly with injury to the spinal cord, and thirdly with peripheral nerve lesions.

Head Injuries

The immediate effects of head injury may be classified into three principal groups which are first, concussion, a temporary and largely reversible disorder of brain function which is not apparently associated with any striking pathological change in the brain; secondly, cerebral contusion or laceration, in which there is direct bruising or tearing of brain tissue; and thirdly, intracranial haemorrhage, either from tearing of the middle meningeal artery or its branches following skull fracture (extradural haemorrhage), subdural haematoma, which results from an injury to veins traversing the subdural space, and intracerebral haemorrhage or traumatic subarachnoid haemorrhage which often accompany cerebral contusion or laceration.

Concussion

There have been many attempts to explain the phenomenon of concussion; this produces the syndrome of impaired consciousness which follows upon a closed head injury. Probably it is due to a transitory disturbance of function in the brain stem reticular substance. Concussion may occur with or without skull fracture. Uncomplicated concussion most often results from blunt head injuries but even these may be found to have caused unexpected areas of focal brain haemorrhage or laceration, particularly in elderly patients suffering relatively minor blows on the head producing little or no impairment of consciousness. Depressed fractures of the skull (such as those produced by sharp, localised blows resulting, say, from a missile) may be associated with severe local brain injury but yet consciousness may not be lost. Extensive linear skull fractures are sometimes found in patients showing only the clinical features of concussion; on the other hand they too can be associated with contusion or laceration (*see below*) of the subjacent brain.

The patient who recovers from concussion is usually unable to recall the actual moment of injury and indeed his memory may be blank for several preceding seconds or much longer. The duration of this **retrograde amnesia** is not a satisfactory guide to the severity of the injury; much more reliable in this respect is the duration of the **post-traumatic amnesia** (i.e. the period for which memory is lost after the accident, corresponding to the duration of the concussion). Usually this period is very much longer than that of observed unconsciousness. After a relatively severe injury the patient may be comatose with shallow, slow respiration, a feeble pulse, and widely dilated pupils; during recovery, after minutes or even several hours the pupils react, the pulse becomes stronger and the patient responsive. For some time, however, he is restless, confused and irritable, complains of headache and may vomit repeatedly, When coma is complete for more than a few hours it is likely that the injury has been more serious than simple concussion. Following a less severe injury the patient may merely be dazed for some minutes or hours and may undertake purposive activities of which he subsequently has no recollection; generalised headache and vomiting are usual at this stage. Most patients recover from mild or moderate concussion within a few days or weeks, but headaches and other symptoms of the post-traumatic syndrome (*see below*) sometimes persist for weeks or months and occasionally for years.

Contusion and Laceration

Cerebral contusion may take the form of localised bruising of the brain directly beneath the point of impact in a closed head injury. Alternatively, a contusion, or a laceration, which can be similarly produced, though it can, of course, result from a penetrating wound, may occur on the side of the brain opposite to the site of injury, due to a sudden thrust of the relatively mobile brain against the inner table of the skull (contrecoup injury). The term contusion has also been applied to a generalised cerebral disturbance more severe than concussion in which there are multiple small intracerebral haemorrhages as well as diffuse cerebral oedema, changes which result at least in part from a sudden violent movement of CSF along perivascular meningeal cuffs which penetrate the brain along the blood vessels. Doubts have indeed been expressed as to whether this form of diffuse pathological change can be distinguished from the wholly reversible phenomenon of concussion. Probably mild and transient concussion on the one hand and this more severe form of pathological change (which may lead to irreversible demyelination in central cerebral white matter and other degenerative changes in the cortex) on the other, represent the two extremes of a continuum of severity. In the more severe cases the diffuse oedema which often develops immediately after the injury can be reduced by drugs (*see* p. 453).

The patient with a severe cerebral contusion is usually unconscious immediately, but becomes progressively more deeply comatose until he dies from respiratory and later cardiac arrest due to brain stem haemorrhage or infarction or medullary compression. Some patients remain unconscious and unresponsive but can nevertheless be kept alive for many weeks or months by careful nursing and sometimes assisted respiration. Usually in patients who show no significant recovery of awareness within a week from the time of injury there has been a degree of damage to the cerebral white matter or to the brain stem reticular substance which is incompatible with complete recovery; in rare instances, however, patients have recovered, though with considerable intellectual impairment, after months of unconsciousness. In less severely injured cases, there is often a period of several days during which the patient is comatose or semicomatose. There may be signs indicating damage to the brain stem (decerebrate posture and spasms, cranial nerve palsies) or to one or other cerebral hemisphere (focal convulsions, or hemiplegia), though these are often difficult to identify while the patient is unconscious. With returning awareness comes the stage of traumatic delirium, in which the patient may be noisy, unco-operative, confused and even violent. It is at this stage that symptoms or signs of focal brain damage often become apparent. Gradually, as improvement continues, the patient becomes more rational and orientated, though headache commonly persists, and symptoms of the post-traumatic syndrome appear. There may also be persisting aphasia, paralysis or cranial nerve palsies if the local injury has been sufficiently severe. If the cranial nerve injuries have been due to tearing of nerve trunks owing to skull fracture involving their exit foramina (as may occur particularly with the facial, auditory, abducent and optic nerves) the injury is often permanent. A sixth-nerve paralysis can occur, however, as a transient phenomenon following a relatively mild head injury, usually being a false localising sign due to cerebral oedema. Occasionally during the recovery phase, a Korsakoff syndrome (*see* p. 120) develops, but soon resolves. In other cases the initial injury has been so severe, and damage so widespread, that permanent intellectual impairment, or traumatic dementia, results. The so-called traumatic encephalopathy or **punch-drunk syndrome** of professional boxers, in which there is usually deterioration of memory and intellect, with tremor and slowness or poverty of movement resembling that of Parkinson's disease, is probably due to the cumulative effect of many episodes of cerebral contusion. In such cases a CAT scan or air encephalography may demonstrate absence of the septum pellucidum. A similar syndrome has been described in steeplechase jockeys.

Intracranial Haemorrhage

Multiple small intracerebral haemorrhages may be due, as already mentioned, to cerebral contusion, and sometimes more extensive and focal bleeding into brain tissue follows injury. It is also common to find bleeding into the subarachnoid space after a closed head injury, particularly if the skull has been fractured. It is, however, those haemorrhages into the extradural and subdural spaces, in which bleeding can continue for some time after injury, that are particularly important to recognise, as these require specific treatment.

An acute **extradural haematoma** can follow any head injury in which there has been a fracture of the skull vault involving one of the channels on the inner table in which lies the middle meningeal artery or one of its branches. Typically in such a case there is a concussive head injury of moderate severity with recovery of consciousness within a few minutes or hours. For an hour or two the patient may then be reasonably alert, but subsequently he becomes increasingly drowsy and lapses into coma. In some such cases, signs of compression of one cerebral hemisphere (contralateral hemiparesis, homolateral fixed dilated pupil or third-nerve palsy, due to cerebral herniation and compression of the third nerve at the edge of the tentorium cerebelli) may develop. There are many cases in which no lucid interval occurs, and in which diagnosis must depend upon progressive deepening of unconsciousness following the injury. Early diagnosis is imperative as operation is usually curative; otherwise death soon results from brain stem compression and infarction.

An acute **subdural haematoma** is another complication of head injury, resulting from rupture of veins which traverse the subdural space. When this condition develops acutely, as it may after severe trauma at any age, the clinical picture differs little from that of extradural haemorrhage, but the prognosis, even after evacuation, is poor. It is cases of subacute or chronic subdural haematoma which more often present baffling diagnostic problems, but their recognition is equally important as the condition may readily be treated neurosurgically; if unrecognised it is eventually fatal. Chronic subdural bleeding generally occurs in elderly patients in whom the subdural veins are fragile; it can follow a trivial injury, such as jarring the head or a minor knock, and sometimes seems to occur spontaneously. 'Spontaneous' subdural bleeding is particularly common in patients receiving long-term anticoagulant therapy or in those with chronic liver disease. Typically the injury has no immediate ill-effects, but over the succeeding days or weeks the patient complains of vague headache, intermittent drowsiness and lapses of memory. There may be episodes of confusion, lack of attention to detail, failure of concentration, and long periods of apathy. Transient severe headache induced by change in posture, coughing or exertion is a notable feature in some cases, but by no means all. Drowsiness, headache and sometimes vomiting become progressively more severe, and the patient eventually lapses into stupor, intermittent mutism or even semicoma. Commonly the conscious level fluctuates, lucid intervals alternating with periods of confusion or stupor. Focal neurological signs, Jacksonian epilepsy, dilatation of the homolateral pupil and papilloedema can result, and eventually respiration and cardiac function are impaired. The CSF is often xanthochromic but contains no blood. The EEG may be helpful, revealing unilateral suppression of the alpha rhythm or else unilateral slow activity, while radiographs of the skull or echoencephalography sometimes demonstrate a shift of the pineal gland and of other mid-line structures. The CAT scan or carotid arteriography give diagnostic appearances. Evacuation of the clot generally leads to complete recovery.

Complications and Sequelae

Infection is an important complication of head injury. When a fracture of the skull is accompanied by scalp wounds, cranial osteomyelitis, which can lead to extradural suppuration, is an important complication, while penetrating wounds carry the risk of infection of the meninges (meningitis) or of the brain tissue itself (suppurative encephalitis, cerebral abscess). Even when there is no wound of the scalp a skull fracture may involve the paranasal sinuses or middle ear. Organisms can then pass through a tear in the dura mater, giving rise to meningitis; this complication should always be considered if there has been bleeding or leakage of CSF from the ears or nose and there may then be an indication for antibiotic therapy, followed later by surgical repair of the dural tear. Such a fistula should be suspected if clear watery fluid drips from the nose, particularly when leaning forwards; the fluid can be shown to contain glucose by appropriate tests and the fistula may then be localised by isotope ventriculography (*see* p. 54). In such cases air may enter the cranial cavity and even the cerebral substance, producing an encysted collection or **aerocele**. This can cause recurrent infection if a communication with the sinus or middle ear persists, Jacksonian epilepsy, or symptoms and signs of an intracranial space-occupying lesion.

The commonest cause of **post-traumatic epilepsy** is, however, a focal cerebral contusion or laceration which, having healed by the formation of a scar, may adhere to the inner surface of the dura. If the scar is large it can produce a cystic evagination of the lateral ventricle (traumatic porencephaly). The incidence of epilepsy is greater after penetrating wounds of the skull; between 25 and 35 per cent of such patients develop fits as a sequel (these figures, however, are derived from cases of gunshot wound, and in civil practice the incidence is lower). After closed head injuries in which there has been no clinical evidence of localised injury to the brain, between 2 and 5 per cent of cases have seizures, but after severe contusion the proportion is probably higher. These usually begin between six months and one year after the injury, but occasionally not for several years. Commonly the fits are of Jacksonian type, and then the clinical features depend upon which area of the brain has been injured; in other cases in which, presumably, the epileptic discharge spreads rapidly throughout the brain, major convulsions are the rule. Usually treatment with anticonvulsant drugs is indicated, but rarely, depending upon its site, surgical excision of a cortical scar can be considered. It is a good general rule to assume that, except in childhood and possibly in the elderly, when fits may occasionally follow a relatively minor head injury, no brain injury giving rise to post-traumatic amnesia of less than 24 hours' duration is likely to be followed by genuine post-traumatic epilepsy. The incidence of late epilepsy is higher in those individuals who have had fits (early post-traumatic epilepsy) in the first week after the injury.

The post-traumatic syndrome is a name applied to a constellation of disabling symptoms which may follow head injury. It is most common and persistent following cases of severe cerebral contusion and in these it may accompany post-traumatic dementia. Following simple concussion it is generally mild and of brief duration, but much depends upon the individual's premorbid personality. Whereas the condition clearly has an organic basis, emotional factors may be responsible for its exaggeration and perpetuation. Patients of good personality may recover quickly even after severe trauma, while those of less stable constitution are often considerably disabled for some time after a relatively trivial injury. The problem of financial compensation can greatly complicate prognosis and management and it is uncommon for a post-traumatic syndrome to improve while a medico-legal action is pending. The characteristic features of the condition are first, headache, which is often persistent or paroxysmally severe; it is generally felt in the frontal and/or occipital regions, is most severe in the mornings, and is accentuated by coughing or by movement. Secondly, defects of memory and concentration and lack of interest are usual, as are periods of depression or anxiety and episodes of fear, panic or depersonalisation. Diminished tolerance of alcohol is common. Commonly, too, there is a complaint of giddiness or instability, which is not always true vertigo though the latter often occurs, particularly after sudden changes in the position of the head. Post-traumatic postural vertigo, a self-limiting disorder which may last for one or two years and which resembles benign positional vertigo, appears to be due to damage to the utricle and saccule of the internal ear. Syncopal attacks, accompanied by hysterical manifestations in some cases, are also frequent and are sometimes difficult to distinguish from post-traumatic epilepsy. These symptoms can persist for many weeks or months, and may even in occasional cases be permanent in some degree, but many patients recover completely in from six months to two years after the injury. The symptoms are nevertheless distressing and many subjects show considerable personality change from their premorbid state; appropriate management is often difficult, but reassurance and confident predictions of eventual recovery are all-important.

The Spinal Cord

The effects of a sudden penetrating injury to the spinal cord and those of cord compression are broadly similar, though certain clinical differences in effect stem from the fact that in the one case the lesion is sudden and in the other it is often more gradual.

Cord Injuries

The spinal cord may be damaged by penetrating wounds resulting from missiles but more often it is injured through indirect violence. Thus severe flexion or hyperextension injuries of the neck can injure the cord, particularly when fracture-dislocation of the spine results. Even without fracture, however, the cord may be contused; this is particularly likely to occur in the cervical region when the anteroposterior diameter of the spinal canal is reduced by cervical spondylosis which may previously have been symptomless. Falls from a height on to the feet or buttocks can also injure the spinal column and secondarily the cord. Sudden cord compression will also result from collapse and angulation of a vertebral body due, for example, to tuberculosis, a haemangioma or myeloma or a spinal metastasis.

The main pathological varieties of spinal cord injury are similar to those which affect the brain. Thus **spinal concussion** is generally a temporary but reversible disorder of function. In **spinal contusion** or bruising there are actual pathological changes including oedema and small focal haemorrhages, and the degree of eventual recovery is less complete as ascending and descending degeneration of spinal tracts takes place. **Laceration of the cord** implies an actual break in continuity which is irremediable, and symptoms resulting from such an injury show no improvement; furthermore, since penetrating wounds may cause laceration, there is the additional complication of possible infection, which may give meningitis or myelitis.

A spinal cord injury usually gives immediate flaccid paralysis and sensory loss in the limbs and trunk below the level of the lesion, with retention of urine and faeces. As spinal shock wears off, movement and sensation gradually return if the lesion is reversible, but if more severe, the patient remains paraplegic and the upper level of sensory impairment fails to recede. In such a case, reflex activity is eventually restored below the level of the lesion, the tendon reflexes become exaggerated, the plantar responses are extensor and automatic bladder and bowel activity are gradually established. Usually contractures of the hamstrings develop and there is a **paraplegia-in-flexion**, as tone is excessive in flexor muscles. Minimal cutaneous stimulation of the lower limbs often evokes painful flexor spasms which are a part of the primitive withdrawal reflex, and these are occasionally accompanied by the so called mass reflex of autonomic activity with profuse sweating below the lesion and evacuation of the bladder and bowels. Paraplegia-in-flexion usually develops after a complete or almost complete cord transection, since the reticulospinal pathways which are responsible for an extensor hypertonus corresponding to that seen in the decerebrate posture, are interrupted. In partial lesions, however, in which the injury involves predominantly the pyramidal or corticospinal tracts, this extensor hypertonus predominates, to give **paraplegia-in-extension**, and the flexor withdrawal reflex, which depends upon short spinal reflex arcs, is partially suppressed. Many other clinical syndromes may result from incomplete spinal injuries. Of these, the Brown–Séquard syndrome, resulting from cord hemisection, is an example (*see* p. 218). The prognosis of spinal cord injuries must of course depend upon the severity of the injury; symptoms of spinal concussion generally resolve within at the most four weeks after the injury. Thereafter comparatively little further recovery of function is to be expected, but remarkable degrees of adaptation are sometimes possible.

Injuries of the **cauda equina** (the spinal roots below the termination of the spinal cord) are relatively uncommon. These usually produce total paralysis of the bladder, bowels and sexual function, with flaccid paralysis of the lower limbs; the actual distribution of muscular paralysis depends upon which roots are involved. Since regeneration of these roots can occur, the prognosis of cauda equina injuries is somewhat better than that of cord injury, provided the continuity of the neurolemmal sheaths of the injured roots is preserved.

Haematomyelia and Central Cord Softening

Haematomyelia is a term which implies bleeding into the substance of the spinal cord. It can occur spontaneously in patients with bleeding disorders, or may result from small vascular malformations or telangiectases within the cord, while it rarely results from haemorrhage into a syringomyelic cavity. More often it is due to relatively minor injury to the spine. It almost always develops in the cervical region and often complicates cervical spondylosis, a condition in which there are multiple chronic central intervertebral disk protrusions. This causes narrowing of the cervical spinal canal, so that sudden hyperextension of the neck, as may occur following a sudden blow upon the forehead, produces sharp but transient compression of the spinal cord, which in turn gives rise to haematomyelia. The haemorrhage recurs as a rule in or around the central canal of the cord and can extend over several segments. Recent evidence suggests that in most such cases there is contusion and central softening of the cord without haemorrhage, but the clinical effects are similar.

As a rule, the patient with cervical haematomyelia or central cord softening experiences sudden weakness or total paralysis of all four limbs; this phase of spinal shock may pass off in a day or two, but spastic weakness of the lower limbs persists, sometimes affecting one leg more than the other if the bleeding is not entirely central and if one pyramidal tract is selectively compressed. As the bleeding or softening in the cervical cord extends into the anterior and posterior horns there is loss of the spinal reflexes innervated by the affected segments as well as atrophy and weakness of lower motor neurone type in the muscles innervated by the affected roots. Wasting of small hand muscles is particularly common. Furthermore, as in syringomyelia, decussating sensory fibres travelling to the spinothalamic tracts may be interrupted so that there is often some dissociated sensory loss in the upper limbs. If the lesion is extensive there will also be damage to the posterior columns of the cord giving impairment of position and joint sense and of vibration sense, particularly in the lower limbs.

Prognostically, much depends upon the severity and extent of the injury; substantial recovery of function can occur in the three months after the injury but some lower motor neurone weakness and dissociated sensory loss in the upper limbs may persist, with residual spasticity in the legs. And if the cervical spinal canal remains narrowed as a result of spondylosis, the spinal cord remains vulnerable and may be injured further by relatively minor trauma.

Spinal Cord Compression

Compression of the spinal cord can result from disease in the vertebral column or in the spinal canal itself. Apart from the injuries of the vertebral column which were described above, the commonest skeletal disorders to compress the cord are intervertebral disk protrusions, either acute or chronic, tuberculous spinal osteitis (Pott's disease), acute staphylococcal osteitis giving rise to extradural abscess, and primary or secondary neoplasms of the vertebral bodies. The commonest situation in which central disk prolapse compresses the cord is in the cervical region; a sudden soft protrusion of the nucleus pulposus may be responsible, but more often there are one or several chronic protrusions which have become calcified to produce bony hard ridges between the vertebrae (cervical spondylosis) and the clinical picture is one of slowly progressive spinal cord disease (**cervical myelopathy**). In patients with Pott's disease, now rare in Western countries but once most common in children and young people, a paraplegia often develops abruptly; this often occurs, too, in older patients when a metastasis in a vertebral body causes a pathological fracture with sudden collapse and angulation. In spinal extradural abscess (*see* p. 282) there is usually acute spinal tenderness and the patient is usually febrile. This condition is a neurosurgical emergency; indeed it must be stressed that any syndrome of rapidly progressive weakness of the lower limbs requires immediate investigation in a specialised neurological or neurosurgical centre. Primary neoplasms of the vertebrae (osteoma, haemangioma, myeloma) and Paget's disease (osteitis deformans) usually give a more slowly progressive clinical picture. Conditions within the spinal theca which may compress the cord include arachnoiditis due to syphilis or to chronic trauma, extra- and intra- medullary neoplasms (*see* Chap. 16), meningeal deposits of neoplastic tissue or of a reticulosis, and exceptionally, congenital fibrous bands or developmental cysts (which are sometimes associated with spina bifida) or parasitic cysts.

The **clinical features** of spinal cord compression depend upon the level of the lesion and its rapidity of development. Not only must one consider the direct effects of pressure but also those which can result from a secondary alteration in blood supply. In general, however, the symptoms and physical signs so produced can be classified into two principal groups which are first, those resulting from compression of nerve roots at the level of the lesion and secondly, those due to interference with the function of long ascending or descending tracts. The principal symptom of root compression is pain, which is generally aching in character, and radiates into the cutaneous area from which the root or roots concerned receive sensory impulses. If the motor roots are also involved there will be weakness, wasting, and sometimes fasciculation of the muscles which they supply. Interruption of the spinal reflex arc gives absence of the reflexes, if any, which are innervated by the segment being compressed. If the pressure develops asymmetrically, these phenomena can occur unilaterally at first. Compression of long tracts may give weakness and dragging of a leg and/or clumsiness of an arm and hand, again depending upon the situation of the lesion, and eventually a spastic paraplegia or quadriplegia will result. When the spinothalamic tract is involved, the patient often experiences unpleasant burning pain in a limb or on the trunk and some hypalgesia is generally found on examination. Similarly, involvement of the posterior columns gives characteristic paraesthesiae below the level of the lesion, often with typical 'electric shocks' radiating downwards on movement of the neck, if the lesion is cervical; there is also impairment of position and joint sense, sometimes of light touch, and generally of vibration sense in the lower limbs. These so-called 'long-tract' symptoms and signs develop especially early when the lesion is intramedullary. As a rule, the pyramidal tract is most sensitive to pressure, possibly because of the comparative vulnerability of its blood supply, while the spinothalamic tracts are most resistant. Hence a slowly progressive lesion generally gives first signs of pyramidal tract dysfunction, next sensory phenomena of 'posterior column' type, and lastly those indicating a spinothalamic tract lesion.

Sphincter disturbances tend to develop late but precipitancy or difficulty in initiating micturition may eventually be experienced. When a severe paraplegia has developed there is often excessive sweating below the level of the lesion. Disturbances of sphincter control appear early, however, in lesions compressing the cauda equina, in which pain in the lower back is usual and there are also symptoms and signs of muscular weakness of 'lower motor neurone' type in the lower limbs. Cutaneous sensory loss is also apparent, its distribution varying depending upon which roots are involved; compression of lower sacral roots, for instance, often produces perianal and perineal anaesthesia. Some of the most difficult lesions to localise accurately on clinical grounds are those which compress both the lower spinal cord (the conus medullaris) and several roots of the cauda equina; in such cases, there are generally severe disorders of sphincter control, along with a combination of 'upper motor neurone' and 'lower motor neurone' signs in the lower limbs.

Accurate **clinical localisation** of the site of cord compression can be greatly helped by the presence of certain specific symptoms and physical signs. The distribution of root pain, or the situation of local spinal pain and tenderness may be valuable, while a 'sensory level' on the trunk, below which sensation is impaired, is also helpful. It must, however, be remembered that the actual site of the lesion may be several segments higher than that suggested by this sensory 'level'. Weakness of lower abdominal muscles, too, or selective absence of lower abdominal reflexes will localise the lesion to approximately the tenth dorsal segment of the cord. Reflex changes are also useful; thus absence or inversion of the biceps and radial jerks with exaggeration of the triceps jerk indicates a lesion of the fifth and sixth cervical segments, while absence of the knee jerks and retention or exaggeration of the ankle jerks indicates usually that the third or fourth lumbar segment is involved. In the lower limbs, too, the distribution of sensory impairment or muscular weakness may clearly indicate disease of specific motor or sensory roots. Thus perianal anaesthesia is diagnostic of lower sacral root involvement. In localising a lesion on the basis of these clinical features one must remember that the spinal cord is much shorter than the spinal column and ends at the lower border of the first lumbar vertebra. Thus the seventh cervical segment of the cord lies beneath the arch of the sixth cervical vertebra, the sixth dorsal segment beneath the fourth dorsal arch; under the tenth dorsal arch are the first and second lumbar segments, under the twelfth the fifth, while the sacral and coccygeal segments are opposite the body of the first lumbar vertebra.

Although these clinical features help to localise a spinal lesion, they are insufficient for the surgeon, should operative intervention be considered. Often when compression has occurred acutely, irreversible damage has taken place before the surgeon can operate. The results of removal of extramedullary tumours are, by contrast, uniformly good, if done sufficiently early. Although there are some causes of cord compression in which the results of surgical decompression are variable (e.g. cervical spondylosis), this is the only effective treatment in some patients. Examination of the CSF is of limited value in diagnosis since although the protein content of the fluid may be raised (*see* p. 47) and Queckenstedt's test may be positive these findings are not invariable and the performance of a lumbar puncture may prejudice subsequent myelography. Radiography of the spine may indicate the cause of the compression, but usually a whole-body CAT scan or myelography are needed for accurate localisation.

Injuries to Peripheral Nerves and Plexuses

A detailed description of the many clinical phenomena which can result from injury to or compression of peripheral nerves or plexuses is outside the scope of this volume, but the salient features of some of the lesions which most often occur in clinical practice will be described briefly. There are two principal types of lesion resulting from injury to nerve trunks. These are first, neurapraxia, a temporary and completely reversible block of nervous conduction which can last for days or even weeks without permanent pathological change; and secondly, neuronotmesis, in which there is interruption in continuity of nerve fibres with subsequent Wallerian degeneration, so that regeneration of nerve fibres is required before recovery can occur. In the early stages these two types of lesion may be indistinguishable, save by specialised methods of investigation (*see* pp. 57–60). Bearing this fact in mind it should be noted that a total lesion of a mixed motor and sensory peripheral nerve gives flaccid paralysis and eventual atrophy of the muscles which it supplies. There is also cutaneous sensory loss, though the area of anaesthesia and analgesia is often less than would be expected, as a result of 'overlap' from nerves supplying adjacent cutaneous areas. Trophic changes (shiny skin, loss of sweating, indolent sores) may be seen in the extremities after complete peripheral nerve lesions. We shall now consider the clinical phenomena which result from lesions of some of the more important nerve plexuses and peripheral nerves. Direct trauma, pressure or irritation are usually responsible, and inflammatory lesions are comparatively uncommon. The condition often referred to in the past as an interstitial neuritis of individual peripheral nerves is generally due to pressure upon or ischaemia of the nerve trunk, although allergic or hypersensitivity neuropathies do occur.

The **phrenic nerve** is derived from the third, fourth and fifth cervical anterior roots; compression or irritation of the nerve can cause an irritating, unproductive cough or hiccup, while a complete lesion gives paralysis of the diaphragm on the affected side. The nerve is usually paralysed as a result of lesions of the anterior horn cells of the cord or the anterior roots, as in poliomyelitis, the Guillain–Barré syndrome and spinal neoplasms, but may be injured in its peripheral course by penetrating wounds, malignant disease in the chest, or an aortic aneurysm.

The **brachial plexus** is formed from the anterior primary divisions of the fifth to eighth cervical and of the first dorsal nerves. Sometimes the plexus is prefixed, receiving contributions from the fourth cervical, or postfixed, with fibres from the second dorsal segment. The divisions split into anterior and posterior trunks which again unite to form three cords. The outer cord is formed from the anterior trunks of the fifth to seventh cervical nerves, the inner or lower cord from the anterior trunk of the eighth cervical and the entire contribution from the first dorsal, while the posterior cord is formed from all the posterior trunks. The lateral head of the median nerve and the musculocutaneous nerve come from the outer cord, the medial head of the median nerve and the ulnar from the inner cord, and the circumflex and radial nerves from the posterior cord. The long thoracic nerve, which supplies the serratus anterior and is derived from the fifth to seventh cervical roots as well as the suprascapular nerve which innervates the spinati, and comes from the fifth and sixth segments, arise proximal to the brachial plexus.

The brachial plexus can be injured or compressed by penetrating wounds, by dislocation of the head of the humerus, by tumours in the root of the neck or by lesions causing compression at the thoracic outlet. Even more commonly it is damaged by traction injuries of the arm, perhaps in an infant during delivery, or in an adult on an operating table while anaesthetised. A common injury is one of the inner cord of the plexus due to hyperabduction of the arm at the shoulder; or alternatively downward compression of the point of the shoulder (as in motor cycle injuries) or a violent pull downward on the arm may tear the outer cord. Severe injuries may forcibly tear the spinal nerves or may even pull the anterior and posterior roots away from their attachment to the spinal cord. When this happens in the cervical region the symptoms and signs are similar to those of brachial plexus injury but the 'flare' response (*see* p. 229) indicates that the lesion in sensory fibres at least is proximal to the posterior root ganglia. Myelography is useful when such an injury is suspected as it shows excessive filling of root 'sleeves' at the appropriate level. It is important to recognise these cases in which no significant recovery is possible; in lesions of the plexus itself, even if severe, some recovery may result from nerve regeneration, even after extensive Wallerian degeneration, provided the damaged nerve trunks remain in continuity.

Injury to the outer cord gives paralysis of the biceps brachii and of the radial flexors of the wrist and fingers. An inner cord lesion, which may be due to shoulder dislocation, gives paralysis of all the small muscles of the hand with sensory loss along the ulnar border of the hand and forearm. The posterior cord is rarely injured. The two common varieties of *birth injury to the plexus* are first, Erb's paralysis, in which the contribution from the fifth cervical nerve is torn; and secondly, Klumpke's paralysis in which the first dorsal nerve is damaged. In Erb's paralysis there is paralysis of the deltoid, spinati, biceps and brachioradialis so that the arm hangs limply by the side, internally rotated with the forearm pronated. Klumpke's paralysis gives a 'claw' hand due to paralysis of small hand muscles with sensory loss down the inner side of the forearm. Whereas about 50 per cent of cases of the Erb type recover, the prognosis of the Klumpke type is less good. Surgical treatment is of no value, but splinting of the arm to prevent overstretching of paralysed muscles can assist partial recovery.

A syndrome with clinical features of inner cord injury can result from compression or angulation of the cord as it crosses a *cervical rib* joining the transverse process of the seventh cervical vertebra to the first rib; a fibrous or cartilaginous band in the same situation may have a similar effect. Commonly in such a case there is aching pain down the inner arm and forearm; this is accentuated by carrying heavy weights in the hand, while weakness and wasting of all small hand muscles and sensory loss on the ulnar side of the hand and forearm develop slowly over months or years. Wasting sometimes begins in the lateral half of the thenar eminence giving difficulty in differentiation from a carpal tunnel syndrome (*see below*) in some cases. An ipsilateral Horner's syndrome due to pressure on the stellate ganglion occurs occasionally. This cervical rib syndrome, which is uncommon (many individuals have cervical ribs visible radiologically which do not give rise to symptoms) is one variety of the *thoracic outlet or costoclavicular outlet* syndrome. Similar compression of the inner cord of the brachial plexus and sometimes of the subclavian artery, leading rarely to aneurysm formation or to ischaemia or embolism of the hand, can be the result of narrowing of the space between a prominent first rib and the clavicle through which the neurovascular bundle to the upper limb must pass. Alternatively, distortion resulting from angulation of the cord as it crosses the scalenus anterior has been implicated. The syndrome has been attributed to drooping of the shoulders, particularly in middle-aged females who customarily carry heavy shopping bags. While it is true that the typical cervical rib syndrome as outlined above can occasionally result from other causes of compression in the costoclavicular outlet, it is evident that many symptoms previously attributed to this cause are due to other lesions, including cervical spondylosis, and, in the case of acroparaesthesiae (*see below*), a common syndrome in middle-aged women, compression of the median nerve in the carpal tunnel. In diagnosing the thoracic outlet syndrome it is important to note that pain and paraesthesiae occur down the *inner* side of the arm and forearm, and that if motor weakness and muscle wasting are present these predominate in the small hand muscles. It is useful to roll the trunks of the brachial plexus beneath the examiner's fingers in the supraclavicular fossa, since this often reproduces the patient's pain and paraesthesiae on the affected side.

Isolated lesions of the **long thoracic nerve** are not uncommon and may result from an inflammatory lesion which is presumed to be auto-immune and which is akin to neuralgic amyotrophy (*see* p. 302). The result is 'winging' of the scapula due to paralysis of serratus anterior. When the patient pushes forward with the arm outstretched horizontally the scapula protrudes backwards like an 'angel's wing'.

When the **axillary** (circumflex) **nerve** is injured, as it may be by direct trauma, shoulder dislocation or 'shoulder girdle neuritis' (*see* p. 302), the deltoid muscle is paralysed and there is often a patch of sensory loss over the belly and insertion of the deltoid.

The **radial nerve** innervates the triceps, brachioradialis, the radial extensor of the wrist and most of the long extensors of the fingers. Hence a lesion of this nerve high up in the spiral groove in the humerus will cause paralysis of extension of the elbow together with wrist-drop and finger-drop. If the lesion is lower the triceps is often spared. Sensory loss is usually slight and is confined to a small area on the dorsum of the hand between the thumb and index finger, even though the nerve has a more extensive cutaneous innervation. The nerve is frequently damaged in its spiral groove when the humerus is fractured, or by pressure, as when the upper arm rests for a long period over the back of a chair (Saturday-night paralysis).

The **musculocutaneous nerve** is rarely injured alone but a lesion will result in paralysis of flexion of the elbow (biceps brachii and brachialis).

A lesion of the **median nerve** at the elbow gives paralysis of the radial flexors of the wrist and also of most of the long flexors of the fingers, except for those which move the ring and little fingers. There is also weakness and wasting of the muscles of the outer half of the thenar eminence (abductor pollicis brevis and opponens pollicis). There is sensory loss over the radial part of the hand and on the palmar aspect of the thumb, index, middle, and half the ring finger. The distal part of the extensor aspect of these fingers may also be anaesthetic. Apart from direct trauma (as by a misplaced injection) the nerve can be compressed at the elbow as it passes through the pronator teres or in relation to the flexor digitorum sublimis; but these disorders are uncommon. A lesion at the wrist gives similar sensory loss, but only the muscles of the lateral half of the thenar eminence are involved. The **anterior interosseous nerve**, a branch of the median, may be constricted by a fibrous band or tendon giving simply paralysis of flexion of the terminal phalanges of the thumb and index finger. Isolated lesions of this nerve sometimes arise spontaneously and recover in a few months.

Lesions of the median nerve are generally due to direct trauma, and causalgia is a particularly common sequel. *Compression of the median nerve in the carpal tunnel* is a common syndrome. It often results from excessive use of the fingers (as in housewives, women who knit a great deal and pianists) and is usually the result of a tenosynovitis of the flexor tendons, causing swelling of their sheaths and increased pressure beneath the carpal ligament. Local injuries of the wrist, rheumatoid arthritis, acromegaly and disorders which give rise to soft tissue swelling (pregnancy, myxoedema, nephrotic syndrome) can have a similar result. The condition is commonest in middle-aged women, but may occur in men. It is often bilateral but worse in the hand which is used more often (usually the right). The most typical symptoms are burning pain, aching or tingling and pins and needles in the fingers (acroparaesthesiae) which are worse in bed at night or in warm surroundings (due to vasodilation and increased nerve compression). Often the patient says that the symptoms affect all fingers until asked to take particular note of this question, when she will admit that the little finger is spared. Not infrequently aching pain and paraesthesiae spread up the arm. Percussion of the median nerve at the wrist sometimes evokes tingling in the affected fingers, while the application of a tourniquet to the arm at above arterial blood pressure gives ischaemic paraesthesiae in the fingers within one to three minutes (an abnormally short period). Often there is some sensory impairment over the tips of the thumb and radial three fingers, while the muscles of the lateral half of the thenar eminence may be weak or even wasted in advanced cases. Nerve conduction velocity studies demonstrate increased terminal latency due to conduction delay beneath the carpal ligament, or a reduced amplitude of sensory nerve action potentials from the median-innervated fingers. The symptoms, which are disabling and can last for many years, may be relieved by rest or by the injection of hydrocortisone into the carpal tunnel; operative section of the carpal ligament will effect a permanent cure.

The **ulnar nerve** at the elbow lies behind the medial epicondyle of the humerus; a lesion at this level, or as it passes between the two heads of the flexor carpi ulnaris (the cubital tunnel syndrome, or 'tardy ulnar palsy'), results in paralysis of the flexor carpi ulnaris, of the ulnar part of the flexor digitorum and of most of the small muscles of the hand save the lateral half of the thenar eminence and the two most lateral lumbricals. The hand is deviated radially, there is inability to flex the ring and little fingers completely and a 'claw-hand' results from paralysis of small hand muscles and from unopposed action of their antagonists. On testing there is inability to abduct the little finger, to adduct the thumb and to separate or oppose the fingers, while lumbrical weakness means that the terminal phalanges of the affected fingers cannot be fully extended. Sensory impairment is found over the palmar and dorsal aspects of the little finger and the ulnar half of the ring finger; it sometimes spreads up the palm as far as the wrist and rarely on to the medial aspect of the forearm. The nerve can be damaged at the elbow by penetrating injuries or fractures of the humerus or it may be subjected to repeated irritation in its groove behind the humerus in patients who have an unusually wide 'carrying angle' or arthritic osteophytes in this area. In such cases, and in those of the cubital tunnel syndrome, the nerve trunk becomes swollen, tender and fibrotic and surgical transposition, bringing it to lie in front of the epicondyle, is necessary. The nerve can also be temporarily compressed through leaning on the elbow for a long period, or by 'sleeping on the arm'. In the region of the wrist the nerve may be injured particularly by penetrating injuries, and it is not uncommon for the median and ulnar nerves and several tendons to be severed, particularly when a hand is thrust through a glass door or window. Atrophy and weakness of the interossei, lumbricals and adductor pollicis, with sparing of the hypothenar eminence and without sensory loss, can result from continuous or repetitive pressure on the medial side of the palm, a hazard of certain occupations, and is due to repeated trauma to the deep palmar branch of the nerve. A similar syndrome occasionally develops spontaneously without a history of trauma and may be found to be due to a ganglion compressing this branch. Nerve conduction velocity studies and measurements of terminal latency are often diagnostic.

The **lumbar plexus** is formed from the twelfth dorsal and first to fourth lumbar nerves, the **sacral plexus** from the fourth and fifth lumbar and first to third sacral nerves. Usually the two together are called the **lumbosacral plexus**. The principal nerves arising from the lumbar plexus are the femoral and obturator, while the greater part of the sacral plexus forms the sciatic nerve. Injuries of the lumbosacral plexus are relatively uncommon, but it can be damaged by undue pressure of the fetal head or by obstetric forceps during delivery (obstetric lumbosacral palsy); a syndrome which may result from this cause is unilateral paralysis of the anterior tibial and peroneal muscles due to a lesion of one lumbosacral cord.

A common clinical syndrome, known as **meralgia paraesthetica**, is due to compression of the lateral cutaneous nerve of the thigh as it passes beneath the lateral part of the inguinal ligament or as it traverses the fascia lata to reach its cutaneous distribution. It usually occurs in the obese, and in middle-age, but not invariably so, and can be unilateral or bilateral. The principal symptoms are an unpleasant burning ache, with superadded tingling or pins and needles, which are accentuated by standing for long periods, and involve much of the lateral aspect of the thigh. In this area there is often some hypalgesia and hypaesthesia. The condition, though benign, is often troublesome. Surgical decompression or division of the nerve may be necessary, but is not always completely effective in relieving symptoms. Repeated injections of local anaesthetic around the nerve at the inguinal ligament occasionally afford relief.

Lesions of the **obturator nerve** are uncommon but can follow hip dislocation or difficult labour. The adductor muscles of the thigh are paralysed, but as a rule there is no sensory loss. Rarely, the **ilioinguinal**

nerve may be injured directly, by a misplaced herniorrhaphy incision, or by hip joint disease, giving pain in the groin and a flexed posture; local anaesthetic injection is the treatment of choice.

The principal effect of a lesion of the **femoral nerve**, which may result from penetrating wounds or compression by pelvic neoplasms, is paralysis of the quadriceps with inability to extend the knee and loss of the knee jerk. There may also be some weakness of hip flexion owing to involvement of the iliacus and sensory impairment is usual over the medial and anterior aspects of the lower two-thirds of the thigh; if the saphenous nerve, a branch of the femoral, is also affected, the analgesia and anaesthesia also extend down the inner side of the leg and foot. In some cases of '*diabetic amyotrophy*' painful wasting of one quadriceps results from a localised ischaemic femoral neuropathy.

The **sciatic nerve** has two principal divisions which form the medial and lateral popliteal (tibial and common peroneal) nerves, respectively, and it divides at a variable point in the back of the thigh. It enters the buttock via the sciatic notch and then passes into the thigh mid-way between the greater trochanter of the femur and the ischial tuberosity. A complete lesion of the nerve gives paralysis of the hamstrings, resulting in inability to flex the knee, as well as paralysis of all muscles below the knee. The foot becomes flail, it cannot be dorsiflexed or plantar-flexed and the toes are immobile. The patient can walk but does so with a drop-foot and cannot stand on his toes. There is sensory loss over virtually the whole of the foot, except for a small area on the medial surface near the heel, and also over the lateral and posterior aspect of the leg below the knee. The ankle jerk and the plantar response are absent. Damage to the sciatic nerve is generally due to gunshot wounds or other penetrating injuries of the buttock or thigh, though it may also be injured by pelvic or femoral fracture or a misplaced injection. Its constituent roots are often compressed by lateral prolapse of an intervertebral disk, giving the syndrome of sciatica.

Lesions of the **lateral popliteal (common peroneal) nerve** are relatively common and usually result from repeated trauma to the nerve as it curls around the neck of the fibula; here it lies just beneath the skin and is particularly vulnerable. Compression by a tight garter or bandage, as a result of repeated crossing of the legs, or in workers who habitually sit with one leg folded beneath them (as in tailors or roofing workers) are common aetiological factors. A complete lesion gives paralysis of the dorsiflexors of the foot and toes and of the peroneal muscles, causing foot drop with some degree of inversion. There is generally sensory impairment over the anterolateral aspect of the leg and foot, extending medially to the cleft between the fourth and fifth toes.

When the **medial popliteal (tibial) nerve** is injured, an uncommon event which is normally seen only after a penetrating wound, the muscles of the calf and of the sole of the foot are paralysed and the foot is partially dorsiflexed and everted. Sensory loss is usually noted on the sole of the foot and the plantar surface of the toes. Very rarely the **posterior tibial nerve** is compressed behind and below the medial malleolus giving sensory loss over almost the entire sole of the foot (the tarsal tunnel syndrome). Rarely, compression of **plantar** and **interdigital** nerves can give similar but less extensive pain and sensory loss.

In this chapter an outline has been given of the effects of trauma upon the central and peripheral nervous system. For more detailed information about the effects of injury to the skull, vertebral column and spinal cord, the reader is referred to textbooks of neurosurgery and orthopaedic surgery. In a case of peripheral nerve injury, a working knowledge of the anatomical relationships of the nerves and plexuses and of the innervation of the skeletal muscles and dermatomes is clearly needed for accurate diagnosis and localisation of the responsible lesion; reference texts which may help in this connexion are listed below.

References

Feiring, E. H., *Brock's Injuries of the Brain and Spinal Cord and Their Coverings*, 5th ed. (New York, Springer, 1974).

Gurdjian, E. S. and Webster, J. E., *Head Injuries* (London, Churchill, 1958).

Guttmann, L, *Spinal Cord Injuries: Comprehensive Management and Research*, 2nd ed. (Oxford, Blackwell, 1976).

Kopell, H. P. and Thompson, W. A. L., *Peripheral Entrapment Neuropathies*, 2nd ed. (Baltimore, Williams and Wilkins, 1976).

Lewin, W., *Management of Head Injuries* (London, Baillière, Tindall and Cassell, 1966).

Medical Research Council, *Aids to the Examination of the Peripheral Nervous System* (London, HMSO, 1976).

Potter, J. M., *The Practical Management of Head Injuries*, 3rd ed. (London, Lloyd-Luke, 1974).

Seddon, H., *Surgical Disorders of the Peripheral Nerves*, 2nd ed. (Edinburgh and London, Churchill Livingstone, 1975).

Sunderland, S., *Nerves and Nerve Injuries*, 2nd ed. (Edinburgh and London, Churchill Livingstone, 1978).

14 Infection and Allergy and the Nervous System

In common with other parts of the human body, the central nervous system, its meningeal coverings and its peripheral ramifications may be invaded by infective agents, of which bacteria, viruses, spirochaetes and parasites of various types are examples. Sometimes a bacterial infection of the nervous system, for instance, is but one part of a more widespread disease process; some viruses, on the other hand, the so-called neurotropic group, have a particular predilection for nervous tissue. In general infective agents produce an inflammatory response; inflammatory changes in the nervous system and particularly in and around its blood vessels can also be the result of an allergic or hypersensitivity response to an infective agent or foreign protein (e.g. serum) which is present elsewhere in the body but which has not invaded nervous tissue. Many nervous complications of general infections are probably due to pathological mechanisms of this nature, involving a number of cell-mediated or humoral immune mechanisms, while others are the direct result of circulating toxins which are produced by the infecting agent.

Bacterial Infections

Bacteria may enter the nervous system by direct spread from an infective focus in the cranial bones or vertebrae, as in patients with suppuration in the middle ear or paranasal sinuses, or osteomyelitis of a vertebra. This spread can be facilitated by injury which has produced a penetrating wound, or a fracture of the cranial vault with a tear of the adherent dura mater. Alternatively the organisms arrive via the blood stream, being derived from a remote focus of infection; commonly this spread is via the arterial system, when it can be assumed that invasion of the nervous system is preceded by a phase of bacteraemia or pyaemia, but an alternative route is via the profuse anastomosis of vertebral veins through which infection may spread directly from the thorax or abdomen to the cranial cavity. The common bacterial infections of the nervous system so produced are meningitis, septic venous sinus thrombosis, intracranial abscess and spinal extradural abscess.

Meningitis

If one excludes meningitis of virus or parasitic origin, most cases are due either to pyogenic infection or to tuberculosis, although traumatic or aseptic meningitis can result from intracranial haemorrhage and some meningeal inflammatory changes occur in spirochaetal infections, in granulomatous processes such as sarcoidosis, and in patients with carcinomatosis.

Pyogenic Meningitis

The commonest variety of pyogenic meningitis is **meningococcal meningitis** or cerebrospinal fever. The disease can occur in epidemic form and the organism is believed to enter the body via the nasopharynx. During epidemics many apparently unaffected individuals carry the organism. There is a preliminary phase of bacteraemia or even septicaemia before meningeal manifestations appear, and in a few cases acute meningococcal septicaemia is rapidly fatal due to adrenal haemorrhage (Friedrichsen–Waterhouse syndrome). More often the phase is asymptomatic but is followed by frontal and occipital headache of mounting severity with fever. Occasionally at this stage there are rose-red or purple spots on the skin of the trunk, but these are infrequent in sporadic cases. As headache worsens and becomes generalised, so drowsiness and confusion supervene and the patient may lapse into semicoma within 12 to 24 hours. Vomiting is frequent and often projectile in type. On examination the patient tends to lie on one side with his eyes away from the light and the knees pulled towards the chin; he is irritable and resents interference, pulling back the bedclothes when an attempt is made to remove them. Generally the pulse rate is slow. Neck stiffness is invariable and in severe and established cases there may even be neck retraction. Kernig's sign is usually positive (restriction of knee extension when the thigh is flexed). Paralysis of one or other sixth cranial nerve is sometimes seen and the patient who is sufficiently conscious then complains of diplopia. Usually the deep tendon reflexes are depressed, but focal neurological signs are rare. Although the inflammatory process affects principally the leptomeninges (arachnoid and pia mater), so that suppuration is mainly confined to the subarachnoid space, there are secondary degenerative changes in the superficial areas of the cerebral cortex, brain stem and cranial nerves in some cases. Hence fits occasionally occur, particularly in childhood; in cases treated late or ineffectively, there may be residual diplopia or nerve deafness, and sometimes communicating hydrocephalus develops giving papilloedema and residual dementia. Other rare complications include spread of infection to the brain or subdural space to give abscess formation.

The CSF is typically under increased pressure and is cloudy or frankly purulent. There are many pus cells present, the protein content of the fluid is increased but sugar is absent. Scanty meningococci may be found on a direct smear of the fluid stained by Gram's stain, and the organisms can be cultured, though they are difficult to grow. If no organisms are isolated in a case of pyogenic meningitis, the infection is probably meningococcal.

The clinical picture of pyogenic meningitis due to other bacteria is similar. That due to the **pneumococcus** can also be due to a blood-borne infection, without clear evidence of an infective focus elsewhere, and the same is true of **Haemophilus influenzae** meningitis. In pneumococcal meningitis the organisms are seen in profusion in direct smears of CSF. Most cases of meningococcal meningitis now survive with appropriate treatment, but the prognosis of pneumococcal meningitis is rather less favourable and there is a significant mortality rate; influenzal meningitis, which is particularly common in childhood, is less ominous, but can run a smouldering course for some weeks even after the initial acute phase has been satisfactorily controlled. Meningitis due to the **streptococcus** or **staphylococcus** is usually due to a spread of infection from the middle ear or elsewhere, although there is a curiously localised variety of spinal staphylococcal meningitis in which the exact method of bacterial entry has not yet been determined. In neonates, a purulent meningitis is often found to be due to infection with **Listeria monocytogenes**.

Tuberculous Meningitis

Tuberculous meningitis can arise as a complication of miliary tuberculosis and meningeal inflammation may smoulder for some weeks before becoming clinically apparent. It is therefore wise to examine the CSF in cases of miliary tubercle in order to determine whether subclinical meningitis is present. The disease can also develop in children with primary tuberculosis or in adults with pulmonary disease and is then usually due to an acute or subacute exudative reaction in the meninges following the rupture of a small cerebral or cerebellar tuberculoma into the subarachnoid space. Cerebral tuberculomas are usually small, although rarely one is of sufficient size to present as a space-occupying lesion; this is commoner in India than in Western countries.

The symptoms of tuberculous meningitis are similar in character but different in tempo from those of the pyogenic variety, although there are rare cases in which the onset is equally abrupt and progression just as rapid. In children and young adults previously vaccinated with BCG the illness is rare, but when it does occur it is often comparatively mild initially and is easily mistaken for benign lymphocytic meningitis. More often, however, there is a period of several days or even weeks of fluctuating premonitory malaise, anorexia, vomiting, vague headache and disinterest, before sustained fever, persistent headache and signs of meningeal irritation become clearly evident. When present, retinal miliary tubercles, yellowish nodules about half the size of an optic disk, are diagnostic. It is important to recognise the disease early, since the longer it exists before treatment, the more probable are complications such as diplopia and communicating hydrocephalus or focal neurological signs (monoparesis or hemiparesis), which can result from cerebral infarction due to associated tuberculous arteritis. Adhesions in the spinal subarachnoid space may cause difficulty in treating the condition with intrathecal remedies, and spinal block sometimes develops; similar adhesions around the brain stem can cause attacks of decerebrate rigidity, which generally imply a gloomy prognosis. The complications and sequelae of tuberculous meningitis are more severe than those of any other variety.

Sarcoidosis

The aetiology of Boeck's sarcoid remains unknown; while its pathological changes resemble those of tuberculosis save for the absence of caseation, it is probably unrelated to tuberculous infection. It is accompanied by a depression of cell-mediated immune mechanisms. While lymphadenopathy in the mediastinum or elsewhere, iridocyclitis and hepatic involvement are its more common manifestations, the nervous system is sometimes involved, resulting usually in a combination of chronic meningitis on the one hand with multiple cranial nerve palsies, a pleocytosis and increased protein in the CSF, and sometimes a peripheral neuropathy or myopathy on the other. However, some patients present simply with features of raised intracranial pressure due to cerebral oedema or communicating hydrocephalus. In the later stages hypothalamic involvement, with obesity, diabetes insipidus, and impairment of recent memory may occur.

Intracranial Thrombophlebitis

Suppurative thrombophlebitis of intracranial venous sinuses most often affects the lateral, cavernous and superior longitudinal (sagittal) sinuses, due to centripetal spread of infection from the middle ear, skin of the face and frontal sinus, respectively. In all three conditions the patients have pyaemia and are acutely ill with high remittent fever. Lateral sinus thrombosis must be suspected in patients with otitis media who show this clinical picture without signs of meningitis or intracerebral spread of infection, while septic thrombosis of the cavernous sinus generally gives unilateral proptosis, chemosis of the conjunctiva and oculomotor paresis. In sagittal sinus thrombosis there may be oedema and tenderness of the scalp over the vertex and spastic weakness of one or both lower limbs; a subdural abscess not uncommonly results. Aseptic thrombosis of the lateral or sagittal sinuses may also complicate middle-ear disease but then causes the syndrome of 'benign intracranial hypertension', or 'otitic hydrocephalus' (*see* Chapter 12, p. 333).

Intracranial Abscess

Localised suppuration within the cranial cavity can occur outside the dura mater, giving an **extradural abscess**. This condition is invariably the result of cranial osteomyelitis which in turn is usually due to infected scalp wounds, otitis media, or paranasal sinusitis. Generally there is a remittent fever and some tenderness over the overlying scalp, but symptoms and signs of increased intracranial pressure are rare and CSF changes, if present at all, are minimal.

A **subdural abscess** or **empyema** is usually a sequel of frontal sinusitis but rarely results from middle ear disease; often the layer of pus extends over the whole of one cerebral hemisphere. Initially there is headache and tenderness over the affected frontal sinus or mastoid bone but subsequently the patient becomes drowsy or stuporose, his fever mounts and neck stiffness develops. Jacksonian seizures are frequent in the contralateral limbs and a hemiparesis or hemiplegia invariably develops. Usually there is a polymorphonuclear pleocytosis in the CSF with a marked rise in protein content. If not treated quickly by surgical evacuation this condition is soon fatal.

Abscess formation in the subarachnoid space is very rare and the commonest site for intracranial suppuration is within the brain substance itself, a **brain abscess**. In about 40 per cent of cases this is due to a direct spread of infection through adherent meninges from the bones of the middle ear, when the principal sites are the temporal lobe (upward spread) or one cerebellar hemisphere (lateral spread); another 10 per cent are due to frontal sinusitis, when the frontal lobe is usually involved. Of the remaining 50 per cent, a few are due to penetrating injuries, but most are metastatic; in many of these the primary focus of infection is in the lung (bronchiectasis, empyema, lung abscess) but it may lie anywhere in the body. Brain abscesses are particularly liable to develop in patients with cyanotic congenital heart disease, even without bacterial endocarditis. The cocci are the organisms usually responsible. Pathologically there is an initial stage of focal necrosis and liquefaction, or suppurative encephalitis, but this is followed by proliferation of glial and fibrous elements, with eventual encapsulation of the abscess.

When a patient with otitis media or sinusitis notes the suppression of a previously profuse discharge and this is followed by headache, vomiting and confusion, it is reasonable to suppose that inflammation has spread intracranially. Often, however, the patient seems to recover from otitis, say, but remains unwell, with depression or irritability, vague intermittent headache and nausea, anorexia, weight loss and mild fever. Even in haematogenous cases, though the onset is occasionally acute, with focal seizures and neurological signs, there may be minimal headache and progressive personality change. If the signs and symptoms of infection have been masked by antibiotic therapy, the patient may be thought to be suffering from an intracranial tumour.

Usually, however, there is intermittent pyrexia, and symptoms and signs of increased intracranial pressure (headache, vomiting, papilloedema, bradycardia) develop steadily. Other manifestations depend upon the localisation of the abscess. There will be aphasia if a frontal or temporal lobe abscess involves the dominant hemisphere; a temporal lobe lesion often gives a quadrantic visual field defect and minimal weakness of the contralateral face and hand, while in frontal lobe abscess, intellectual impairment may be prominent and a contralateral hemiparesis is common. When the cerebellum is involved, headache is often suboccipital, nystagmus is seen and signs of cerebellar dysfunction (ataxia, dysemtria, etc.) are usually present in the ipsilateral arm and leg.

In the early stages, examination of the CSF can be helpful but this test is not without risk, and is contraindicated if the intracranial pressure is clearly raised. Usually its pressure is increased and it contains up to 100 white cells/mm^3, of which many are lymphocytes, though some are usually polymorphonuclear; there is a moderate rise in protein, while the sugar content of the fluid is normal. The EEG may be helpful, revealing a striking focus of delta activity over the affected cerebral hemisphere, but the CAT scan is usually diagnostic. Where this technique is not available, gamma encephalography may be suggestive, but angiography, often followed by ventriculography, may be needed. Treatment, apart from systemic antibiotic therapy, is then neurosurgical. Where possible the abscess is excised; in other instances it is aspirated and antibiotic solutions are instilled into the cavity. About 30 per cent of patients die; many survivors suffer from headaches, epilepsy (up to 50 per cent) and residual limb weakness or ataxia according to the situation of the lesion.

Intraspinal Suppuration

An **intramedullary spinal abscess** is a very rare condition of metastatic origin; it usually presents with initial paraesthesiae in the lower limbs followed by a flaccid paraplegia of rapid progression. Generally there is suppuration elsewhere in the body, but few cases are diagnosed in life, and the condition is difficult to distinguish from other forms of acute myelopathy and from rapidly-growing intramedullary neoplasms. It should be considered in patients presenting with signs of an acute spinal cord lesion, as improvement may follow surgical drainage.

Much more common and particularly important to diagnose is **spinal extradural abscess**. This can be due to tuberculous caries of the spine (Pott's disease), but a staphylococcal aetiology is now much commoner. In about a third of all cases the condition is secondary to osteomyelitis of a vertebral body but in the remainder the infection, of metastatic origin, develops primarily within the extradural space. Suppuration and exuberant granulation tissue may extend over several segments of the spinal cord and eventually spread into the spinal muscles and soft tissues of the back. Compression of the cord and interference with its circulation are the most important complications.

The initial symptom is usually an ache in the affected area of the spine, followed by root pain and fever. Intense spinal tenderness follows, particularly in osteomyelitic cases, and paraesthesiae in the lower limbs followed by ascending paralysis subsequently develop. The diagnosis must be made early as paralysis, once present, may be irreversible, while surgical exploration and drainage of the abscess, combined with appropriate antibiotic therapy, can be curative. Lumbar puncture (which usually demonstrates complete spinal block) and myelography are usually essential for diagnosis and localisation, but should not be performed close to an area of spinal pain or tenderness in view of the risk of introducing organisms into the subarachnoid space. When clinical evidence suggests that such a lesion is present in the lumbar region it is wiser to introduce contrast medium cisternally. Even in osteomyelitic cases, spinal radiographs are often normal initially.

Leprosy

Leprosy, an infectious disease due to *Mycobacterium leprae*, is endemic in some tropical countries, particularly Africa and India. It is characterised by a long incubation period, a prolonged remittent course and involvement of the skin, mucous membranes and peripheral nerves. The more acute and infectious or lepromatous form affects particularly the nasal mucosa and the skin; it is in the chronic tuberculoid form that the peripheral nerves are generally involved. In the beginning there are generally thickened, pigmented and anaesthetic areas of skin; later the areas of numbness extend, many peripheral nerves are thickened and tender and eventually there is destruction of the distal phalanges in the hands and feet with painless ulcers of the extremities.

Virus Infections of the Nervous System

The neurotropic viruses have in common the fact that they are visible only under the electron microscope, that they generally pass through filter candles and that they are intracellular parasites. They attack principally nerve cells and hence the main brunt of the pathological changes which they produce falls upon the grey matter of the central nervous system. Recent work has suggested that the distinction between neurotropic and non-neurotropic viruses according to whether or not the nervous system is the primary or secondary site of attack by the disease process is largely artificial. Most viruses which attack the nervous system do so after

Table 6   Viral Infections of the Nervous System*

	Some representative viruses causing neurological disease in man and animals
RNA viruses	
Picornavirus	Poliovirus
	Coxsackie virus
	Echo viruses
Arbovirus	Equine encephalomyelitis
	St Louis encephalitis
	Japanese B encephalitis
	California encephalitis
	Tick-borne encephalitis (including louping-ill)
Myxovirus	Influenza
Paramyxovirus	Measles (and subacute sclerosing panencephalitis)
	Mumps
	Canine distemper
Arenavirus	Lymphocytic choriomeningitis
Rhabdovirus	Rabies
Unclassified	Rubella
DNA viruses	
Herpes viruses	Herpes simplex
	Varicella-zoster
	Cytomegalovirus
	Epstein-Barr virus (infectious mononucleosis)
Papova virus	Progressive multifocal leucoencephalopathy
Poxvirus	Vaccinia
Unidentified presumed viral illnesses	Encephalitis lethargica
	Kuru
	Creutzfeldt-Jakob disease
	Scrapie

*Reproduced, with permission, from *Brain's Diseases of the Nervous System*, 8th edition, ed. Walton, J. N., 1977.

multiplying in other organs; involvement of the nervous system results from haematogenous spread or retrograde dissemination along nerve fibres after endocytosis at axonal terminals. Viruses are classified according to their nucleic acid content, size, sensitivity to lipid solvents, morphology and method of development in cells. The commoner viruses which may attack the nervous system are listed in Table 6, from which it will be seen that viruses certainly account for acute anterior poliomyelitis, various forms of encephalitis and encephalomyelitis, rabies, lymphocytic meningitis, herpes zoster and probably also for encephalitis lethargica. Others which are not normally neurotropic, such as those of mumps and glandular fever (infectious mononucleosis) may attack the nervous system, giving rise to an encephalitic or meningitic illness.

In recent years the concept of **'slow virus' infections** of the nervous system has aroused interest. Kuru, a progressive disorder characterised initially by cerebellar ataxia and confined to the natives of New Guinea, has been transmitted to the chimpanzee; the same is now true of subacute spongiform encephalopathy (Creutzfeldt–Jakob disease). Both conditions appear to be due to filterable viruses and show affinities with scrapie, a disorder of sheep, which has an incubation period, after inoculation, of at least nine months. In another rare disorder, progressive multifocal leucoencephalopathy (PML), which usually complicates Hodgkin's disease or other reticuloses, polyoma virus has now been identified in cerebral lesions. It has been suggested, without, as yet, good evidence, that some commoner conditions (e.g. multiple sclerosis) will eventually prove to be due to viral infection. Subacute sclerosing panencephalitis (SSPE) (*see below*) now appears to be due to the prolonged persistence of measles virus in the brain.

Acute Anterior Poliomyelitis

Three principal strains of poliomyelitis virus have been identified and are known as the Brunhilde, Lansing and Leon strains, of which the Lansing is probably the most virulent. Other closely-related viral agents (e.g. the Coxsackie A7 virus) may occasionally produce a clinical picture like that of poliomyelitis. The virus attacks particularly the anterior horn cells of the spinal cord, around which collections of inflammatory cells are generally found in fatal cases, but the cells of motor brain stem nuclei and even those of the cerebral cortex may be invaded. The virus appears to enter the nervous system by travelling along peripheral and autonomic nerves. The usual portal of entry into the body is the alimentary tract, although in some cases it may be via the nasopharynx, particularly after recent tonsillectomy. In cases of the latter type there is a particular tendency for the bulbar nuclei to be involved.

As alimentary infection is derived from contaminated water or food, and flies are a common vector, epidemics are particularly liable to occur in summer and early autumn, though sporadic cases occur all the year round. The disease was once virtually confined to young children (hence the name 'infantile paralysis'), but in the 1940s and 1950s, particularly in countries like the United States, Britain and Scandinavia, in which standards of hygiene had been steadily improving, there was a tendency for more older children and young adults to be afflicted. This change was probably accounted for by the fact that fewer children were acquiring immunity as a result of sub-clinical infections in early life. The pattern has now changed even further as most children and young people have been effectively protected by inoculation and the incidence of the disease has declined sharply.

The incubation period of the illness is usually between seven and 14 days. During epidemics many individuals are infected and acquire immunity without developing symptoms **(subclinical cases)**. A second group of patients experience a mild febrile illness without clinical evidence of nervous system involvement **(abortive cases)**; in a third group there is a meningitic illness with headache, fever, neck stiffness and a CSF pleocytosis but no muscular paralysis ensues **(non-paralytic cases)**. The fourth group of patients in whom paralysis develops **(paralytic cases)** constitute a relatively small proportion of the whole. Excessive physical exertion or localised trauma to a limb (e.g. a prophylactic inoculation) during the pre-paralytic phase can promote paralysis of the affected member.

In non-paralytic cases or in the pre-paralytic phase of the paralytic form, headache, fever, neck stiffness and Kernig's sign are usually present and there may be abdominal pain and widespread muscular pain and tenderness. Attempted spinal flexion is often particularly painful. Sometimes after two or three days of fever there is apparent improvement for from 24 to 48 hours followed by a recrudescence of fever and the onset of paralysis, with muscle pain and tenderness. The distribution of muscular weakness is very variable from case to case. Typically it is asymmetrical, affecting perhaps one arm and the opposite leg, but any muscle group may be involved. Occasionally the weakness increases in an ascending manner with danger to life through respiratory paralysis. In a small group of cases the main brunt of the disease falls upon the brain stem (polioencephalitis), giving paralysis of the facial, pharyngeal and/or laryngeal muscles. The combination of pharyngeal and respiratory paralysis which occurs in some such bulbar bases is particularly sinister because of the danger of inhalation of secretions or vomit, and tracheotomy and assisted respiration are then required. Once paralysis has appeared, it usually reaches its maximum distribution within 24 hours, but in a few cases it continues to progress for two or three days. Fortunately the extent of the muscular weakness at the height of the illness is not always an indication of the degree of permanent paralysis which will remain; some anterior horn cells are only temporarily affected, recovery occurring subsequently. This is the principal justification for using assisted ventilation in this disease. Nevertheless there is nearly always some residual paralysis, followed by muscular wasting and often fasciculation, contractures of paralysed muscles, bony deformity and failure of growth in the affected member. Rarely, progressive muscular weakness and atrophy develop many years later to give a clinical picture like that of progressive muscular atrophy (*see* p. 363).

It is very difficult to assess accurately the mortality of the disease, in view of the many subclinical and abortive cases which occur. Furthermore, the mortality varied from epidemic to epidemic, having been as high as 25 per cent of paralytic cases in some, but this was an exceptionally high figure and 10 per cent was more usual. Respiratory paralysis and/or infection are generally the cause of death, which is now less common with modern management.

The CSF in the first two to three days of the illness generally shows an increase of polymorphonuclear leucocytes, but these are soon replaced by a lymphocytic pleocytosis, up to 200 or more cells per mm³. A substantial rise in the protein content of the fluid persists much longer than the pleocytosis.

Prevention of this disease is more satisfactory than any form of treatment. Passive immunisation with γ-globulin gives temporary protection during an epidemic, but permanent immunity is only achieved either by acquiring a natural infection or by active immunisation. The Salk and British vaccines were partially effective, particularly in reducing the incidence of paralytic cases; these have now been supplanted by the Sabin type oral vaccine, utilising live but attenuated virus.

Encephalitis Lethargica

This disease is probably due to a neurotropic virus, although no organism has ever been isolated. The principal site of pathological change is in the grey matter of the mid-brain, and particularly in the substantia nigra. The disease appeared in Europe in 1915 and occurred in epidemic proportions up to the early 1920s, when its frequency began to wane. No epidemics have occurred subsequently, but some believe that sporadic cases still occur. Thirty years ago the illness was usually acute, beginning with headache, vomiting, convulsions and confusion; nowadays the condition probably presents, if indeed it occurs, in a more subacute or chronic form, with manifestations of post-encephalitic Parkinsonism (*see* p. 249).

In the acute cases, there was characteristic lethargy and somnolence, sometimes amounting to stupor, during the day, but the patient was often awake, though confused and perhaps delirious, at night (reversal of sleep rhythm). Ocular palsies and pupillary changes were always present, giving blurring of vision and diplopia. Choreiform movements of the limbs, tremor and tics involving the facial and respiratory muscles were also seen. Sometimes Parkinsonian features (mask-like face, festinant gait, tremor, oculogyric crises) were observed in the early stage, but more often did not appear until several years after the acute illness. Nevertheless, it is probable that in such cases, even after an interval of many years, the causal organism persisted in the central nervous system. Indeed many patients with postencephalitic Parkinsonism gave no history of a previous recognisable encephalitic illness. Not only were neurological abnormalities common sequelae; in children particularly, after partial recovery from the acute disease, there were often severe behaviour disturbances, including cruelty, violence and moral and intellectual degeneracy. Many such individuals required permanent institutional treatment.

Only about 25 per cent of patients afflicted by this disease in its acute form seemed to recover completely. About one-third died within four weeks of the onset, but the remainder were usually disabled in the end by Parkinsonism.

The CSF in this disease was often normal, but there was sometimes a minimal pleocytosis and increase in protein.

Other Forms of Virus Encephalitis and Encephalomyelitis

Several specific varieties of encephalitis occurring in various parts of the world have been found to be due to viruses. In this group are the Japanese type B, St Louis, Russian spring–summer and Murray Valley varieties, in which infection is transmitted by the mosquito or by a tick. Equine encephalomyelitis, which occurs in the USA, is transmitted by the mosquito from a reservoir of virus in birds or in the wood-tick. Louping ill, a virus disease of sheep, has also been known to cause an encephalitic illness in man in Great Britain. Although all these forms of encephalitis show differences from one another in clinical presentation, course and mortality, each gives an encephalitic illness characterised by headache, fever, a period of confusion, stupor or semicoma and/or rigidity or tremor of the limbs. In equine encephalomyelitis particularly there may be spastic paresis of the limbs, fits and permanent mental deterioration. Each of these conditions (and there are probably many more varieties as yet unrecognised) is likely, after an acute onset, to result in a relatively protracted illness, with fluctuating levels of consciousness; and the mortality can be as much as 60 per cent in some epidemics. Though some patients recover completely, a number show intellectual and physical residua which persist when the acute illness is over. In each type the CSF is abnormal; there is a lymphocytic pleocytosis in the Japanese B and St Louis types, and in louping-ill, but polymorphs predominate, often in large numbers, in the early stages of the equine variety.

Similar, though generally less severe, encephalitic illnesses occur in Great Britain and only rarely is the causal virus identified except perhaps in the small proportion of cases of infectious mononucleosis in which an encephalitic illness develops, in mumps, in some Coxsackie or Echo virus infections and in herpes simplex encephalitis (*see below*). In Western Europe post-infective encephalitis (*see* p. 308) may be as common as the viral variety, although a mild and transient encephalitic illness sometimes occurs in influenza.

Herpes Simplex Encephalitis

While an encephalitic illness rarely complicates disseminated herpes simplex infection in infancy, in patients of all ages an explosive cerebral illness characterised by coma, hyperpyrexia and features (fits, hemiparesis) suggesting a lesion in one temporal lobe, may be due to infection with the virus. Subacute cases also occur. Often, because of the clinical picture, cerebral haemorrhage or abscess are suspected. Herpes simplex virus may be cultured or identified on electron microscopy in biopsy specimens obtained from the necrotic temporal lobe; because of the focal features many such cases are explored neurosurgically. While operative decompression alone may save life and recovery may in the end be remarkably complete, good results have been achieved in some cases with massive dosage of steroid drugs (e.g. dexamethasone 5 mg four times daily) and many authorities now favour antiviral chemotherapy with idoxuridine, cytosine arabinoside, or newer antiviral agents such as adenine arabinoside.

Benign Myalgic Encephalomyelitis

This name has been given to an encephalomyelitic illness which has occurred in outbreaks throughout the world. It has also been called 'epidemic neuromyasthenia'. It may be due to a virus infection, but no organism has been isolated, even from the many cases which occurred in the Royal Free Hospital, London, in 1955. The illness usually begins with lassitude and malaise, headache, neck stiffness and generalised muscular pain. Vertigo, vomiting and diplopia are common, as are bizarre disorders of concentration, behaviour and gait, with inordinate fatigue, suggesting hysteria. Indeed some believe that the condition is due to 'epidemic hysteria', as it has often occurred in closed communities (schools, convents, nurses' homes), especially in females. Paraesthesiae are frequent and there is variable paralysis and sensory loss in the limbs with, however, preservation of deep reflexes. The EMG often demonstrates a curiously intermittent pattern of voluntary muscular contraction. Rarely, there is an associated hepatitis. There is little or no fever and the CSF is always normal. The illness may run a prolonged relapsing course of many weeks or months, and during this period persistent fatigue and depression are common.

Subacute Sclerosing Panencephalitis

This subacute variety of encephalitis, which was previously called subacute inclusion body encephalitis (Dawson) and subacute sclerosing leuco-encephalitis (van Bogaert), is clearly due to virus infection. Recent serological and other evidence has confirmed that it is usually a late effect of measles, and that the measles virus has persisted in the brain and has undergone modification to make it behave like a 'slow virus'. The disease is commonest in infancy and childhood but can occur in adult life; nerve cell degeneration, gliosis and inflammatory changes occur in the cerebral cortex and many nerve cells and astrocytes contain inclusion bodies. The disease is characterised clinically by progressive dementia, spastic paralysis of the limbs and myoclonus, and generally runs a fatal course, usually within nine to 12 months. Retinal degeneration and pigmentation with visual failure occur in some cases. Rarely, partial remissions are seen and in exceptional cases incomplete recovery has occurred. The EEG is virtually diagnostic, revealing bizarre generalised repetitive slow wave complexes separated by periods of comparative electrical silence and the CSF shows increased measles specific immunoglobulin.

Rabies

Rabies in man follows a bite from an infected animal, usually a dog, which excretes the virus in its saliva. The virus enters the nervous system along peripheral nerves and attacks nerve cells in which the characteristic acidophilic inclusions (Negri bodies) are eventually demonstrated. Rabies in animals is characterised first by a change in behaviour with perversion of appetite, excessive excitement, salivation and progressive paralysis with muscular spasms. The incubation period in man is from 28 to 60 days or even more; during this asymptomatic period, protective inoculation can prevent the development of the disease. The first symptoms are usually apprehension, depression and restless sleep. These are followed by pharyngeal spasm (hydrophobia) which soon extends to the muscles of respiration and then to those of the trunk and limbs, producing opisthotonos. Any attempt to drink brings on the spasms which are accompanied by profuse salivation and later succeeded by profound paralysis. Death may occur during the spasms or later, and is usually due to respiratory or cardiac failure.

Lymphocytic Meningitis

This benign disorder is often due to a virus which also afflicts mice, and the house mouse may be the source of the human disease which can occur sporadically or in small epidemics. The condition is commonest in childhood but also affects adults. The prodromal symptoms are those of fever and are rapidly succeeded by headache, drowsiness and neck stiffness. Severe disturbance of consciousness is uncommon and many patients are alert throughout; diplopia is an infrequent complication. The illness usually lasts for about a week but complete recovery is the rule. The CSF is usually under increased pressure and may contain 1,000 or more cells per mm^3, of which most are mononuclear, though an occasional polymorph may be seen; the protein content of the fluid is raised and a 'cobweb clot' may form on standing. The sugar content of the fluid is generally normal; this helps in the differential diagnosis from tuberculous meningitis with which the condition is most often confused. It is impossible clinically to distinguish this condition from a non-paralytic case of poliomyelitis or from the meningeal illness which can complicate mumps or infectious mononucleosis (glandular fever). In glandular fever, while a meningitic illness is the commonest neurological complication, encephalitis sometimes occurs, a picture resembling transverse myelitis (*see* p. 307) is occasionally seen and, uncommonly, some patients develop isolated palsies of individual cranial or peripheral nerves or even an acute polyneuropathy. A similar picture is also seen in some cases of canicola fever (*see below*) and as a result of infection with one of the Coxsackie or Echo viruses; another form of Coxsackie A_2 virus infection causes epidemic myalgia (Bornholm disease).

Herpes Zoster

In herpes zoster or shingles, the principal sites of pathological change are the posterior root ganglia and the sensory ganglia of the cranial nerves, but occasionally the grey matter of the spinal cord and brain stem is damaged. Intranuclear inclusions have been demonstrated in cases of this disease and the causal virus is larger than many others in the neurotropic group; it appears to be identical with that of varicella (chicken-pox). The condition can develop without apparent precipitating cause, and usually does so in elderly people, but it may follow spinal cord trauma, intervertebral disk prolapse, spinal tumour, subarachnoid haemorrhage, or radiotherapy to the nervous system. This course of events suggests some excitation by the precipitant concerned of a virus which was previously lying dormant in the nervous system.

The incubation period of the illness is about 14 days; the first symptom is usually continuous dull burning pain in the distribution of the affected nerve root or roots, and this mounts in severity. There is often cutaneous hyperaesthesia. Within three to four days an erythematous rash appears in the affected region and is followed by a vesicular eruption which dries within a few days leaving pigmented scars which may itch for a time. The pain and skin eruption are always unilateral. Persistent severe pain may persist for weeks, months or even years after the initial illness, particularly in elderly people (post-herpetic neuralgia). Often the affected skin area becomes permanently anaesthetic and sometimes the anterior horn cells of the same segment of the spinal cord are also damaged, giving muscular weakness and wasting. Rarely there is evidence of damage to long tracts (pyramidal and spinothalamic), indicating a 'zoster myelitis'. Zoster of the ophthalmic division of the fifth cranial nerve is particularly unpleasant; the vesicles in the supraorbital region may spread to the cornea, leaving permanent scars. Oculomotor paresis can also occur. Herpes of the geniculate ganglion produces vesicles on the tympanic membrane or soft palate; often there is a watery or sanguineous discharge from the ear, homolateral deafness and facial paralysis and loss of taste on the anterior two-thirds of the tongue (the Ramsay Hunt syndrome). Sometimes there is also sensory loss on the affected side of the face. Rarely in severe herpes zoster there is some headache and neck stiffness indicating meningeal inflammation, and a herpes zoster encephalitis has been described but is uncommon.

Behçet's Syndrome

This is an uncommon syndrome of unknown aetiology, although it has been suggested that it may be due to a virus. The condition is characterised by ulceration of the mouth and genitalia, often with iritis, and runs a remittent course. When the nervous system is involved the picture may be that of indolent meningitis with variable headache, while Parkinsonian features and cranial nerve palsies or fluctuating spastic weakness of the legs may occur, sometimes suggesting multiple sclerosis. The CSF usually demonstrates a lymphocytic pleocytosis (up to 100 or more cells/mm^3) and a rise in its protein content. When nervous manifestations arise the ultimate prognosis is poor and treatment of little avail, although steroids have been recommended.

Spirochaetal Infections of the Nervous System

The principal spirochaetal agents which may invade the nervous system are first, and most important, the *Treponema pallidum* of syphilis, and secondly the leptospirae of Weil's disease and of canicola fever.

Neurosyphilis

Invasion of the nervous system accounted in the past for many deaths due to syphilis. The three main types of pathological change resulting from the neurological effects of the spirochaete can be classified as meningeal, vascular and parenchymatous. Meningeal and vascular symptoms appear relatively early in the course of the disease, often during or just after the secondary stage and within one to five years of the primary infection; these can generally be treated effectively. Manifestations of parenchymatous cerebral and spinal cord disease, which usually develop in the tertiary and quaternary stages of the illness, do not appear for some 10 to 20 years, or exceptionally even later; treatment of these conditions is less effective, though considerable improvement can nevertheless be expected in many cases. The secondary manifestations of syphilis are more acute and florid, and tertiary manifestations (gummata, skeletal involvement) more common, in populations and communities in which syphilis is a relatively recent acquisition. When the disease has been present in a community for hundreds of years the quaternary or parenchymatous neurosyphilitic manifestations are commoner. Tertiary syphilis is comparatively rare nowadays in Great Britain, but quaternary neurosyphilis is seen more often. However, because of early and effective identification and treatment of primary infections, the overall incidence of neurosyphilis has declined in most developed countries.

Asymptomatic neurosyphilis is not uncommon. This term identifies cases in which there are no symptoms or signs indicating disease of the nervous system but nevertheless there are changes in the CSF (pleocytosis, raised protein, positive VDRL or equivalent reaction) indicating activity of the disease. In addition to the VDRL test, the treponema immobilisation test and fluorescent treponemal antibody absorption (FTA-ABS) tests are now used in many laboratories, and the IgM and IgG immunoglobulin fractions are usually increased. The positive serological reactions reveal that the nervous system has been invaded, while the cell count usually parallels the degree of activity. Marked abnormality of the CSF usually heralds the eventual development of clinical neurosyphilis. If the fluid is normal in every respect it can be assumed with reasonable confidence that affection of the nervous system has not occurred or that it is no longer active.

An acute **meningitic illness** (luetic meningitis) can occur in the secondary stage of the illness, within two years of the primary infection. This is characterised by fever, headache and neck stiffness, sometimes with confusion or semicoma and even papilloedema. There are usually many hundreds of lymphocytes per mm^3 in the CSF, the VDRL reaction is strongly positive and the Lange curve is meningitic in type. The condition can resemble lymphocytic or early tuberculous meningitis; it usually responds well to anti-syphilitic treatment.

The term **meningovascular syphilis** is applied to a group of clinical manifestations of luetic infection which generally appear between two and five years after the primary infection. They result from a subacute or chronic inflammatory change in the leptomeninges (arachnoiditis) on the one hand or from a syphilitic endarteritis of cerebral and/or spinal cord arteries on the other. There may be symptoms of subacute meningitis with intermittent headache, low fever and neck stiffness, but more often the arachnoiditis at the base of the brain results in strangulation of one or more cranial nerves to give clinical signs of a cranial nerve palsy. The third and sixth nerves are particularly vulnerable; sometimes affection of the eighth nerve gives unilateral or bilateral deafness, while an optic chiasmal arachnoiditis can occur giving progressive bilateral, but often asymmetrical, visual failure. Manifestations of communicating hydrocephalus are also sometimes seen and convulsions are not uncommon. The arterial changes, if involving cerebral, brain stem or cerebellar arteries, may cause infarction, particularly if a vessel is suddenly occluded, and the clinical effects are indistinguishable from any episode of cerebral 'thrombosis' (*see* pp. 345–352). Hemiplegia, monoplegia, aphasia and vertigo can all occur. Syphilis was once the commonest cause of cerebral 'thrombosis' in relatively young people, but this is no longer so. The arteries of the spinal cord may also be involved; one mode of presentation is with an acute transverse cord lesion or so-called luetic transverse myelitis. Sometimes the arterial changes are more insidious and the pyramidal tracts, which are supplied by the peripheral branches of the anterior spinal artery, suffer increasing ischaema so that a gradually progressive spastic paraplegia develops (Erb's syphilitic spastic paraplegia). Often arachnoidal and vascular lesions are combined in the cervical region; as a result of strangulation of nerve roots produced by the arachnoiditis there is weakness and wasting of muscles in the upper limbs, while in the lower limbs there is a spastic paraplegia, due to ischaemia of long tracts. This condition, which can resemble motor neurone disease (*see* p. 361) has been called luetic amyotrophic lateral sclerosis, or, because of macroscopic changes in the cervical meninges, pachymeningitis cervicalis hypertrophica. The CSF in meningovascular syphilis is always abnormal, showing a lymphocytic pleocytosis, an increase in protein, a positive VDRL reaction and a Lange curve which is usually of luetic or meningitic type due to changes in the immunoglobulins (*see* p. 48).

Tabes Dorsalis

Tabes dorsalis (locomotor ataxia) is the name given to one quaternary or parenchymatous form of neurosyphilis, in which the spirochaetes have invaded nervous tissue, though they cannot always be demonstrated at autopsy. The principal pathological change is degeneration at the entry zone of the posterior spinal roots, with secondary involvement of ascending fibres in the posterior columns of the cord. Typically patients with this disease experience 'lightning pains' which are probably due to gliosis in the posterior roots. These are often described as 'like red hot needles sticking into the legs'. Generally, too, there is a severe sensory ataxia, and the unsteadiness in walking which patients describe is therefore worse in the dark. Paraesthesiae, particularly in the lower limbs, and subjective numbness are also common. Sometimes transient episodes or 'crises' occur whose aetiology is not fully explained. In laryngeal crises there is spasm of the vocal cords with stridor and difficulty in breathing; in gastric crises acute upper abdominal pain and vomiting occur, lasting perhaps for several days, while renal (like renal colic) and rectal (rectal pain and tenesmus) crises have also been described. Urinary symptoms (delayed or difficult micturition) are not infrequent and the normal sensation indicating a need to micturate may eventually be lost, while impotence is also frequent.

On physical examination, tabetic patients show a characteristically ataxic, high-stepping gait, and Romberg's sign is positive. The Argyll Robertson pupil is almost invariable. The pupils are small, irregular and unequal, they fail to react to light but do so on accommodation–convergence; there is atrophy of the iris and loss of the ciliospinal reflex (dilatation of the homolateral pupil on pinching the skin of the neck). Bilateral optic atrophy, with pallor of the disks and concentric constriction of visual fields, is seen in about 10 per cent of patients. Some degree of ptosis is usual, contributing to the characteristic long, drooping, 'tabetic facies'. There is often some loss of superficial pain sensibility (i.e. to pinprick) over the bridge of the nose, the centre of the sternum, the perineum, and in variable degree over the lower limbs. Deep pressure over the Achilles tendons is often painless. Generally the deep tendon reflexes, and certainly those in the lower limbs, are depressed or absent and there is severe impairment of position and joint sense and of vibration sense in the legs. Loss of pain sensation can lead to the development of a degenerative arthropathy (Charcot's joint) in the feet, ankles or knees.

In early cases of tabes dorsalis the Wassermann, VDRL, and treponema immobilisation reactions are usually positive in the blood and CSF and the latter shows a pleocytosis and luetic Lange curve. In 20 per cent of late or so-called 'burnt-out' cases, the Wassermann, VDRL, and even the treponema immobilisation tests are negative, and the CSF is normal in all respects. These investigations are nevertheless important in distinguishing between tabes dorsalis and various forms of peripheral neuropathy; in so-called diabetic pseudotabes there may actually be pupillary changes as well as involvement of peripheral nerves. Tabes dorsalis is the least satisfactory of all syphilitic conditions to treat, as there is often little or no improvement. Nevertheless, treatment should certainly be given (*see* Chapter 20, p. 438).

General Paresis
General paresis (general paralysis of the insane or GPI) is a form of progressive dementia, in which there are extensive inflammatory and degenerative changes throughout the cerebral cortex, and the treponema pallidum can generally be found in the brain at autopsy. In the beginning the symptoms can consist of little more than impairment of memory and concentration, and undue fatigue. Subsequently, however, judgement and personality deteriorate and there is increasing neglect of responsibility and personal hygiene. Often the patients are confused, apathetic and show a poor memory for recent events, combined with a singular lack of insight and concern. A grandiose variety of the disease is relatively uncommon, but such patients are often euphoric, hypomanic and have delusions of great personal power or ability. They may confabulate wildly, describing in detail personal experiences which have no foundation in fact. It seems that these manifestations occur particularly in individuals of previously ex-traverted personality. In due course even patients of this type become grossly demented and bed-ridden. There are a few individuals in whom the disease presents more acutely with headache, sudden confusion, convulsions and focal neurological signs (aphasia, hemiparesis, etc.) but this variety of the illness is relatively uncommon. Physical examination reveals evidence of a clear-cut dementia; Argyll–Robertson pupils are usual but not invariable. There are commonly tremors of the lips, tongue and out-stretched hands, the tendon reflexes are generally exaggerated, and often the plantar responses are extensor. Occasionally the lower limb reflexes are absent and there are other features reminiscent of tabes dorsalis, in which case the condition is usually called **taboparesis**. **Juvenile paresis** is general paresis due to congenital syphilis, and developing usually

in adolescence. The clinical manifestations are similar to those in the disease of late onset, except that the pupils, though unresponsive to light, are often dilated; the prognosis of juvenile paresis is poor despite treatment. General paresis must be distinguished from other causes of dementia arising in the presenium (*see* p. 241). This is most readily achieved by means of CSF examination. The fluid is always abnormal in untreated cases; the VDRL and treponema immobilisation reactions are positive, there is a lymphocytic pleocytosis, the protein content is raised, and the Lange curve is paretic in type (*see* p. 48). The condition, if untreated, is fatal within a few years, but most cases improve with treatment and 50 per cent or more may recover completely.

Leptospirosis

In leptospirosis icterohaemorrhagica (Weil's disease) the organism, de-rived usually from rat's urine, attacks principally the liver (giving hepatitis and jaundice) and the kidneys (giving nephritis) but occasionally there are also symptoms and signs of a lymphocytic meningitis. A meningitic illness, clinically, indistinguishable from other varieties of lymphocytic meningitis may, however, be the predominant or sole manifestation of canicola fever, which is due to *Leptospira canicola*, an organism which is generally carried by dogs. Hence this diagnosis should be considered in all cases of lymphocytic meningitis, particularly if the patient has been in contact with a sick dog.

Fungal Infections

Fungal disorders of the central nervous system are rare. **Actinomycosis** has been known to cause a subacute purulent meningitis of invariably fatal termination in certain cases, and in others vertebral involvement has resulted in extradural abscess formation with spinal cord compression. **Torulosis**, due to *Cryptococcus neoformans (Torula histolytica)*, a yeast-like organism, is the commonest fungal infection of the nervous system but is also rare. It gives the clinical picture of a subacute or chronic and fluctuating meningitic illness which sometimes lasts for many months with increasingly severe headaches, confusion and neck stiffness. There is usually papilloedema and sometimes cranial nerve palsies occur. The condition often develops in patients with reticulosis or debilitating ill-nesses, but can arise *ab initio* in the apparently healthy. This diagnosis should always be considered when the clinical picture suggests tuberculous meningitis, intracranial sarcoidosis, or carcinomatosis of the meninges. Although in the past the condition was generally fatal, effective treatment, in the form of amphotericin B or 5-fluorocytosine, is now available. The organism may be recognised in direct smears of the CSF or it can be grown on Sabouraud's medium or identified by a specific antibody reaction.

Parasitic Disorders of the Nervous System

Malaria

Cerebral symptoms are not uncommon in malignant tertian malaria (due to *Plasmodium falciparum*), particularly in children. The manifestations are probably due to blockage of cerebral capillaries by parasites. Commonly the onset is abrupt with high fever (up to 40°C), severe headache, neck stiffness and sometimes focal neurological signs (hemiplegia, aphasia). In some cases there is papilloedema, and clinical differential diagnosis from cerebral tumour or abscess may be difficult. The prognosis of cerebral malaria is grave, the mortality being as great as 50 per cent.

Toxoplasmosis

This condition, due to the protozoan toxoplasma, is usually congenital, being transmitted from the mother *in utero*. Often the infection in adults is asymptomatic, though some experience an acute or subacute illness with fever, headache and a skin rash when first affected. The encephalomyelitis which is the commonest manifestation of this disease in infancy usually causes fits, hydrocephalus, intracerebral calcification and chorioretinitis. In some babies the disease runs an acute and fatal course, in others it becomes arrested leaving permanent mental defect with a recurrent tendency to convulse, but some few children survive with minimal disabilities. The diagnosis may be confirmed serologically; no effective treatment is available.

Trypanosomiasis

This disease occurs in African (*Trypanosomiasis gambiense* and *rhodesiense*) and South American (*Trypanosomiasis cruzi*) forms. The African form, sleeping sickness, is transmitted by the tsetse fly. After a long incubation period, there is a febrile illness followed by meningitic symptoms, irritability, indifference, somnolence and eventually after some months by coma and death. The South American form (Chagas disease) is a more acute illness, commoner in children and less grave in outlook, but often followed by mental defect and residua like those of cerebral palsy; it may also cause myositis.

Trichiniasis

This disease is contracted usually through eating inadequately-cooked pork containing the larvae of the *Trichina spiralis*. The larvae are released in the intestinal tract, mature and produce further larvae which penetrate the intestinal wall and enter the blood stream. The common clinical features at this stage are fever, puffiness of the eyelids, and severe generalised muscular pain and often weakness, indicating invasion of the muscles. Respiratory difficulty due to diaphragmatic involvement is common. Sometimes fits or paraplegia result from blockage of cerebral or spinal blood vessels. Though the disease is occasionally fatal the illness usually resolves within a few days or weeks and the larvae become encysted. During the acute stage there is usually a striking eosinophilia and the parasites can be identified in muscle biopsy sections.

Cysticercosis

This disorder is contracted by eating food which has been contaminated with tapeworm ova, usually those of *Taenia solium*. The ova are converted into the larval form of the parasite which then penetrates the intestinal wall and enters the circulation to reach the brain, muscles and subcutaneous tissues. The larva becomes encysted to form a cysticercus which may then calcify and often has a characteristic oval shape which can be recognised on radiographs. Rarely, a hypertrophic myopathy results. Cysticercosis of the brain often causes epilepsy but a racemose form has also been described in the cerebral ventricles (particularly the fourth) which can result in either repeated attacks of lymphocytic meningitis or in intermittent or progressive hydrocephalus suggesting the presence of a posterior fossa tumour.

Bilharzia

Involvement of the nervous system in bilharzia or schistosomiasis, which results, especially in the Middle East, from bathing in infested water, is rare, but paraplegia has been described.

Neurological Complications of Specific Infections

Disorders due to Specific Exotoxins

The principal infecting organisms which produce exotoxins with an affinity for nervous tissue are diphtheria, tetanus and botulism.

Diphtheritic Polyneuropathy
The exotoxin of the diphtheria bacillus gives a polyneuropathy which generally begins in the musculature nearest to the point where the infecting organism is located. Since this is usually the tonsillar fossa, larynx or nasal mucosa, the muscles most often paralysed initially are those of the pharynx, larynx and soft palate, with resulting dysphagia, dysarthria or aphonia, or nasal speech. Sometimes the external ocular muscles are affected. When the organism has contaminated a limb wound, then the weakness may begin in the muscles of that limb. Whatever the site of infection, the weakness may remain localised, but in other instances it

spreads to involve the muscles of all four limbs and those of the trunk. The physical signs of generalised muscular weakness with absent deep reflexes and variable sensory impairment are typical of any polyneuropathy, save for the almost constant involvement of bulbar muscles. Frequently the initial manifestations of diphtheritic polyneuropathy are observed within seven to 10 days of the onset of the infection, and weakness can be profound and generalised in two to four weeks. Recovery soon begins to occur spontaneously and is often complete, though variable muscular weakness and depression of deep reflexes sometimes persist. Fortunately, as a consequence of prophylactic inoculation, diphtheria is now a rare disease.

Tetanus

This condition is due to the exotoxin of the tetanus bacillus, which, being an anaerobic organism, flourishes only in deep penetrating wounds. The exotoxin enters the central nervous system by travelling along the sheaths of the peripheral nerves from the site of the injury. If the amount of toxin produced is large there is also rapid dissemination via the blood stream. This toxin interferes with the activity of the reflex arc in such a way that intense muscular spasms are produced by minimal sensory stimulation. The incubation period of the illness varies from three or four days to as long as several weeks after the injury. The longer the incubation period, the better the prognosis, as the development of symptoms within a few days after the injury usually implies a massive infection. Usually the first symptom is one of trismus or inability to open the jaw; this is followed by stiffness of the neck, dysphagia, spasm of the facial muscles (risus sardonicus) and eventually by rigidity of the abdominal muscles and of all the limbs. Noise or minimal sensory stimulation of any kind may then provoke intense and generalised muscular spasms, with arching of the back (opisthotonos). Between spasms the muscles remain rigid and the tendon reflexes are brisk. Hyperpyrexia often develops; death can result from heart failure, asphyxia or exhaustion. If the patient survives the first critical days the spasms gradually lessen in frequency and severity and recovery eventually occurs, though some stiffness may persist for several weeks. The disease can occur in a less severe or localised form when bacteria are present in fewer numbers, or when the patient has previously received prophylactic inoculations. In such cases the rigidity and spasms may remain localised to the limb or part of the body in which the original injury occurred and can persist for several weeks or months. In cephalic tetanus, following a facial wound, in addition to spasm of facial and jaw muscles, facial paralysis and ophthalmoplegia often develop on the side of the face nearest to the injury.

Botulism

This condition follows ingestion of the exotoxin of *Clostridium botulinum* and is always acquired from infected foodstuffs, particularly tinned food. The toxin has a direct effect upon the neuromuscular junction, inhibiting acetylcholine release. Symptoms usually develop within 24 to 48 hours after eating the tainted food. The first symptoms are usually vomiting and diarrhoea, followed by blurring of vision (due to pupillary dilatation), diplopia, ptosis, dysphagia, dysarthria and weakness of jaw muscles. Death is due to respiratory paralysis or bronchopneumonia. Between 20 and 60 per cent of cases are fatal; paralysis is lessened if antitoxin is administered quickly, and guanidine hydrochloride or other remedies which increase acetylcholine output (*see* p. 449) have been found to be helpful. The toxin can be destroyed by cooking tinned food for a few minutes and prophylaxis is much more satisfactory than treatment.

Other Neurological Complications of Specific Infections

In certain cases of **typhus fever** and other disorders due to rickettsial infection, nervous symptoms are prominent. Headache, sleeplessness and delirium may indicate an encephalitic element of the general infection but in addition, focal neurological signs (hemiplegia, aphasia, dysarthria, facial paralysis) occasionally develop and are most probably due to occlusion of cerebral vessels by so-called typhus nodules (foci of perivascular inflammation). In **typhoid fever,** delirium and confusion are common, but meningitis or cerebral abscess can rarely result from direct invasion of the nervous system by the typhoid bacillus. Rarely, too, the bacillus of **dysentery** or even the *Entamoeba histolytica* of amoebic dysentery are responsible for intracranial abscess formation. A form of **encephalopathy** can also complicate whooping cough; in such cases multiple cerebral petechial haemorrhages may be demonstrated and are possibly due to violent bouts of coughing. The clinical manifestations include convulsions, which may be repetitive and fatal, and focal neurological signs such as aphasia and hemiplegia. A similar syndrome, of unknown aetiology, but occasionally following non-specific or banal infections, has been called **acute toxic encephalopathy** and may be related more closely to post-infectious encephalitis (*see* p. 308). It occurs chiefly in young children, sometimes in small epidemics and is characterised by delirium or coma, convulsions, variable paresis of the limbs, and signs of meningeal irritation. The condition may be fatal but when recovery does occur it is often complete. A specific sub-variety is called **acute toxic encephalopathy with fatty degeneration of the viscera (Reye's disease)** and causes similar clinical manifestations in childhood along with hypoglycaemia and evidence of hepatic dysfunction; it is probably of viral origin. Yet another variant may be associated with opsoclonus (jerky spontaneous ocular movements) and myoclonus and is called **subacute myoclonic encephalopathy**. The CSF is usually normal in such cases.

While a depressive syndrome of considerable severity is a common sequel of **influenza**, cases of post-influenzal encephalomyelitis have been described; most are probably due to viral invasion of the brain, but others may be allergic in origin and related to the forms of encephalomyelitis which may complicate childhood exanthemata (*see* p. 308). The principal neurological complication of **acute rheumatism** is **rheumatic chorea**, which has already been mentioned in Chapter 9 (p. 202). Probably this condition is a form of rheumatic encephalitis, although the pathological changes in the brain in such cases are non-specific and the condition is not usually a complication of acute rheumatism but rather an alternative manifestation of rheumatic disease. It can affect the face and all four limbs or may be hemiplegic in distribution. In severe cases there are also mental confusion, restlessness and emotional lability. The involuntary movements of characteristic type sometimes persist for some months or years and may recur, especially in pregnancy (chorea gravidarum), but as a rule recovery is complete. One further neurological symptom which deserves mention is the **meningism** or occipital headache and neck stiffness which occasionally complicates infective illnesses and particularly pneumonia in childhood. Under such circumstances, lumbar puncture may be necessary to exclude meningitis, but the CSF is normal and the neck stiffness is difficult to explain.

Allergic or Hypersensitivity Disorders

It is now evident that many disorders of the central and peripheral nervous systems which were once thought to be due to unidentified infective agents result from an allergic or hypersensitivity response occurring within the nervous substance but affecting particularly the blood vessels and connective tissue elements. The pathological changes in such cases can be regarded as inflammatory in the broadest sense and often occur as the secondary effect of an infective agent which has not invaded the nervous system itself but has precipitated a cell-mediated or humoral immune response. In other instances the neurological manifestations are but one element of a clinical syndrome resulting from a generalised disorder of blood vessels and connective tissue. The neurological sequelae of prophylactic inoculation and the nervous complications of the common childhood exanthemata constitute an important group of disorders falling into this category; in most instances the neurological syndrome so produced is one of encephalomyelitis. This condition is generally considered with the group of so-called demyelinating disease, and will be described in Chapter 15. The principal conditions which warrant consideration here are serum neuropathy, 'shoulder girdle neuritis', postinfective polyneuritis and the neurological complications of the 'collagen', 'collagen-vascular' or 'connective tissue' diseases.

Serum Neuropathy

Serum neuropathy or neuritis is a condition which can follow the injection of foreign serum (e.g. antitetanic serum, antidiphtheritic serum). It is usually but one manifestation of the syndrome of serum sickness which may follow some days or weeks after such an injection, and in which fever, nausea and joint pains are usually the most prominent clinical features. The neuropathy generally affects cervical nerve roots and gives weakness and wasting of a group of muscles around the shoulder girdle, sometimes with localised sensory loss. Though some cases recover, in others, particularly when a single peripheral nerve seems to be involved (e.g. the nerve to serratus anterior), the weakness is permanent. The condition of so-called **shoulder-girdle neuritis** or **neuralgic amyotrophy** is similar and must be distinguished from the clinical syndrome designated by the outmoded term **brachial neuritis**; most cases so diagnosed in the past were the result of prolapse of a cervical intervertebral disk (*see* p. 367). True shoulder-girdle neuritis is a disorder of sudden onset which can follow an acute non-specific infection (e.g. influenza) or may complicate any febrile illness (e.g. pneumonia); occasionally it develops during pregnancy, after relatively minimal trauma or without apparent precipitating cause. The first symptom is a severe burning pain which generally develops over the shoulder and spreads down the arm to a variable extent. It can persist for several days making sleep impossible except with the aid of powerful analgesics and sedatives. Within a few days the patient becomes aware of muscular weakness and certain muscles (deltoid is a typical example) are found to be completely paralysed. The weakness may be limited to a single muscle (e.g. serratus anterior) but is sometimes much more extensive. Areas of sensory loss are often found, but are much less striking than the motor deficit. Gradually the pain improves and some return of muscular function occurs during the succeeding weeks or months; in most cases recovery is eventually complete, but some permanent weakness occasionally persists. No treatment, apart from analgesics, and later, remedial exercises and splinting where necessary, appears to be of any value.

Postinfective Polyneuritis

Postinfective polyneuritis or polyneuropathy is the term now used to describe the condition once entitled infectious polyneuritis. It is also known as the Guillain–Barré syndrome and is one of the commonest causes of the clinical syndrome of ascending paralysis (Landry's paralysis). The principal pathological change in such cases is an auto-immune inflammatory response within multiple spinal roots, so that strictly the disorder is a radiculopathy (polyradiculitis) as well as a peripheral neuropathy. Thus, lymphocytic infiltration is often found in peripheral nerves as well as in the roots. There is now good evidence to suggest that the nerves are attacked by lymphocytes which have become specifically sensitised to peripheral nerve protein, but humoral factors also play a part. The neuropathy is demyelinating in type although in long-lasting cases some secondary axonal degeneration occurs.

The condition can follow a preceding infective illness or may develop without apparent antecedent infection. Sometimes the first symptom is one of weakness in the feet and legs, which within a few hours or days spreads up the lower limbs and trunk giving an ascending flaccid paralysis. In acute cases the motor weakness ascends rapidly to involve the upper limbs, muscles of respiration and bulbar musculature; assisted respiration and tracheotomy may be necessary. More often weakness begins in the proximal muscles of the limbs. In some cases there are accompanying paraesthesiae and sensory loss with an ascending sensory 'level' on the trunk but usually motor symptoms and signs predominate. There are subacute cases in which the paralysis increases slowly over the course of several weeks or even months, in which despite a complaint of paraesthesiae sensory loss cannot be demonstrated, and in which the march of the disease process apparently becomes arrested when the weakness and sensory loss has reached the mid-dorsal or lower cervical level. In occasional cases weakness begins in the muscle innervated by the cranial nerves (cranial polyneuritis), again without significant sensory impairment.

Eventually there is usually spontaneous remission and the motor and sensory changes regress, until complete recovery occurs within the course of a few months, but in the more acute cases the condition constitutes a severe danger to life. Typically all the tendon reflexes in the affected limbs are lost and the paralysed limbs remain flaccid throughout; the plantar responses, when obtainable, are flexor. Though sensory loss is often minimal or absent, when present it usually affects all modalities of sensation; sphincter control is sometimes impaired, though not usually so early or as completely as in transverse myelitis (*see* p. 307) which may present a similar clinical picture but in which the plantar responses are extensor. In the occasional cases of cranial polyneuritis it may be difficult to distinguish the disorder from bulbar poliomyelitis and from neoplasms or granulomas of the basal meninges. In postinfective polyneuritis, after the first few days of the illness the CSF typically shows a substantial increase in protein content (0.1–1.0 g/l) but there is generally no pleocytosis (*dissociation albuminocytologique*). Slowing of nerve conduction is found early in the course of the illness. Although many patients with this disease recover completely, residual weakness and sensory impairment of some degree persist in some; some patients but not all appear to respond to prednisone or ACTH, and immuno-suppressive agents are often used in steroid-resistant cases. Many authorities, however, believe that these remedies are of no value and treatment, except with appropriate supportive measures, remains controversial.

Neurological Complications of the 'Collagen' Diseases
Many of the 'neurological' complications of the 'collagen' diseases using

neurological in its broadest sense to imply those disorders which fall into the province of the neurologist, affect the voluntary muscles. The principal conditions of this type, namely polymyositis and dermatomyositis, occurring alone or in combination with other conditions such as rheumatoid arthritis or scleroderma, are considered in Chapter 18. Polyneuropathy also occurs occasionally in association with rheumatoid arthritis. Chorea, as a form of rheur··ntic disease, has already been mentioned and cranial arteritis as well as other auto-immune arteritides are discussed in Chapter 17. The major disorders of the collagen group which remain are **systemic lupus erythematosus and polyarteritis nodosa** and so-called **mixed connective tissue disease**. Each of these disorders can give symptoms and signs of nervous disease by producing pathological changes in small blood vessels in the central or peripheral nervous system. Thus in systemic lupus erythematosus, focal lesions in the brain or brain stem may cause epilepsy, limb paresis, vertigo or cranial nerve palsies, while paraplegia due to spinal disease has been described. In occasional cases, too, a symmetrical polyneuropathy develops. Polyneuropathy (*see* Chapter 18) is even more common in polyarteritis nodosa, but can be asymmetrical or may give a clinical picture suggesting multiple peripheral nerve lesions (mononeuritis multiplex). More rarely, there are symptoms and signs indicating multiple lesions of the brain, brain stem or spinal cord. Whether systemic lupus or polyarteritis is the cause, there will usually be associated clinical features in such cases (including fever, multiple arthropathy, albuminuria, increased serum immunoglobulins, raised ESR) to indicate the nature of the underlying disease, but these features are sometimes unobtrusive and 'collagen' disease should always be considered in patients with obscure neurological syndromes which run a subacute or remittent clinical course.

References

Adams, R. D. and Petersdorf, R. G., 'Pyogenic infections of the central nervous system', in *Harrison's Principles of Internal Medicine*, Ed. Isselbacher, K. J., *et al.*, 9th ed., Chapter 368 (New York, McGraw-Hill, 1980).

Aita, J. A., *Neurologic Manifestations of General Diseases,* 2nd ed. (Springfield, Ill., Thomas, 1972).

Behan, P. O. and Currie, S., *Clinical Neuroimmunology,* Vol. 8 in Major Problems in Neurology, Ed. Walton, J. N. (London, Philadelphia, Toronto, W. B. Saunders, 1978).

Holmes, K. K., 'Syphilis', in *Harrison's Principles of Internal Medicine,* Ed. Wintrobe, M. M., *et al.*, 7th ed., Chapter 159 (New York, McGraw-Hill, 1974).

Kakulas, B. and Adams, R. D., 'Viral infections of the nervous system', in *Harrison's Principles of Internal Medicine,* Ed. Isselbacher, K. J., *et al.*, 9th ed., Chapter 369 (New York, McGraw-Hill, 1980).

Menkes, J. H., *Child Neurology,* 2nd ed. (Philadelphia, Lea and Febiger, 1980).

Merritt, H. H., *A Textbook of Neurology,* 5th ed., Chapter 1 (London, Kimpton, 1973).

Pennybacker, J. B., 'Abscess of the brain', in *Modern Trends in Neurology,* Ed. Feiling, A., 1st series, Chapter 10 (London, Butterworth, 1951).

Russell, W. R., *Poliomyelitis,* 2nd ed. (London, Arnold, 1956).

Spillane, J. D. (ed.), *Tropical Neurology,* (London, Oxford University Press, 1973).

Walton, J. N., *Brain's Diseases of the Nervous System.* 8th ed. (London, Oxford University Press, 1977).

15 Demyelinating Diseases

The demyelinating diseases are a group of disorders of the nervous system characterised pathologically by a destructive process affecting the myelin sheaths of nerve fibres within the brain and spinal cord. Although grey matter can be secondarily involved, these are primarily white matter diseases. The principal conditions which fall into this group are acute disseminated encephalomyelitis, acute haemorrhagic leucoencephalitis, neuromyelitis optica, multiple sclerosis and diffuse cerebral sclerosis. Whereas it now seems likely that autoimmune mechanisms within the nervous system account for most cases of acute encephalomyelitis, and similar factors may play a part in multiple sclerosis, the exact aetiology and pathogenesis of these disorders remains obscure, so that an aetiological classification of the separate disease entities within the group is still impossible. Clinical differentiation may also be difficult; although the natural history of a chronic relapsing case of multiple sclerosis is quite different from that of encephalomyelitis following measles, in other instances there may be no means of distinguishing between an acute episode of multiple sclerosis on the one hand and an encephalomyelitic illness on the other. Pathologically, too, there are similarities between the changes in the nervous system in each of these diseases. Between the acute perivascular inflammatory and demyelinating lesions which occur in en-cephalomyelitis, and the massive confluent areas of demyelination of diffuse cerebral sclerosis, there exists a spectrum of pathological change which can occur in varying permutations and combinations in each of these conditions. Sometimes the axis cylinders within areas of demyelination are destroyed early, in others they survive for some time, but the overall pattern of pathological reaction is broadly similar; this does not imply identity of aetiology, as the nervous system has only a limited repertoire of pathological responses and myelin destruction may result from many noxious agents. Thus no clear-cut definition of the demyelinating diseases is at present possible, and some of the clinical syndromes customarily identified (of which neuromyelitis optica is a good example) may be artificially defined. Certainly several conditions traditionally classified as forms of cerebral diffuse sclerosis (such as metachromatic leucodystrophy due to aryl sulphatase deficiency) are now known to be due to specific inborn metabolic abnormalities.

Acute Disseminated Encephalomyelitis

Acute disseminated encephalomyelitis is an acute inflammatory disorder of the brain and/or spinal cord of variable clinical course and severity, in which the principal pathological changes are perivascular cellular infiltration and perivenous demyelination in the white matter of the brain or spinal cord. Pathologically the condition differs from the various viral forms of encephalitis (*see* pp. 283–290) which are essentially polioclastic (i e. involving grey rather than white matter). The syndrome can follow smallpox vaccination, inoculation against rabies or other protective inoculations, or a non-specific 'influenzal' infective illness; alternatively it may develop during one of the childhood exanthemata, while on occasion such an illness occurs without there being any clinical evidence of preceding or concurrent infection. Probably this is an autoimmune response of the nervous system to many antigenic agents, some viral; the disorder closely resembles experimental allergic encephalomyelitis which can be produced in animals by injecting brain emulsion or purified encephalitogenic factor with Freund's adjuvant. Recent work suggests that the distinction between this condition and the viral encephalitides is less absolute than was once thought as in some such cases active virus can be isolated from brain tissue.

The clinical picture of the illness is variable; sometimes it is primarily encephalitic with headache, drowsiness, confusion and possibly convulsions, but in other cases the disease process appears to be confined to the spinal cord and a syndrome of transverse or ascending myelitis results. Indeed at the present time, when neurosyphilis is comparatively rare, post-infective encephalomyelitis and multiple sclerosis are the most common causes of **transverse myelitis**. Less commonly the clinical features indicate that the disease process is involving brain-stem structures or cerebellar connexions, to give ataxia, nystagmus, vertigo and cranial nerve palsies. In such a case, differential diagnosis from an acute episode of multiple sclerosis is difficult if not impossible, and may depend wholly upon follow-up studies. In yet other cases there may be involvement of motor and sensory roots as well as the spinal cord and the condition resembles the closely-related acute post-infective polyneuritis (the Guillain–Barré syndrome). Often the question as to whether or not the spinal cord is involved depends upon the plantar responses. It will now be convenient to consider the clinical features of the different varieties of encephalomyelitis.

Post-vaccinal encephalomyelitis and the disorder which may follow **rabies inoculation** are broadly similar. The post-vaccinal condition is most common after primary smallpox vaccination in children of school age, and has been known in epidemics to affect as many as 1 in 2,500 vaccinated individuals though its incidence at the present day is very much less. Many patients have a relatively mild encephalitic illness which begins with headache, neck stiffness, drowsiness, fever and vomiting and lasts for only a few days. In others convulsions occur and there is stupor and later deepening coma. The condition must be distinguished from post-vaccinial encephalopathy which, particularly in infants and young children, causes transient drowsiness and convulsions, often lasting for no more than 24 to 48 hours. Often symptoms and signs of spinal cord involvement are seen; hemiplegia is comparatively rare but often there is ascending flaccid weakness of the limbs with loss of tendon reflexes and paralysis of the bladder and bowels. Indeed, in occasional cases, a myelitic picture of this nature can occur without headache, neck stiffness or clouding of consciousness. The disease may be fatal in up to 30 per cent of cases, although the prognosis is probably influenced favourably nowadays by steroid therapy. In the remaining cases eventual recovery is often complete, although neurological signs, intellectual deterioration and personality change may persist for some years and are rarely permanent. A similar illness is seen less often after prophylactic inoculation against pertussis and more rarely still after diphtheria or tetanus vaccine.

The commonest variety of **post-exanthematous encephalomyelitis** is that which complicates *measles*, though a similar disorder may also occur following *chicken pox* (varicella) or *German measles* (rubella), and very rarely in *scarlet fever* (scarlatina). The neurological complications of mumps and glandular fever are probably due to direct invasion of the nervous system by the causal virus, giving a lymphocytic meningitis and occasionally encephalitis, while those of whooping cough (pertussis encephalopathy) are more probably due to repeated episodes of cerebral anoxia developing during bouts of coughing. The encephalomyelitis of measles usually develops some two to four days after the rash appears but can even antedate it; it has been known rarely to develop in contacts who do not develop a rash. The usual pattern of the illness is one of encephalitis which, if mild, gives headache, neck stiffness, drowsiness and confusion for a few days, but if severe there are convulsions and deepening coma. Less commonly an acute hemiplegia develops, or a cerebellar ataxia of acute onset, while some few cases develop a transverse myelitis or polyradiculitis. About 10 per cent of cases end fatally; many recover completely but a few remain disabled by hemiplegia, paraplegia, fits or dementia. In chicken pox the clinical picture is broadly similar but most cases of encephalitis complicating this illness are mild and recover completely, while cerebellar ataxia occurs in an unusually large proportion. An explosive encephalomyelitic illness can occasionally complicate rubella, but more often in this disease the encephalitic or myelitic illness, if it occurs, is mild and transient.

The form of **postinfective encephalomyelitis** which can follow non-specific infective illnesses or which may occur without clinical evidence of preceding infection, is even more protean in its manifestations. Sometimes the picture is that of severe disseminated encephalomyelitis with deepening coma, convulsions and flaccid paraplegia, or the illness may be mild with headache, drowsiness, fever and transient limb or bulbar pareses. Alternatively, a transverse myelitis may be the presenting feature, while in many cases the disease process affects the brain stem, giving nystagmus, impairment of conjugate ocular movement, dysphagia, facial weakness and variable long-tract signs. As mentioned above the clinical features may be indistinguishable from those produced by an initial episode of multiple sclerosis. There may also be difficulty in diagnosis from viral encephalitis. While herpes simplex encephalitis (*see* p. 288) usually gives a hyperacute clinical picture suggesting a focal lesion in one temporal lobe, some patients show a non-specific acute encephalitic picture and the diagnosis may depend upon fluorescent antibody studies. Other specific varieties of viral encephalitis (e.g. the St Louis type) occur in endemic areas. The view that many cases previously regarded as examples of postinfective encephalomyelitis may result from viral infection is gaining ground. In early childhood the condition which has been called 'acute cerebellar ataxia of infancy' is probably a variant of encephalomyelitis and can also occur in a subacute form.

The changes in the cerebrospinal fluid in all varieties of encephalomyelitis are similar, though by no means diagnostic. There is a variable pleocytosis, usually lymphocytic, but in acute cases polymorphonuclear leucocytes are present for a few days; the protein and immunoglobulin content of the fluid is invariably raised.

Acute Haemorrhagic Leucoencephalitis

This condition, which in the United States is often called acute necrotising haemorrhagic leucoencephalopathy, is a fulminating form of acute encephalomyelitis. A closely related condition is brain purpura which can be fatal within a few hours and is probably due to an acute hypersensitivity reaction affecting cerebral blood vessels. In haemorrhagic leucoencephalitis the pathological changes are those of widespread vascular necrosis with perivascular haemorrhage in the cerebral white matter and with large areas of demyelination which may be confluent. The onset of the illness is often apoplectiform, with headache, convulsions and coma which deepens rapidly. The physical signs are often unilateral in the first instance so that an onset with hemiplegia is not infrequent. Death often occurs within 24 to 48 hours; comparatively few cases are recognised during life, but a polymorphonuclear reaction in the CSF with a moderate rise in protein can be a valuable guide to the diagnosis, even though the clinical features may mimic those of massive cerebral infarction or cerebral abscess. This clinical picture is similar to that of herpes simplex encephalitis, although pathologically the two conditions are quite different. Recent evidence suggests that the herpetic condition is the commoner of the two and that haemorrhagic leucoencephalitis is now very rare. Possibly in some cases of myelitis of exceptionally acute onset, the pathological process in the spinal cord is similar.

Neuromyelitis Optica

It is doubtful whether neuromyelitis optica (Devic's disease) should be considered as a separate disease entity, as the clinical features which are typical of this syndrome can occur as one episode in the course of multiple sclerosis. Rarely, too, cases of postinfective encephalomyelitis present in this way. The symptoms of the condition, which is relatively common in Japan, are, however, sufficiently distinctive for it to be regarded as a separate syndrome even though its pathogenesis and nosological status remain uncertain. The condition may develop at any age and in either sex. Typically it begins with pain in the eyes and visual loss which may be unilateral at first but usually involves the other eye within hours or days. Blindness may rapidly become complete with subsequent slow regression but in other cases some useful vision is retained throughout. Usually the optic disks are swollen and the visual fields show bilateral central scotomas, though one eye is often more severely affected than the other. Soon afterwards the typical picture of a transverse myelitis appears with flaccid paralysis of the limbs, loss of sphincter control, absence of tendon reflexes, extensor plantar responses, and an ascending sensory 'level' below which all forms of sensation are impaired. Sometimes the spinal cord symptoms precede the visual loss, and it is possible that some cases of bilateral retrobulbar neuritis without neurological signs are abortive examples of this syndrome. The CSF shows simply a non-specific rise in protein and mononuclear cells with raised IgG. The disorder is fatal within a few weeks in some cases, others make a slow but complete recovery; in this instance one may assume in retrospect that the pathological process was probably one of acute encephalomyelitis. However, a number of patients have residual visual loss and optic atrophy with paraplegia, and many of these eventually turn out to be suffering from multiple sclerosis. Probably all cases of this syndrome should be treated initially with ACTH or prednisone.

Multiple Sclerosis

Multiple or disseminated sclerosis is a disease of obscure aetiology characterised clinically by symptoms which indicate the presence of multiple lesions in the white matter of the brain and spinal cord. In most cases the disease process extends episodically, with remissions of variable duration separating the relapses, but in other individuals it presents as an intermittently progressive disease with spastic paraparesis and/or signs of cerebellar or brain-stem disease. Although there are many relatively mild cases in which relapses occur at intervals of several years and even then are comparatively transient and only slightly incapacitating, it is equally true that in others the disease is inexorably progressive, producing almost total disability and rarely death within one to two years of the onset. Eventually most patients are disabled by progressive paraplegia and/or ataxia. Pathologically there are multiple plaques of demyelination and gliosis of varying age throughout the nervous system; these mainly involve the white matter of the brain and cord and are often perivenous or periventricular in distribution, but the grey matter is sometimes involved as well.

The **aetiology** of the disease remains obscure. It is commonest in temperate climates, being rare in the tropics, and although it is principally a disease of the white races it does appear sometimes in Negroes living in Europe or North America. It occurs equally in the two sexes and usually begins between the ages of 20 and 40, although it occasionally develops in the first and second decades or in the fifth and sixth. Its prevalence in temperate zones is between 50 and 150 per 100,000 population. It certainly occurs more often in several members of a family than could be accounted for by chance, but rarely afflicts more than one of a pair of identical twins, so that the genetic factor cannot be very powerful. Probably there is an inherited susceptibility to the agent or agents which account for the demyelinating process. Recent evidence suggests that this susceptibility may be related to the presence of certain histocompatibility antigens. The determinants HLA–A3 and HLA–B7 are significantly more common in MS patients than in controls; the increased frequency of these may be related to a high incidence of the mixed-leucocyte culture determinant HLA–DW2. These relationships may account at least in part for the geographical distribution of the disease. The rarity of conjugal cases is against an infective theory of aetiology, and there is no concrete evidence to indicate that the disease is due to infection by a virus or spirochaete. However, recent work has revived the view that the condition may be due to a 'slow virus' infection or alternatively that it may represent an abnormal hypersensitivity response on the part of the nervous system to the presence of one or more common viral agents. Antibody studies have suggested that the measles virus may sometimes play such a role. Other theories implicating excessive dietary animal fat, heavy-metal poisoning, vasospasm or venous thrombosis also have adherents. Current opinion favours the view that the disease is due to a recurrent allergic response of the nervous system to various allergens. Although evidence in favour of the allergic hypothesis is much less convincing in this disease than in acute encephalomyelitis, it receives modest support from the fact that the total γ-globulin and oligoclonal IgG are generally increased in the CSF. It is also apparent that relapses can repeatedly follow infective illnesses in some individuals, and they have also been described following prophylactic inoculation. The fact that onset or relapse may also follow trauma and/or emotional stress is much less easy to explain.

The **clinical manifestations** of the disease can be very variable, depending upon the situation and intensity of the pathological changes. A single discrete lesion occurring at the outset may be responsible for many individual symptoms and signs depending upon its site, but if multiple lesions occur simultaneously in eloquent areas of the nervous system a much more specific clinical picture will result. This variation in spatial distribution of the areas of demyelination is responsible for the remarkable clinical pleomorphism of the disease. Symptoms due to a single localised lesion almost always remit within a few days or weeks as do those attributable to multiple lesions which have developed acutely. In such cases, numerous relapses may occur, each followed by a partial remission, but each leaving in its wake further evidence of permanent neurological deficit upon which each succeeding manifestation is superimposed. In the end the clinical picture is often indistinguishable from that observed in cases which from the beginning are recognised as harbouring multiple and widespread lesions, all progressing inexorably at much the same rate. The relapsing type with multiple acute or subacute episodes is commoner in young patients, whereas in cases with an onset in middle life the course of the disease is more often slowly progressive and the brunt of the disease process usually falls upon the spinal cord. Although it is possible that in a few cases the disease becomes arrested, and that in fewer still a remission may be complete and permanent, most cases eventually follow a final common path of increasing ataxia and/or spasticity, immobility, respiratory or urinary infection and death.

Although it is a truism that almost any symptom of neurological disease can at some time be observed in cases of multiple sclerosis, there are certain symptom-complexes which occur particularly often, usually as the presenting features of the disease.

One of the most frequent initial symptoms is *visual failure*, which is generally unilateral but occasionally bilateral, and is the result of *retrobulbar neuritis*. There is often pain in the eye with progressive blurring or dimming of vision over a period of several hours or days. Often vision is totally lost but spontaneous improvement generally occurs and recovery may be complete within a few weeks or months, although a central scotoma sometimes remains. In the acute stage the optic disk is usually swollen, but subsequently waxy pallor of the temporal half of the disk or optic atrophy is seen. An alternative presenting symptom, which can also antedate other neurological manifestations by several years, is *diplopia*, lasting for several hours or days. Occasionally this is due to involvement of the nucleus of one of the oculomotor nerves, but more often it is of central or internuclear type, occurring without an objective ocular palsy. A sign almost pathognomonic of this disease is Harris's sign, or ataxic nystagmus, in which, on lateral gaze, there is gross nystagmus in the abducting eye and failure of medial movement of the adducting eye.

An alternative mode of onset is with *transient weakness or loss of control of the limbs.* The weakness can take the form of a monoparesis or hemiparesis, but paraparesis is more common. There is weakness and clumsiness of the affected limb or limbs with difficulty in walking. Frequently, the weakness is asymmetrical so that even in the presence of clear-cut signs of pyramidal tract dysfunction in both legs the patient may complain that one leg only 'drags' and often insists that the other is normal. In mild or early cases the weakness may only become apparent after walking or standing for long periods. Physical examination during the episode reveals either spasticity with increased reflexes and extensor plantar responses, or cerebellar ataxia. These initial manifestations may resolve over a few days or weeks to be succeeded by other manifestations in the subsequent months or years.

Sensory symptoms are also common as primary manifestations. Paraesthesiae in a limb lasting for a few days can easily be overlooked; often these spread in a typical manner, indicating centrifugal spread of a plaque of demyelination in the posterior columns of the cord. In such a case the tingling and numbness may spread up one leg and down the other or from an arm to the trunk and then to the face and leg on the same side of the body. Often there are 'tight-band' sensations or feelings of swelling in the affected member (*see* p. 213). The so-called 'useless hand' syndrome is often due to such a lesion which so impairs proprioceptive sensation in one hand that the patient is virtually unable to use it even though motor power remains intact. On examination there is impairment of position and joint sense, of vibration sense and two-point discrimination in the affected limb or limbs, while if the legs are involved, Romberg's sign will be positive. Lhermitte's sign is often present too. Less frequently the patient observes, particularly on entering a hot bath, that pain and temperature sensation is diminished in one leg, and examination reveals the clinical features of a partial Brown–Séquard syndrome, indicating the presence of a plaque of demyelination in one lateral column of the spinal cord. Sensory symptoms almost invariably remit over the course of a few weeks or months.

Symptoms indicating primary *involvement of brain-stem structures* are also common. One mode of presentation is with an acute episode of vertigo and vomiting due to involvement of vestibular centres; evidence of sensory or motor long-tract lesions is occasionally seen in such cases. More often as the vertigo abates the patient also complains of diplopia and ataxic nystagmus is often found. Alternatively, there is sometimes an ataxia of relatively acute onset with signs of cerebellar disease affecting the co-ordination of all four limbs; this is generally associated with severe nystagmus on lateral gaze and with dysarthria (Charcot's triad). A similar constellation of signs may also develop at a later stage in established cases. Combined lesions involving cranial-nerve nuclei and long tracts are also seen occasionally in bewildering variety. Unilateral facial paralysis is seen rarely and may be difficult or impossible to distinguish from Bell's palsy unless there are other signs. Some patients develop a unilateral facial anaesthesia which is followed months later by tic douloureux on the same side of the face and later still by evidence of spinal cord disease. Tic douloureux (*see* p. 88) can also develop in patients who have suffered from the disease for some years.

As already mentioned, many patients demonstrate a *slowly-progressive weakness and clumsiness of the limbs.* When this occurs in younger patients there is usually clinical evidence of widespread lesions. Thus it is common to find in such individuals temporal pallor of the optic disks (even without a previous history of retrobulbar neuritis), nystagmus, cerebellar ataxia, and spastic weakness of the limbs with absent vibration sense at the ankles. In the common intermittently-progressive form of multiple sclerosis which begins in middle life the main brunt of the disease falls upon the pyramidal tracts in the spinal cord, and the signs are those of a spastic paraparesis or quadriparesis with impaired or absent perception of vibration in the lower limbs, but without any evidence of cranial nerve involvement. A transient increase in the severity of both symptoms and signs may occur due to vasodilatation as after a hot bath or physical exertion (Uhthoff's symptom).

Acute episodes of multiple sclerosis can involve almost any area of the central nervous system. Thus the onset may be explosive with headache, vomiting, vertigo and facial pain and with a succession of symptoms indicating severe involvement of the brain stem, optic nerves or spinal cord. Indeed an episode indistinguishable from other forms of transverse myelitis may occur. Rarely a cerebral illness with mental changes, convulsions, aphasia, hemiplegia or hemianopia develops at the onset. Even in subacute or chronic cases, plaques of cerebral demyelination occasionally cause recurrent focal or major fits. Under such circumstances, differentiation from acute encephalomyelitis is difficult or impossible.

Mental symptoms are not infrequent. Often features of emotional elaboration of symptoms suggesting hysteria are present at the outset and may mask the organic nature of the illness. Euphoria is the prevailing mood of many patients, but some are depressed; in the late stages a progressive dementia sometimes develops.

Sphincter involvement is common; urgency or precipitancy of micturition is a constant feature in most established cases, but as the paraplegia advances, urinary retention with overflow is common and even faecal incontinence occasionally develops.

The **prognosis** of the disease is variable. Many patients live for as long as 30 to 50 years from the onset, while a few die within one to two years. The prognosis is much more favourable in patients who are not significantly disabled within five years of the onset or in those presenting with sensory symptoms or with relapses followed by complete remission. An onset with cerebellar ataxia or the development of cerebellar signs at any stage imply a more serious outlook. However, the disease runs a very indolent or benign course in almost 20 per cent of patients. A few who suffer episodes of retrobulbar neuritis or other attacks strongly suggestive of multiple sclerosis even remain symptom-free indefinitely. The average duration of the disease is from 20 to 30 years; the final state of the bedridden incontinent patient, racked by painful flexor spasms of the lower limbs and shaken by febrile episodes of intercurrent infection, is one of the most distressing in medicine.

The **cerebrospinal fluid** may be normal, particularly in chronic or advanced cases. During an acute episode there is occasionally a moderate mononuclear pleocytosis of up to 50 cells/mm^3 and the protein content of the fluid is often raised to between 0.5 and 0.9 g/l. In about 25 per cent of cases the colloidal gold (Lange) curve is paretic in type. However, this abnormality is seen in less than 50 per cent of cases. Over 50 per cent show an increase in the total γ-globulin content of the fluid, but between 70 and 90 per cent have an increased percentage (in relation to the total protein) of oligoclonal IgG, especially in acute cases or during relapses.

Electrophysiological techniques have recently been shown to be of considerable diagnostic value. Delay in the conduction of pattern-evoked visual potentials from the eye to the cerebral cortex may give evidence of subclinical optic nerve demyelination, even in the absence of a history of retrobulbar neuritis. Measurement of auditory evoked potentials and of both cerebral and spinal somatosensory potentials have proved of lesser value but are helpful in detecting unsuspected conduction delay indicative of demyelination in some cases. The **CAT scan** shows in some cases areas of reduced density, presumed to be plaques of demyelination, in the cerebral white matter.

The **diagnosis** in a typical case in which there has been a remittent course and the clinical features indicate the presence of lesions widely disseminated throughout the central nervous system, is not difficult. It is indeed a useful axiom that this disease should not be diagnosed when all the symptoms and signs can be accounted for by a single lesion. Whereas this rule must often be ignored in the presence of one of the typical symptom-complexes described above, it is a useful guide. Acute episodes may mimic epidemic vertigo, meningovascular syphilis and even encephalitis; the first of these can only be recognised by the course of the illness and then not with certainty, but the other two conditions will generally be identified by means of CSF examination. Distinction from acute encephalomyelitis may also be particularly difficult but the latter is usually a monophasic self-limiting disease. In the more chronic cases, diagnosis from the familial ataxias is made by virtue of the consistent pattern of inheritance and stereotyped clinical pattern of the latter group of diseases, while motor neurone disease is identified by the presence of muscular wasting and fasciculation, features which are very rare indeed in multiple sclerosis, in which the lower motor neurones are hardly ever involved. Subacute combined degeneration can occasionally be mimicked and when 'posterior column' and 'pyramidal' symptoms and signs predominate, examination of the blood and estimation of the serum B_{12} are obligatory. In patients who present with a progressive spastic paraplegia it is sometimes impossible to exclude spinal tumour and cervical spondylosis with certainty except by myelography, and in such individuals the diagnosis of multiple sclerosis may have to be made by exclusion, although a raised IgG in the CSF will give valuable confirmatory evidence.

The **treatment** of this and other conditions will be considered in Chapter 20, but it may be said that no single form of therapy is uniformly successful, though there is some evidence that ACTH or steroid therapy may favourably influence acute relapses of the disease in a few cases and that others may obtain temporary benefit from physiotherapy. Drugs such as diazepam, dantrolene or baclofen may be helpful in reducing spasticity, while propantheline and related remedies sometimes help to diminish urgency and incontinence of micturition. In advanced cases with painful and disabling extensor spasticity or flexor spasms, intrathecal phenol injections may be of great value. It is usually wise not to reveal the nature of the illness to patients who have had one or two transient episodes of disability, and to use terms such as 'neuritis' in explaining the nature of their symptoms, but when the disease process is established and progressive, there is little advantage in withholding the true facts of the situation; in appropriate cases it is useful to stress how benign the disorder can often be.

Diffuse Cerebral Sclerosis and the Leucodystrophies

Diffuse cerebral sclerosis was first described by Schilder in 1912 under the title of **encephalitis periaxalis diffusa**. Pathologically it was thought to be characterised by a progressive massive demyelination of the cerebral white matter, usually beginning posteriorly and spreading more or less symmetrically throughout the two hemispheres but sparing the arcuate fibres of the occipital lobes. Macroscopically the affected white matter became greyish, rubbery and translucent, and microscopically there was accumulation of sudanophilic lipid derived from the degenerating myelin so that the condition was sometimes called **sudanophilic diffuse sclerosis**. Clinically the condition was described as beginning usually in childhood with progressive visual failure, focal or generalised fits, aphasia, mental deterioration and variable degrees of paresis of the limbs, leading eventually to total blindness, dementia and spastic quadriplegia. Rarely the onset was sudden with headache, stupor and convulsions. The condition was progressive, uninfluenced by treatment and usually ended fatally in the first decade within one to three years of the onset. The CSF commonly showed an increase in its protein content, the EEG diffuse slow activity.

The nosological status of Schilder's disease has become confused over the years because the condition has not been properly distinguished either clinically or pathologically from a number of other progressive white matter diseases, often occurring in infancy and childhood, which have in the past been classified as diffuse cerebral sclerosis but which are now known to be disorders of the metabolism of myelin or to be the result of storage of abnormal chemical substances in the cerebral and spinal white matter and sometimes even in peripheral nerves. These are now classified as the **leucodystrophies**. Another important development has been the discovery that many male patients previously diagnosed as examples of Schilder's disease also show adrenal atrophy pathologically and some also have the clinical features of Addison's disease. This condition, now known to be due to an X-linked gene, is known as **adrenoleucodystrophy** (Addison–Schilder's disease). It has also become evident that many other cases of what was once called Schilder's disease are due to acute cerebral multiple sclerosis. Whether there is a form of Schilder's disease which is sporadic and not X-linked and not associated with adrenal dysfunction, and which is not due to cerebral multiple sclerosis, is still uncertain.

Of the other leucodystrophies, there is one of infantile onset and X-linked recessive inheritance which usually presents with disorganised ocular movements and cerebellar ataxia; in this condition, **Pelizaeus–Merzbacher disease**, the pathological changes are similar to those of Schilder's disease but the adrenals are spared. In autosomal recessive **metachromatic leucodystrophy** (p. 243) due to aryl-sulphatase deficiency, there is diffuse demyelination with the accumulation of metachromatically staining granules in the white matter of the brain and peripheral nerves. In childhood, dysarthria, spasticity, athetoid movements and dementia begin at about the age of two years and there are signs of polyneuropathy with slowing of peripheral nerve conduction. Death occurs within six months to three or four years after the onset. The CSF protein is usually raised and peripheral nerve biopsy may give diagnostic findings. An adult-onset form occurs giving rise to progressive dementia, spasticity and subclinical polyneuropathy. The features of **globoid cell leucodystrophy** (Krabbe's disease) are not very different except that the onset is usually in the first six months of life with irritability, convulsions, spasticity, optic atrophy and progressive dementia, death occurring as a rule within a few months. There is a substantial rise in the CSF protein and marked slowing of nerve conduction. Large globoid cells containing cerebroside are found in areas of degenerating white matter in the brain, spinal cord and peripheral nerves. The condition is due to an autosomal recessive gene causing a deficiency of galactocerebroside beta-galactosidase.

References

Acheson, D., Matthews, W. B., Batchelor, J. R. and Weller, R., *McAlpine's Multiple Sclerosis* 3rd ed. (Edinburgh and London, Churchill Livingstone, 1981).
Adams, C. W. M., *Research on Multiple Sclerosis* (Springfield, Ill., Thomas, 1972).

Behan, P. O. and Currie, S., *Clinical Neuroimmunology,* Major Problems in Neurology, Vol. 8 (London, Philadelphia, Toronto, W. B. Saunders, 1978).

Dawson, D. M., *Multiple Sclerosis Update,* Section II in *Current Neurology,* Vol. 2, Ed. Tyler, H. R. and Dawson, D. M. (Boston, Mass., Houghton Mifflin, 1979).

Menkes, J. H., *Textbook of Child Neurology,* 2nd ed. (Philadelphia, Lea & Febiger, 1980).

Millar, J. H. D., *Multiple Sclerosis: A Disease Acquired in Childhood* (Springfield, Ill., Thomas, 1971).

Walton, J. N., *Brain's Diseases of the Nervous System,* 8th ed. (London, Oxford University Press, 1977).

Wood, J. H. (Ed.), *Neurobiology of the Cerebrospinal Fluid,* Vol. 1 (New York and London, Plenum Press, 1980).

16 Neoplasms and the Nervous System

About 1 per cent of all deaths are due to intracranial tumours. These occur in great variety; most are locally malignant, and constitute about 15 per cent of all malignant tumours occurring in man. Of these, most arise primarily within the cranial cavity and, being invasive, can rarely be removed surgically, but many are metastatic from a malignant neoplasm growing elsewhere in the body which has given secondary deposits within the brain or in the bones of the cranial cavity. There are, however, a number of benign neoplasms which may grow within the skull, and it is particularly important that these should be recognised as they can generally be removed in whole or in part at operation, with excellent results. The proportion of intraspinal tumours which compress the spinal cord and are benign is very much higher, and diagnosis of these removable growths is even more imperative. The symptomatology of intracranial neoplasia is very variable, as it depends not only upon the character of the neoplasm but also upon its situation and rate of growth, There are limitless permutations and combinations of these three factors which may influence the clinical picture. However, intracranial tumours generally produce a number of general symptoms, upon which the specific features produced by different varieties of tumour arising in individual situations are superimposed. Before considering these general symptoms and some of the more common and important tumour syndromes, it is first necessary to formulate a working classification of tumours of the nervous system, in order to provide an understanding of the basic pathological features of intracranial and intraspinal new growths, and to give an approximate outline of their relative incidence.

Classification of Neoplasms in the Nervous System

In the absence of any convincing evidence about the aetiology of intracranial or intraspinal tumours, they are at present classified according to their cells of origin. Of the **primary neoplasms**, those arising from the nerve cells and fibres themselves or from their cells of embryonic origin (neuroblastomas and neurocytomas) are rare. Commonest are the gliomas, of which the most malignant is the glioblastoma multiforme, the least invasive the astrocytoma. According to the popular Kernohan classification all gliomas are called astrocytomas and are graded in Groups I to IV according to the characteristics of the predominant cells in the tumour; Group I is the least, and Group IV the most anaplastic and malignant. Accurate grading can be difficult, as in a single tumour it may be possible to find certain cells characteristic of glioblastoma and others which are those of a typical slowly-growing astrocytoma. The rapidly-growing medulloblastoma, a common malignant tumour of the posterior fossa in infancy and childhood, which tends to metastasise, usually in the subarachnoid space, but sometimes to long bones, is probably best classified with the gliomas, although its predominant cell is very different from the astrocyte and its precursors. Other tumours of the nervous supporting tissues are first, the relatively slow-growing and benign oligodendroglioma, which has a particular tendency to calcify, and the ependymoma, which, because of the cells from which it originates, grows in relation to the cerebral ventricles or to the central canal of the spinal cord.

Of the primary neoplasms which arise in the meninges, the benign meningioma is the most common, but occasionally a fibrosarcoma, a reticulum cell sarcoma, or a melanoma may arise in this situation. In considering growths which arise from organs which are attached to or lie in close relationship to the brain, though not strictly a part of it, there are the adenomas of the pituitary gland (the hypophysis), pinealomas, papillomas of the choroid plexus and glomus tumours which arise from the glomus jugulare. Neoplasms of developmental origin ('rest cell' tumours) include: the craniopharyngioma which arises from remnants of Rathke's pouch; haemangioblastomas which are usually found in the cerebellum; arteriovenous angiomas or hamartomas (which are more properly regarded as vascular malformations rather than tumours); chordomas, which are generally found either in relation to the brain stem or in the sacral region and grow from primitive remnants of the notochord; lipomas in the corpus callosum or spinal canal; epidermoid (cholesteatoma) and dermoid cysts, some of which are teratomas; and an uncommon tumour called a colloid cyst which is generally found in the third ventricle and arises from vestiges of the primitive paraphysis. Primary neoplasms of the cranial or vertebral bones which secondarily involve the brain or spinal cord are relatively uncommon. These include osteomas, osteogenic sarcomas, osteoclastomas, and haemangiomas of vertebral bodies. Lastly, in considering primary tumours, one must remember those which grow from or in relation to nerve trunks, as these may form upon cranial nerves or spinal nerve roots to give symptoms and signs indicating the presence of an intracranial or intraspinal tumour. By far the commonest is the neuroma, neurolemmoma, neurinoma, or neurofibroma (as it is variously called), which grows from the sheath of Schwann; usually a neoplasm of this type takes the form of an encapsulated swelling upon a nerve, but occasionally it infiltrates between nerve fibres, with which it becomes inextricably intermingled to give a plexiform neuroma. This latter type of growth is seen particularly on peripheral nerves. Neurofibromas sometimes grow in relation to nerve plexuses or single peripheral nerves outside the central nervous system, when they give a clinical picture indicating a peripheral nerve or plexus lesion (*see* Chapter 13) and there is usually a palpable swelling over the nerve trunk. Fibrosarcomas also occur occasionally on or in peripheral nerves.

When one comes to consider **secondary tumours**, those which are most common are secondary carcinomas, arising as blood-borne metastases from tumours in other sites, of which the lung, breast, kidney, ovary and colon are the most frequent. Sarcomas of bone and other tissues and malignant melanomas also sometimes metastasise to the brain. Another common group of cases is that in which malignant tumours involve the cranial bones, vertebral bodies or extradural tissues and subsequently involve the brain or spinal cord. Of these the most prominent are carcinoma of the nasopharynx or paranasal sinuses, metastatic carcinoma involving the bone (lung, prostate, breast, thyroid) and multiple myelomatosis; cranial (particularly orbital) and spinal myelomas are often single and unaccompanied, at least for some time, by diffuse myelomatosis. Deposits of lymphadenoma (Hodgkin's disease), of the other reticuloses and leukaemic infiltrates occasionally involve the brain, more often the cranial and spinal meninges.

Lastly it is important to remember that certain conditions which are not strictly neoplastic can give a clinical picture suggesting the presence of a space-occupying lesion within the skull or spinal column. That this is true of cerebral abscess has already been mentioned (*see* p. 281) but in such individuals there is usually clinical evidence of infection. In others, however, an intracranial or intraspinal mass of inflammatory origin develops in an indolent manner without such clear clinical evidence. This is true of certain granulomas (gumma, tuberculoma, sarcoidosis) and parasitic cysts (e.g. cysticercosis). Arachnoidal cysts of developmental origin are rare in the cranial cavity, more common in the spinal canal.

There is much evidence to suggest that the relative incidence of these tumours has changed considerably over the years. Thus the once common granulomas (gumma, tuberculoma) are now rare in Western Europe and in the USA (though not in parts of Asia) and the incidence of metastatic tumours is increasing. The most common intracranial tumours are gliomas, metastases and meningiomas in that order. In adult life, most gliomas are supratentorial, and over half are glioblastomas; more males than females are affected. In childhood, most gliomas occur in the posterior fossa and are generally either medulloblastomas, cerebellar astrocytomas or pontine gliomas. Gliomas developing in adult life are most common in middle-age; but in women, with increasing age there is an increasing probability that a supratentorial neoplasm will be a meningioma. In the spinal canal, gliomas are comparatively rare, and neurofibromas, which occur at any spinal level and equally in the two sexes, are much more common. Spinal meningiomas usually occur in the dorsal region, and nearly always in women. An outline of this classification with approximate figures of incidence are given in Table 7.

Intracranial Tumours

The Pathophysiology of Increased Intracranial Pressure

We must first consider the means by which intracranial tumours alter brain function and so give rise to symptoms and signs. The brain and its membranes are contained within the rigid bony skull; any increase in volume of the intracranial contents means that CSF is displaced from the cranial cavity, so that the pressure of this fluid within the spinal theca, which can usually be regarded as giving a reasonably faithful indication of the intracranial pressure, rises. As would be expected from the principles elucidated in Chapter 4 (pp. 83–85), headache is an almost invariable accompaniment. In extreme cases the pressure is raised to such a degree that there is increased resistance to the entry of blood into cerebral arteries, so that the cerebral blood flow is reduced. This increased arterial resistance leads in turn to a reflex raising of arterial blood pressure in an attempt to overcome it, so that temporary hypertension develops. Rarely blood flow may nevertheless be reduced sufficiently for infarction to occur. The local cerebral oedema which is almost invariable in the immediate vicinity of an intracranial tumour contributes to the increasing intracranial tension. Not only is the pressure of the CSF increased in the spinal theca but in all extracranial extensions of the subarachnoid space. Thus the pressure in the meningeal sheaths around the optic nerves also rises; this in turn leads to diminished venous return from the retinae, with engorgement of retinal veins, swelling of the optic nerve heads or disks (papilloedema) and in severe cases, retinal haemorrhages and exudates around their edges. Another effect of increased intracranial pressure is compression of the respiratory and cardiac centres in the brain stem so that both respiration and the heart rate become slower; a full, slow pulse is characteristic. In severe cases with progressive deterioration, brain-stem centres (the reticular substance) can be so compressed as to cause coma. In these later stages, respiration becomes irregular or of Cheyne–Stokes type and eventually ceases altogether, while a terminal tachycardia, rather than bradycardia, is common.

The severity of the symptoms of increased intracranial pressure depends not only upon the size and rapidity of growth of the tumour but also upon its situation. Thus a slowly-growing meningioma in one or other frontal region will produce few pressure symptoms, at least initially, when manifestations of focal cerebral dysfunction predominate. Growths in the posterior fossa, however, which interfere with the free circulation of CSF

Table 7   Classification of Intracranial and Intraspinal Tumours

	Approximate incidence in cranium
I. *Primary tumours*	
1. Neuroblastomas and neurocytomas.	Rare
2. Gliomas and other supporting cell tumours.	
(*a*) Glioblastoma.	
(*b*) Astrocytoma.	
(*c*) Medulloblastoma.	40 per cent
(*d*) Oligodendroglioma.	
(*e*) Ependymoma.	
3. Meningeal tumours.	
(*a*) Meningioma.	15 per cent
(*b*) Fibrosarcoma and reticulum cell sarcoma.	
(*c*) Melanoma.	Rare
4. Tumours of secretory or glandular tissues.	
(*a*) Pituitary adenomas	
(*b*) Pinealoma.	8 per cent
(*c*) Papilloma of choroid plexus.	
(*d*) Glomus tumours.	
5. Tumours of developmental origin.	
(*a*) Craniopharyngioma.	
(*b*) Haemangioblastoma.	
(*c*) Arteriovenous angioma.	10 per cent
(*d*) Chordoma.	
(*e*) Epidermoid and dermoid cysts.	
(*f*) Colloid cyst of third ventricle.	
6. Primary tumours of cranial vertebral bones.	
(*a*) Osteoma.	
(*b*) Osteogenic sarcoma.	Rare
(*c*) Haemangioma of vertebral body	
7. Tumours of nerves and nerve roots.	
(*a*) Neurinoma (neurofibroma) and plexiform neuroma.	10 per cent
II. *Secondary tumours*	
1. Intracranial and intraspinal metastases.	
(*a*) Carcinoma (lung, breast, kidney, thyroid, ovary, colon).	15 per cent
(*b*) Sarcoma.	
(*c*) Melanoma.	
2. Tumours involving cranial bones, vertebral bodies and meninges.	
(*a*) Carcinoma of nasopharynx and paranasal sinuses.	
(*b*) Metastatic carcinoma of bone (lung, prostate, breast, thyroid).	
(*c*) Multiple myelomatosis and solitary myelomas.	
III. *Granuloma* (gumma, tuberculoma, sarcoid, parasitic invasion).	2 per cent

at an early stage, either through aqueductal pressure, or through blockage of foramina in the fourth ventricle, give symptoms or raised pressure very early. Additional complications may arise as a result of herniation of brain tissue under the free edge of the falx cerebri, through the tentorial notch, or the foramen magnum. The falx is the longitudinal and vertical fold of dura mater which separates the medial surfaces of the two cerebral hemispheres, while the tentorium is the horizontal fold whose curved free edge encircles the upper brain stem, and which separates cerebrum from cerebellum. A mass in either cerebral hemisphere can cause a gradual extrusion of a part of the hemisphere across the free edge of one of these folds. Downward displacement of the medial aspect of the temporal lobe through the tentorial notch is particularly important. As the third (oculo-motor) cranial nerve crosses this notch, it is often compressed, and the first sign of herniation may be a fixed dilated pupil, ptosis or later a complete third-nerve palsy on the side of the lesion. Subsequently there is compression of the upper brain stem with stupor or coma and occasionally homolateral pyramidal signs develop due to compression of the contra-lateral crus cerebri against the opposite free tentorial edge. If tentorial herniation is allowed to increase or to persist unchecked then tearing of small perforating arteries and veins can cause haemorrhages in the mid-brain (median raphe haemorrhages); when such lesions occur, damage is generally irreversible. Reduction of the pressure below the tentorium, say by lumbar puncture, will increase the herniation, giving a rapidly fatal termination to the illness owing to brain-stem compression. The risks of lumbar puncture are equally great when there is a tumour in the posterior fossa, but then it is herniation of the cerebellar tonsils through the foramen magnum (a pressure cone), with compression of the medulla oblongata, which is responsible.

General Symptoms

Since all cerebral tumours, whatever their character and situation, can be expected to increase the intracranial pressure, the characteristic symptoms and signs so produced appear eventually in almost every case. They are headache, vomiting and papilloedema.

The **headache** is of little localising value, although it is sometimes unilateral and then generally affects the side of the head upon which the tumour is situated. More often it is frontal or occipital or both. It may be more severe posteriorly in patients harbouring posterior fossa tumours, but this is not invariable. It is often intermittent and usually 'throbbing' or 'bursting' in character. It is generally most severe on waking and tends to improve as the day wears on; typically it is made worse by coughing, stooping or straining at stool. But these features are not invariable and in some cases the pain is vague and indefinite.

The **vomiting** experienced by patients with intracranial neoplasms often has no specific characteristics, though it tends to be worse in the mornings, like the headache, and is sometimes precipitate and projectile, occurring without preceding nausea.

Papilloedema, though a characteristic physical sign, does not as a rule produce symptoms in the early stages. Typically the retinal veins are distended, the optic disk is pinker than normal, the physiological cup is obliterated, and the edges of the disk (including its temporal edge) are blurred. There is, of course, some blurring of the nasal edge of the disk in many normal persons. As papilloedema increases, haemorrhages may be seen in 'flare' formation around the disk and the patient will often complain of some visual obscuration, or of seeing haloes around lights. These are ominous symptoms, as is transient blindness occurring in one or other eye, say on stooping, since although gross papilloedema can exist without apparent impairment of visual acuity, visual failure, when it comes, is often rapid, complete and irreversible, due to occlusion of the central retinal artery.

The increased intracranial pressure and/or hydrocephalus produced by a tumour in any site can cause mental symptoms and false localising signs. **Mental symptoms** may take the form of progressive apathy leading in the end to stupor and coma, but earlier there is often evidence of mild dementia with impairment of memory, intellect and social adaptation. Later there may be incontinence of urine and faeces. Confusion and disorientation in time and place are common and occasionally there is a fully-developed Korsakoff syndrome (*see* p. 120). The commonest **false localising signs** are a unilateral or bilateral sixth-nerve palsy (due to pressure upon the nerve trunks in their long intracranial course), a partial third-nerve paralysis (due to tentorial herniation) or an extensor plantar response on one or both sides due to brain-stem compression.

It will next be appropriate to describe the various **modes of clinical presentation** of intracranial tumours. As in most nervous diseases the physical signs are generally of most assistance in localising the lesion, whereas one is dependent upon the clinical history in attempting to identify the nature of the growth. As a rule the onset is relatively rapid when the tumour is a glioblastoma, a medulloblastoma or a metastasis, but when it is an astrocytoma, an oligodendroglioma, a meningioma, an acoustic neuroma or pituitary adenoma, the symptoms usually develop insidiously. In many cases, and particularly when the tumour is a supratentorial glioma or meningioma, the clinical picture is one of progressive focal symptoms and signs indicating cerebral compression or destruction, combined with features of increased intracranial pressure. In other instances, particularly when the tumour is slow-growing, the focal symptoms progress insidiously but there are no clinical features indicative of raised pressure when the patient attends for examination. Another common history is one of focal or generalised epileptiform seizures. When the fit has focal or Jacksonian features the suspicion that it may be the result of a focal lesion such as a tumour is immediately raised, but if the seizures are generalised from the start, they may have occurred intermittently for months or exceptionally for several years before symptoms (headache, vomiting) or physical signs (papilloedema, monoparesis or hemiparesis) arise to indicate that they are not idiopathic. Another common group of cases is that in which there are symptoms and signs clearly indicating raised pressure, but there is no clinical evidence whatever to indicate the situation of the neoplasm. While this may be the case in a patient harbouring a glioblastoma, even in one cerebral hemisphere, it is particularly common in children with medullo-blastomas and in adults with tumours in the posterior fossa or in the upper brain stem or third or fourth ventricle. A final but important group of cases is that in which the symptoms of indefinite headache, intermittent giddi-ness, vague memory loss and lack of concentration are ill-defined but nevertheless progressive. These are the most difficult cases of all, as the clinical picture is easily confused with that of emotional illness. Under these circumstances it is often difficult to decide how far investigations should be pursued in an attempt to demonstrate an intracranial neoplasm. Cases of this type are unfortunately common and it is in just such an individual that diagnostic errors are particularly easy. Hence before discussing specific tumour syndromes it will be appropriate to consider a number of cardinal points of value in the management of patients in whom the diagnosis of intracranial tumour is suspected.

Management of the Tumour Suspect

When the patient's history suggests that an intracranial tumour may account for his symptoms, a careful physical examination is of course imperative. If papilloedema is observed as well as a hemiparesis in a patient with a few weeks' history of increasing headache and drowsiness, it is not difficult to conclude that a glioblastoma in one cerebral hemisphere is the most probable diagnosis, while, alternatively, unilateral ataxia will point to one lateral cerebellar lobe as the most likely site. Jacksonian epilepsy, too, suggesting the presence of a lesion near to the motor or sensory cortex, is of great localising value. It is when the physical signs are minimal or indefinite that difficulties arise. In such a case the importance of palpation, percussion and auscultation of the skull should not be overlooked. A localised area of bony tenderness or hyperostosis is sometimes present in the skull overlying a meningioma, while in young children with tumours in the posterior fossa, there may be separation of the cranial sutures and a typical 'cracked-pot' note on percussion, as in hydrocephalus from any cause. Similarly, a cranial bruit or enlarged arteries in the scalp may suggest the presence of an intracranial arterio-venous angioma.

If clinical examination is uninformative, the next investigations indicated are radiography of the skull and chest. The plain films of the skull may reveal a shift of the pineal gland from the midline, enlargement of the sella turcica (due to a pituitary tumour), flattening of the sella and erosion of the clinoid processes (due to raised intracranial pressure), intracranial calcification, or erosion of the internal auditory meatus on one side (in a patient with an acoustic neuroma). In the chest film a shadow indicating the presence of a silent bronchogenic neoplasm will suggest that the intracranial lesion is probably a metastasis. If available, then a CAT scan is next performed and this, in most cases, will not only localise the neoplasm but will often suggest a pathological diagnosis, whether it be in a cerebral hemisphere, a ventricle or in the posterior fossa. If no CAT scan can be performed, then an EEG may localise the lesion to one cerebral hemisphere. Gamma-encephalography is another useful and harmless method which may demonstrate an area of increased uptake of radioactive material in a tumour. This investigation is particularly helpful in patients with suspected cerebral metastases, as two or more foci are sometimes outlined.

The advisability of lumbar puncture is a matter of debate. This investigation is certainly contraindicated in the presence of papilloedema or other evidence of raised intracranial pressure. Indeed it is best avoided whenever there is a strong clinical presumption that an intracranial tumour is present. In occasional doubtful cases, however, it can be helpful. The CSF pressure is usually raised in a patient with an intracranial neoplasm, unless it is slow-growing or infiltrating in character, and in most cases there is also an increased quantity of protein in the fluid. The protein level is often exceptionally high (up to several grams per litre) if the tumour is an acoustic neuroma, while it is in general higher in patients with extracerebral lesions such as meningiomas than in those with gliomas. If the pressure is normal, and suspicion of an intracranial neoplasm persists, and no CAT scan is available then air encephalography (*see* p. 70) may be performed using the fractional technique if a posterior fossa lesion is suspected. However, this procedure should not be carried out in a patient in whom there are reasonable grounds for suspecting the presence of an intracranial tumour unless neurosurgical aid is close at hand and the neurosurgeon, duly warned in advance, is ready to act should evidence of tentorial or cerebellar herniation appear.

When the pressure is raised, however, and certainly in the presence of papilloedema, the next investigation (again when no CAT scan is possible, or rarely when it has given negative findings) must depend upon the presence or absence of localising signs, either clinical or in the EEG or gamma scan. If there is clinical evidence that a tumour is likely in one cerebral hemisphere, the appropriate investigation is carotid angiography, as this technique will not only localise the tumour but the vascular pattern may indicate its nature. When there are no localising features, however, and particularly if a neoplasm in the posterior fossa is suspected, air ventriculography may be needed, and in occasional cases it is necessary to inject contrast medium into the cerebral ventricles for accurate localisation of the neoplasm. Although it is difficult to generalise, surgical exploration should be considered in all cases in which a tumour appears to be at all accessible, and particularly if there is any possibility, however remote, that it may be benign. On the other hand, if the presence of a glioma is confirmed and unless the pressure is greatly raised, indicating that decompression is necessary as a life-saving procedure, exploration, biopsy and partial removal for internal decompression may be better avoided as many patients deteriorate rapidly after this procedure. Temporary but prolonged improvement may be achieved with high doses of steroids (e.g. dexamethasone 5 mg four times daily at first with subsequent lower maintenance doses) which reduce cerebral oedema. Radiotherapy may prolong life and improve its quality in some patients (*see* Chapter 20).

Tumour Syndromes

Having considered the general symptomatology and the management of cases of suspected intracranial tumour, it will now be appropriate to describe briefly a number of the syndromes which may result from specific tumours in different parts of the cranial cavity.

Glioma

Between the rapidly-growing glioblastoma on the one hand, and the insidiously invasive astrocytoma on the other, many types of gliomatous tumour are seen, each with its own pathological characteristics and rate of growth. As the clinical history of the illness produced by such a lesion depends upon its rate of development, it is impossible to describe fully all the possible variations in clinical presentation and course which can be observed in such cases. Typically, however, the patient with a glioblastoma gives a history of increasingly severe headache, drowsiness, nausea and vomiting, with or without focal or generalised epileptic attacks and often with recent disorders of memory, of speech or of movement of the limbs; usually in such a case the duration of the illness is measured in weeks. By contrast, in the patient with a slowly-growing astrocytoma, it is common to obtain a history of occasional major seizures and of vague headache or failure of concentration, beginning some years previously and not causing undue alarm until some new symptom (aphasia, monoparesis, vomiting) made its appearance. Much depends, of course, upon the situation of the tumour. Those in the **frontal lobe** often produce progressive dementia without other localising features until the motor cortex or speech area is irritated or invaded, when Jacksonian epilepsy, or hemiparesis or aphasia will result. Rarely there are episodes of turning of the head or eyes away from the side of the lesion (adversive attacks). Occasionally a contralateral grasp reflex can be elicited. Lesions in the anterior part of the **temporal lobe** may produce initially any of the features of temporal lobe epilepsy (attacks of fear, *déjà vu*, unreality, hallucinations of smell or taste, and lip-smacking or chewing) while the proximity of the face and arm areas of the motor cortex means that Jacksonian seizures affecting the contralateral face and hand or else weakness of the hand and arm often occur. Should the lesion extend more posteriorly, there may be an upper quadrantic visual field defect, or sensory aphasia if the dominant hemisphere is involved. Lesions of the **parietal lobe** generally result in impairment of the appreciation of the finer and discriminative aspects of sensibility in the opposite limbs, while disorders of the body image (*see* p. 104) may occur in non-dominant, and apraxia and agnosia in dominant hemisphere lesions. Formed auditory or visual hallucinations can be experienced if a tumour is present in the auditory or visual association areas of the cortex, but when, as rarely happens, it involves the **occipital lobe**, visual hallucinations are generally crude (e.g. unformed flashes of light) and a contralateral homonymous hemianopia, either partial or complete, is invariable. Involvement of the **thalamus and basal ganglia** usually leads to contralateral patchy impairment of all forms of sensation, somnolence and a dense hemiplegia due to damage to the internal capsule, while tumours of the **corpus callosum** are characterised particularly by progressive apathy, disorders of memory and ultimately dementia, followed usually by generalised convulsions and later still by unilateral and then bilateral pyramidal signs.

When a glioma develops in the **mid-brain**, symptoms and signs of increased intracranial pressure develop early owing to hydrocephalus due to aqueductal compression, but in addition there is generally impairment of conjugate ocular deviation upwards or laterally or both, with bilateral ptosis and/or ophthalmoplegia and variable long-tract signs. Gliomas of the **pons or medulla** tend to be particularly slow-growing ('benign hypertrophy of the pons') and are commonest in children; diplopia is usually the first symptom and is followed by other cranial nerve palsies, often combined at first with contralateral sensory or pyramidal signs ('crossed paralysis') but subsequently the 'long-tract' signs are bilateral. Perhaps remarkably, it is well-recognised that temporary remission of symptoms and signs, often for weeks but rarely for months, sometimes occurs in such cases. Gliomas rarely develop in an **optic nerve or the chiasm**, again usually in children, or in adults with neurofibromatosis, and cause progressive unilateral visual failure with optic atrophy and a visual field defect which tends to be unusual in outline. Astrocytomas of one **cerebellar hemisphere** are particularly common in childhood but do occur in adult life. In such cases the intracranial pressure is increased early, but there is usually evidence of cerebellar ataxia in the limbs on the side of the tumour with nystagmus on lateral gaze to the same side. When the growth involves central cerebellar structures (the vermis and roof nuclei) the patient's gait is grossly ataxic ('truncal ataxia') but there may be no nystagmus and no clear evidence of ataxia in the limbs when these are tested individually.

Occasionally multiple areas of gliomatous infiltration can develop, apparently simultaneously, throughout the brain and brain stem (**gliomatosis cerebri**). In such a case the clinical picture, indicating the presence of multiple lesions, may suggest a diagnosis of multiple metastases. Microgliomatosis cerebri is a name sometimes given to the rare diffuse **reticulum cell sarcoma** of the brain which presents similarly.

Medulloblastoma

This common tumour of infancy and early childhood grows almost invariably in midline cerebellar structures and has the property of seeding throughout the meningeal space so that tumour cells may be discovered in the CSF. Metastases outside the nervous system (e.g in bone) sometimes develop, particularly after operative treatment. The characteristic clinical picture is one of progressive ataxia, with frequent falls, followed by drowsiness and vomiting in a young child. Papilloedema is almost invariable and the cranial sutures are separated at an early stage.

Oligondendroglioma

These uncommon tumours, which usually grow in one cerebral hemisphere, and particularly in the temporal lobe, are remarkably benign, and most patients experience intermittent focal or generalised seizures for several years before additional symptoms appear. They often calcify and a punctate area of calcification seen on a skull radiograph can be virtually diagnostic.

Ependymoma

This rare intracranial tumour is most often found in the fourth ventricle; it rapidly produces symptoms and signs of raised intracranial pressure and other signs are rare although there may be evidence of cerebellar dysfunction or of compression of long tracts in the brain stem. Positional vertigo, occipital headache and morning vomiting are common in the early stages, and may indeed be the only symptoms, while nystagmus with variable neck stiffness or vertigo provoked by attempted neck flexion are often the only physical signs.

Meningioma

A meningioma compressing one cerebral hemisphere may produce a clinical picture indistinguishable from that resulting from an astrocytoma arising in a similar situation, although Jacksonian epilepsy seems to be particularly common with these benign neoplasms. There are, however, several specific syndromes which have been recognised as being due to meningiomas arising in particular situations. The **olfactory groove meningioma** which lies beneath one frontal lobe typically gives unilateral anosmia and dementia, often with inappropriate jocularity (*Witzelsucht*) due to frontal-lobe compression. As it extends posteriorly it can compress the homolateral optic nerve to give unilateral optic atrophy, and when this is combined with contralateral papilloedema, this combination of signs is known as the Foster Kennedy syndrome. A **parasagittal meningioma,** growing between the two cerebral hemispheres, typically compresses the foot and leg areas of the motor or sensory cortex in both cerebral hemispheres, giving Jacksonian seizures in one or rarely both legs and/or a spastic paraplegia. Urinary retention or incontinence sometimes occur. A meningioma in the **cerebellopontine angle** can cause a clinical picture indistinguishable from that resulting from an acoustic neuroma (*see below*), while a similar tumour growing above the sella turcica (**parasellar meningioma**) typically produces progressive unilateral and later bilateral visual failure with a visual field defect indicating chiasmal compression. The meningiomas which arise from the **sphenoidal ridge**, on the lesser wing of the sphenoid, protrude into the orbit to produce unilateral proptosis, optic atrophy (due to compression of the optic nerve), ptosis and diplopia (due to involvement of the oculomotor nerve). Rarely a growth arising from the basal meninges may gradually involve multiple cranial nerves as they approach the exit foramina by which they leave the skull (**meningioma en plaque**). Meningiomas occasionally recur after apparently total surgical removal and rarely show sarcomatous malignant change.

Pituitary Adenomas

There are two principal varieties of pituitary adenoma which produce similar neurological signs but have different endocrinological effects. An adenoma of the acidophil cells gives rise to gigantism if it develops before puberty and to acromegaly afterwards, while most chromophobe adenomas eventually produce signs of hypopituitarism. However, recent evidence has revealed that some contain a few active acidophil or basophil cells but that many more secrete prolactin, causing galactorrhoea and amenorrhoea (prolactinomas). Basophil adenomas are uncommon and do not usually grow sufficiently large to give symptoms or signs of an intracranial space-occupying lesion. They produce the endocrine features of Cushing's syndrome which is, however, more often produced by over-activity of the adrenal cortex. Both the acidophil and chromophobe tumours are generally large enough to cause expansion of the sella turcica (which can be recognised radiologically) and also tend to extrude above the sella to compress the medial aspect of both optic nerves and the chiasm. A bitemporal hemianopia is the typical field defect but many variations are seen. Occasionally a chromophobe adenoma expands rapidly due to infarction when it outstrips its own blood supply; it may then compress one third nerve and the optic nerve to give sudden severe headache, unilateral blindness, a third-nerve palsy and sometimes subarachnoid haemorrhage (the syndrome of 'pituitary apoplexy').

Pinealoma, Papilloma and Glomus Tumour

The *pinealoma* is an uncommon tumour of children or young adults which usually presents solely with symptoms of increased intracranial pressure due to aqueductal compression and hydrocephalus; however, compression of the corpora quadrigemina and upper mid-brain can give a characteristic impairment of upward conjugate gaze. Many so-called pinealomas are teratomas or gliomas. Those uncommon tumours which arise from pineal parenchymal cells may cause precocious puberty or diabetes insipidus in addition. *Papillomas* of the choroid plexus, too, are usually responsible for recurrent subarachnoid haemorrhage or for a hydrocephalus without other specific features. The characteristic manifestations of the rare *chromaffinoma of the glomus jugulare* are multiple lower cranial nerve palsies (deafness, facial palsy, dysphagia, hemiatrophy of the tongue), combined sometimes with a vascular polyp in the inner ear or a palpable mass anterior to the mastoid bone.

Craniopharyngioma

This relatively common tumour, arising from developmental remnants of Rathke's pouch, may be solid, but more often produces a cholesterol-containing cyst which is suprasellar in situation. It compresses the optic chiasm to give unilateral or bilateral optic atrophy and progressive visual-field defects, and also extends upwards into the hypothalamus. In childhood it can give delayed physical and sexual development (pituitary infantilism), or diabetes insipidus; in some cases symptoms do not develop until early adult or even middle life, when diminished libido, mental dullness and signs of hypopituitarism develop. The sella turcica is generally enlarged but shallow, unlike the typical ballooning produced by a pituitary adenoma, and there is often calcification in the tumour, visible radiologically in up to 50 per cent of cases.

Haemangioblastoma

This tumour occurs almost invariably in one cerebellar hemisphere in children or young adults and gives symptoms indistinguishable from a cerebellar astrocytoma. It may be familial and is often associated with angiomatosis of the retina or abdominal organs (Lindau-von Hippel disease). Polycythaemia is often present.

Arteriovenous Angioma

The characteristic clinical features produced by these vascular malformations, which will be further considered in Chapter 17, are epilepsy, subarachnoid haemorrhage, focal neurological signs, depending upon their situation, and a cranial bruit. Small vascular malformations (hamartomas) may remain silent for many years before producing epileptic attacks as their only clinical manifestation.

Chordoma

This soft jelly-like tumour usually grows either between the basisphenoid and the anterior aspect of the brain stem, or in the sacral canal. When it develops intracranially there are typically multiple cranial-nerve palsies; in the sacrum it produces signs of involvement of multiple roots of the lower cauda equina.

Epidermoid or Dermoid Cysts

These rare pearly tumours or cholesteatomas are most commonly found in the posterior fossa, and are usually indistinguishable clinically from other posterior fossa tumours. Diagnosis is generally made at operation.

Colloid Cyst of the Third Ventricle

This uncommon tumour arises within the third ventricle from vestigial remnants of the primitive paraphysis. Usually it produces clinical features indicating merely a progressive increase in the intracranial pressure, but the presence of such a lesion may be suspected when the patient experiences intermittent hydrocephalus with attacks provoked by change in posture; in such cases it seems that the pedunculated cyst may act as a ball-valve, giving intermittent blockage of the foramina of Monro.

Neurofibroma (Neurinoma)

This relatively common intracranial neoplasm is sometimes single, sometimes multiple; in the latter case the patient is usually suffering from neurofibromatosis, and other stigmata of the disease will generally be apparent. Thus there may be a family history of the disease and careful examination will reveal cutaneous neurofibromas and pigmentation. Whereas in the cranial cavity these neoplasms can grow upon the fifth or seventh nerves, the commonest site by far is the eighth or acoustic nerve (the acoustic neuroma). This tumour is commonest in middle-aged and elderly patients (except in individuals with neurofibromatosis). Unilateral nerve deafness is almost invariable and may be associated with some indefinite giddiness, but true paroxysmal vertigo is uncommon. Next in frequency as signs are nystagmus and unilateral facial sensory loss (an absent corneal reflex is sometimes the initial sign); later as a rule comes homolateral facial paresis or twitching due to compression of the facial nerve. Minimal cerebellar ataxia on the side of the lesion is often observed and there may be pyramidal signs which are usually contralateral but occasionally ipsilateral. The protein content of the CSF is often greatly raised and radiographs commonly demonstrate erosion of the internal auditory meatus. Neuro-otological studies (audiometry and caloric tests— see p. 78) are valuable aids to early diagnosis in such cases.

'Pseudotumour Cerebri' (Benign Intracranial Hypertension)

The clinical picture of this condition, which has also been called toxic hydrocephalus or serous meningitis, can closely resemble that of cerebral tumour, as the predominant symptom is headache and bilateral papilloedema is discovered on examination. CAT scanning, however (or ventriculography which is needed if no CAT scan is possible), reveals that the cerebral ventricles are either normal in size and situation or more often are unusually small. The condition can complicate otitis media, pregnancy, or cachexia, or may follow head injury; it is particularly common in plump young or middle-aged women. It is due either to aseptic thrombosis of one or more intracranial venous sinuses or more often to diffuse brain swelling of unknown cause. It is a self-limiting condition which recovers completely in a few weeks or months, but during the acute stage the papilloedema constitutes a danger to vision and urgent treatment is necessary, usually with steroid drugs (*see* p. 453) to reduce cerebral oedema; surgical decompression was rarely required in the past. Most such patients are surprisingly well considering the severity of the papilloedema; bilateral sixth-nerve palsies are sometimes present as false localising signs.

Intracranial Metastases

Intracranial deposits secondary to extracranial malignant disease are generally carcinomatous, and the most common sites of primary growths which spread to the cranial cavity are the lung, breast, kidney, ovary and colon, although occasionally the primary tumour may be in some other organ. Sarcomas too may metastasise to the brain, as may malignant melanomas, while rarely a reticulum cell sarcoma appears to arise primarily within the cranial cavity, either in the meninges or within the substance of the brain itself. The clinical picture produced by one or more intracranial metastases can be very variable, but does not appear to be dependent in any sense upon the nature or situation of the primary growth. Subarachnoid haemorrhage is a rare complication of intracranial metastases except that it frequently occurs in cases of malignant melanoma when the metastatic deposits are very numerous and very vascular; cytological study may then demonstrate melanin-containing cells in the CSF. In many cases the manifestations of intracranial disease precede those attributable to the primary tumour and the symptoms and physical signs usually resemble closely those produced by a glioblastoma in one or other cerebral hemisphere, or by a rapidly-growing tumour in the posterior fossa. Thus while the syndrome of morning headache and vomiting with postural vertigo and nystagmus, if occurring in a young person, may suggest an ependymoma of the fourth ventricle (*see* p. 330), in the middle-aged or elderly patient this clinical picture is more likely to be due to a metastasis (often from a bronchial carcinoma) in this situation.

The discovery of an opacity in a chest radiograph may be the first indication that the tumour is metastatic. Although cerebral metastases are frequently multiple it is comparatively uncommon, though not unknown, for the symptoms or physical signs to indicate the presence of more than one lesion. On occasion the clinical picture is even more indefinite, with vague headache, forgetfulness, lack of concentration, depression and intermittent confusion, and a diagnosis of presenile dementia may be seriously considered. Rarely, too there are widespread carcinomatous deposits in the leptomeninges and the clinical picture is then one of headache, severe neck stiffness, confusion and sometimes paresis of one or more cranial nerves (*carcinomatosis of the meninges*). In such a case there is generally a moderate pleocytosis and rise in protein in the CSF, the sugar content of the fluid is greatly diminished and malignant cells can be recognised by cytological techniques.

Carcinomatous deposits in the bones of the skull may produce headaches and tenderness of the scalp, but only rarely do neurological signs result from involvement of the underlying brain. It is not uncommon, however, for a *nasopharyngeal carcinoma* to erode the base of the skull and to destroy multiple cranial nerves in succession, at first unilaterally and later bilaterally. Hence in any case in which there is progressive paralysis of the third, fourth, fifth, sixth or seventh nerves and later perhaps of those arising from the lower part of the brain stem, this diagnosis should be strongly suspected. A tumour mass may be felt in the nasopharynx but often nasopharyngeal biopsy is necessary in order to confirm the diagnosis. A somewhat similar picture, in which deafness and involvement of multiple lower cranial nerves on one side develop gradually over a period of months or years, may be the result of invasion of the cranial cavity by a *glomus tumour* arising from the glomus jugulare. A carcinoma in the maxillary sinus can also involve multiple cranial nerves, while a malignant neoplasm in the ethmoid sinus more often gives an asymmetrical proptosis with lateral displacement of the eye. Proptosis is also occasionally seen as a result of a *myeloma* of the orbit, although in general, multiple myelomatosis involving the skull does not give rise to neurological symptoms and signs. Deposits of *lymphoma, lymphosarcoma* and of *leukaemic cells* may involve the cerebral substance giving clinical manifestations similar to those of single cerebral tumours or multiple metastases, but more often develop in the meninges, compressing the brain or spinal cord or giving a clinical picture like that of meningeal carcinomatosis.

Intracranial Granulomas and Parasitic Cysts

A *gumma* is now a rare lesion, although this diagnosis should be suspected when a patient with proven syphilis develops clinical features suggesting the presence of an intracranial space-occupying lesion. *Tuberculomas* are also uncommon, except in parts of Asia, and while the rupture of such a lesion into the subarachnoid space can cause tuberculous meningitis, they are rarely of sufficient size to give symptoms of focal brain disease. Cysticerci within the brain are an occasional cause of epilepsy, and in Britain were once seen particularly in those who had served in the Forces in India; typical calcified 'oval' lesions were sometimes recognised radiologically. Occasionally cysticerci of racemose type form in the cerebral ventricles and are then responsible for repeated attacks suggesting lymphocytic meningitis, followed by a progressive or intermittent hydrocephalus of the type which occurs in any patient with an intraventricular tumour.

Endarteritis with single or multiple infarction of the brain can be the result of meningovascular syphilis, connective tissue disease (Chapter 14) or other forms of arteritis (Chapter 17). However, *sarcoidosis* is another well-recognised cause of granulomatous meningitis which often presents with either hydrocephalus or multiple cranial nerve palsies.

Spinal Tumours

The tumours which arise within or encroach upon the spinal cord can be divided into three groups. These are: first, those which arise in the bones of the spinal column or in the extradural space (extradural tumours); secondly, those which lie within the dura mater but outside the spinal cord (intradural–extramedullary); and thirdly, those which grow within the substance of the spinal cord itself (intramedullary). In a general hospital, about 40 per cent of all spinal space-occupying lesions are extradural, and of these the majority are **metastases**, although deposits of a reticulosis, extradural granuloma (due, for example, to tuberculous spinal caries), chordoma (in the sacral region) or a haemangioma or myeloma of a vertebral body can produce similar effects. Intradural–extramedullary tumours constitute about 50 per cent of all spinal growths and intramedullary neoplasms about 5 per cent. The common intradural–extramedullary tumours are first, the **neurofibroma**, and secondly the **meningioma**. A neurofibroma may occur at any level of the spine and in either sex. It grows from a spinal root or nerve to give a mass which lies partly inside and partly outside the spinal canal, eroding generally the intervertebral foramen and adjacent vertebral pedicles (a 'dumbbell' tumour). Meningiomas are nearly always found in the dorsal region and usually in women. The commonest intramedullary tumours are the **glioma** and the **ependymoma**, though arteriovenous angiomas, or other small and discrete vascular malformations of small blood vessels (telangiectases) occur from time to time. Intramedullary metastases are very rare.

Although the clinical presentation of a spinal tumour will clearly depend upon its character and situation, the initial symptoms are usually those of compression of one or more spinal roots, of the spinal cord, or more often of both. If the tumour is intramedullary there is progressive destruction or distortion of long tracts resulting in motor and sensory change in the limbs and trunk below the level of the lesion, depending upon which pathways are principally involved; impairment of sphincter control usually appears comparatively early. Extradural growths are particularly liable to give pain of a persistent aching character in the back at the level where the tumour is situated; sometimes, if spinal roots are compressed, the pain radiates along the dermatomes innervated by the roots concerned. These symptoms are often present for some time before symptoms and signs of spinal cord compression appear, but this is not invariable and if a carcinomatous deposit causes collapse of a vertebral body, a sudden paraplegia may result. Pain in root distribution is also a characteristic symptom of an intradural–extramedullary tumour, particularly the neurofibroma, but is not invariable, and the clinical picture may be predominantly that of progressive spinal cord compression, as described in pp. 266–269. If the tumour is situated in the cervical region there will often be muscular wasting, weakness and sensory loss in one or both arms, indicating a lesion of one or more spinal roots or nerves, in addition to the evidence of spinal cord disease, but if it is dorsal in situation these signs are unobtrusive and it may be impossible clinically to determine whether the lesion is intramedullary. A Brown–Séquard syndrome can be an early result of an extramedullary tumour, but a clinical picture suggesting syringomyelia of unusually rapid progression generally implies that the lesion is intramedullary, and very probably an ependymoma. When the neoplasm lies below the termination of the spinal cord, the characteristic clinical features of involvement of one or more roots of the cauda equina are seen and there is often some pain over the lumbosacral region. Urinary retention and impotence usually develop and if the lower sacral roots are involved there is generally perianal or 'saddle' anaesthesia. A tumour at the eleventh and twelfth dorsal or first lumbar level can compress not only the roots of the cauda equina but also the conus medullaris to give a combination of upper and lower motor neurone signs. The commonest tumours involving the cauda equina are a neurofibroma, an ependymoma of the filum terminale, or a chordoma which may produce massive erosion of the sacrum, clearly visible radiologically. Rarely a solitary sacral myeloma produces similar effects.

The accurate diagnosis of spinal tumours is of the greatest importance, as so many are benign and can be successfully removed; if irreversible damage due to restriction of blood supply to the cord has not occurred, most patients recover completely. On suspicion that a tumour may be present, the first obligatory investigation is radiography of the spine, which may reveal excessive separation of the pedicles or bony erosion. Lumbar puncture may be helpful, especially if the protein content of the CSF is raised, but when there is a strong suspicion of the presence of a spinal neoplasm it is better to proceed direct to opaque myelography which would in any event be needed if the preliminary lumbar puncture gave suggestive findings. Some patients with spinal tumours deteriorate rapidly after lumbar puncture and myelography is often more difficult to perform if attempted soon after lumbar puncture, as the spinal theca distal to a block may collapse after CSF has been withdrawn. Unfortunately the diagnosis of an intramedullary neoplasm cannot always be substantiated by myelography, even though in many such cases the spinal cord is seen to be expanded. It is, however, the extramedullary lesions which are particularly important to recognise, as these are so eminently treatable, and in this myelography rarely fails. The whole body CAT scanner is likely to be used increasingly in the detection and identification of spinal tumours.

Neurological Complications of Malignant Disease

It is now well recognised that a number of specific neurological manifestations may develop in patients with malignant disease which are not dependent upon the development of metastases within the brain or spinal cord. The symptoms of nervous disease can indeed antedate those attributable to the primary growth. The aetiology of these disorders is obscure; nutritional, toxic and autoimmune processes have been proposed to explain these reactions of the nervous system to the presence of a neoplasm elsewhere in the body, but up to the moment none has been substantiated. Current evidence suggests that many of these complications are due either to a hypersensitivity reaction on the part of the nervous system to the presence of the neoplasm, or to a concomitant 'slow virus' infection (*see* p. 285) to which patients with malignant disease appear to be peculiarly susceptible. It must be stressed that clinical evidence of the neurological complication may appear months or rarely even years before the manifestations of the neoplasm responsible become apparent. The primary neoplasm is often a bronchogenic carcinoma but neurological complications of this type have now been described in occasional cases of malignant disease in many different sites and also in some patients with reticulosis. The two principal syndromes have been entitled **carcinomatous neuropathy** and **carcinomatous myopathy**. In patients suffering from a neuropathy the most common features are those of a progressive polyneuropathy (*see* p. 372) affecting principally the lower limbs and sometimes involving motor function predominantly, sometimes sensory function. Unilateral and subsequently bilateral footdrop may be the initial manifestation, or alternatively the patient complains of aching pains in the legs on exertion; gradually over a period of weeks or months the tendon reflexes become depressed and are eventually lost. Peripheral sensory impairment often develops subsequently but occasionally a severe sensory neuropathy is present from the beginning. In some cases there is also a symmetrical **cerebellar ataxia**, affecting all four limbs, and a typical spinocerebellar degeneration has been demonstrated pathologically in such individuals. More often this cerebellar syndrome occurs alone. Occasionally, too, the neuropathy is associated with a severe depressive psychosis or else this emotional disturbance may be the sole manifestation. Other rare disorders which may complicate malignant disease include **subacute encephalomyelitis**, **subacute necrotic myelopathy**, and **multifocal leucoencephalopathy**; the latter disorder, which typically occurs in patients with a reticulosis such as

Hodgkin's disease, has been shown to be due to the presence of polyoma virus in the brain. Hypercalcaemia and hyponatraemia (due to inappropriate ADH secretion), each giving rise to an encephalopathy, have also been described.

Carcinomatous myopathy causes progressive weakness and atrophy of proximal limb and girdle muscles without sensory loss. In some such cases the clinical and pathological features are those of polymyositis (*see* p. 383). In others the myopathy is non-specific biochemically and histologically and there may be associated evidence of peripheral nerve involvement so that the condition is a **neuromyopathy**. In yet others a partial response to edrophonium may suggest a diagnosis of myasthenia gravis, but the tendon reflexes are depressed or absent and there may be a paradoxical increase rather than a decrease in muscle power after repeated contraction (the Eaton-Lambert syndrome). This so-called myasthenic-myopathic syndrome which has relatively specific electrophysiological features (*see* p. 61) may be temporarily improved by treatment with guanidine hydrochloride.

References

Adams, R. D. and Sidman, R. L., *Introduction to Neuropathology* (New York, Blakiston–McGraw-Hill, 1968).

Adams, R. D., Hochberg, F. and Webster, H. de F., 'Neoplastic disease of the brain', in *Harrison's Principles of Internal Medicine*, Ed. Isselbacher, K. J., *et al.*, 9th ed., Chapter 367 (New York, McGraw-Hill, 1980)

Brain, the late Lord and Norris, F., *The Remote Effects of Cancer on the Nervous System* (New York, Grune and Stratton, 1965).

Elsberg, C. A., *Tumours of the Spinal Cord* (New York, Hoeber, 1925).

Hankinson, J. and Banna, M., *Pituitary and Parapituitary Tumours*, Major Problems in Neurology, Vol. 6 (London, Philadelphia, Toronto, W. B. Saunders, 1976).

Hughes, J. T., *Pathology of the Spinal Cord*, 2nd ed. (London, Lloyd-Luke, 1978).

Northfield, D. W. C., *Surgery of the Central Nervous System* (Oxford, Blackwell, 1973).

Russell, D. S. and Rubenstein, L. J., *Pathology of Tumours of the Nervous System*, 4th ed. (London, Arnold, 1977).

Thompson, R. A. and Green, J. R. (Eds.) *Neoplasia in the Central Nervous System*, Advances in Neurology, Vol. 15 (New York, Raven Press, 1976).

Walton, J. N., *Brain's Diseases of the Nervous System*, 8th ed., Chapters 3 and 17 (London, Oxford University Press, 1977).

17 Vascular Disorders of the Nervous System

The effects of disease in the cranial and/or spinal blood vessels upon the functioning of the nervous system may be profound. Indeed the clinical syndromes or 'strokes' produced by disorders of the cerebral circulation are the most common of nervous diseases. In 1952, 170,000 people in the United States died of cerebral vascular accidents, and many more were left crippled in body or in mind by a stroke or series of strokes which were not sufficiently severe to end their lives. While many of the patients so afflicted are elderly, the effects of cerebral vascular disease are nowadays seen with increasing frequency in patients under the age of 60 and even in relatively young adults. Although cerebral vascular disease is usually manifest through symptoms and signs indicating a disorder of brain function, 'stroke syndromes' cannot be regarded as specific diseases, but rather as stereotyped combinations of clinical features which can be produced by many different diseases of the cerebral arteries and veins and which only secondarily affect the behaviour of the nervous system. Most of these disorders are complications of hypertension and atherosclerosis, while other cardiovascular factors, including disease of the heart and great vessels, and variations in the systemic blood pressure, may play a part in their genesis. Hence it is important always to bear in mind the possibility in any patient manifesting a cerebral vascular syndrome, that the primary abnormality may lie in the heart or kidneys. In this chapter, the common vascular disorders of the brain will first be considered and then brief references will be made to the much less common vascular syndromes of the spinal cord.

Cerebral Vascular Disease

The commoner cerebral vascular accidents fall into two principal categories, namely spontaneous intracranial haemorrhage on the one hand and cerebral infarction or ischaemia on the other. The word spontaneous is taken to exclude intracranial haemorrhage resulting from an obvious traumatic cause, which is usually evident in cases of extradural haemorrhage and in subdural haematoma (*see* pp. 261–262), though the latter condition masquerades in many guises and is a common pitfall for the unwary. Probably about 70 per cent of cerebral vascular accidents are the result of infarction or ischaemia (50 per cent 'thrombotic', 20 per cent 'embolic') while primary cerebral haemorrhage accounts for approximately 20 per cent and subarachnoid haemorrhage for about 8 per cent of all cases.

Spontaneous Intracranial Haemorrhage

The two principal varieties of intracranial haemorrhage are first, primary intracerebral haemorrhage, which is usually of hypertensive origin, and secondly, subarachnoid haemorrhage, which generally results from the rupture of an intracranial aneurysm or angioma. The term 'subarachnoid haemorrhage' is in many cases a misnomer, since in 50 per cent of cases at least the haemorrhage involves brain tissue and is not purely subarachnoid in situation; furthermore, in many cases of primary cerebral haemorrhage the bleeding extends into the cerebral ventricles or subarachnoid space. As will be seen, this can cause considerable diagnostic difficulty in some cases.

Primary Intracerebral Haemorrhage

This condition is responsible for the classical stroke or apoplexy. It usually arises as a result of rupture of small perforating arteries, either in the putamen and internal capsule (the territory of the lenticulostriate artery), in one cerebellar hemisphere, or in the pons. Hypertension is the most important cause and the condition often begins during exertion or emotional stress when the blood pressure is at its height. Little is known of the pathological changes in the blood vessels which finally account for the arterial rupture, though recent work confirmed the 'classical' view that microaneurysms on small arteries are frequently present within the brain in hypertensive patients; it seems that rupture of such a microaneurysm frequently initiates the haemorrhage. The condition is commonest in the elderly (60–80 age group) but can occur in severely hypertensive individuals at any age. There is a rapid outpouring of arterial blood and, after ploughing up the brain tissue surrounding the site of origin of the haemorrhage, this often enters the ventricular system; if the bleeding is massive, death may occur within a few hours. More often the patient, without prodromal symptoms, complains of a sudden ill-defined sensation that something is wrong within the head. Within a few moments the face becomes twisted, weakness of one arm and leg and headache develop and consciousness is soon lost. The period of evolution of the stroke is rarely as brief as that seen in cases of cerebral embolism and onset is usually less abrupt than in subarchnoid haemorrhage; the full clinical picture can take up to half or one hour to develop. By this time the patient is usually deeply comatose, with stertorous respiration, neck stiffness, a slow, bounding pulse, deviation of the head and eyes away from the side of the lesion, and a dense, flaccid hemiplegia. Vomiting and incontinence of urine and faeces are usual. Occasionally 'decerebrate attacks', or generalised or focal convulsions occur at the onset. When the cerebellum is the site of the haemorrhage, the clinical picture may be indistinguishable from that produced by a severe cerebral haemorrhage, but if the bleeding is less quick to develop or is not too extensive, the early clinical features are vertigo, repeated vomiting and ataxia, often of truncal or central type; sometimes, however, unilateral ataxia confirms that the bleeding has involved one cerebellar hemisphere. When the primary site of bleeding is the pons, the patient is as a rule comatose from the beginning, but in addition there are often inequality of the pupils, of which one may be pinpoint in size, with hyperpyrexia and a quadriplegia rather than hemiplegia.

About 80 per cent of patients die, some within the first 24 hours, the remainder during the next few days. A fluctuant clinical course, and clinical features indicative of recurrent bleeding, are not usually observed; deterioration is generally remorseless in the severe cases. Of the patients who survive, about half remain helpless neurological cripples, but there are some in whom the haemorrhage is relatively small, loss of consciousness brief, and residual disability comparatively slight. These cases are, however, difficult to recognise clinically, and are easily confused with examples of cerebral infarction.

Unfortunately, cerebral haemorrhage presents a gloomy picture therapeutically. Save in exceptional cases little, apart from nursing and other supportive care, can be done, though steroids may be used to reduce cerebral oedema (*see* p. 453). In selected cases surgical evacuation of the intracerebral clot, after localisation by CAT scan and/or angiography or ventriculography, can occasionally be of benefit, but this procedure is only justifiable in less severe cases and in younger patients. It is especially helpful in patients with cerebellar haemorrhage who survive the first few days. Lumbar puncture is of no therapeutic value and carries considerable risks of tentorial or cerebellar herniation. The administration of powerful hypotensive agents after the haemorrhage has occurred is not indicated, as lowering the blood pressure, in the presence of widespread vascular spasm (which is an almost invariable concomitant of intracranial haemorrhage) may give rise to the further complication of infarction. Clearly, prevention of cerebral haemorrhage (through the effective treatment of hypertension), rather than treatment, must be the aim.

Subarachnoid Haemorrhage
This is the second major category of spontaneous intracranial bleeding and therapeutically it is much more hopeful. In about 85 per cent of cases the condition results from rupture of an intracranial aneurysm on a major artery of the circle of Willis, while in about 10 per cent an arteriovenous angioma is present. The remaining 5 per cent of cases include patients with intracranial neoplasms, cerebral venous sinus thrombosis, blood diseases,

and other conditions of which the subarachnoid bleeding is symptomatic. The so-called berry aneurysms, which are the commonest cause, are probably due to the coexistence of a congenital defect in the media of a cerebral artery with an early atheromatous lesion in the intima which breaches the internal elastic lamina. Mycotic aneurysms are now rare and syphilitic arterial dilatations virtually non-existent. Aneurysms are particularly common at arterial bifurcations and are multiple in about 16 per cent of cases. Their commonest sites are upon the internal carotid artery, below or near its bifurcation, the region of the anterior communicating, and the middle cerebral artery, but they can arise upon any intracranial artery.

The patient, who may be a young adult or even a child, but who is usually between 40 and 60 years of age, is suddenly struck down by an intense and catastrophic headache. Consciousness may be lost at the outset, and convulsions are common, but often the senses are retained, though the patient is drowsy and confused and complains bitterly of headache. The headache, which is usually frontal or occipital in situation at first, then mounts in severity and becomes generalised, severe neck stiffness and other symptoms and signs of meningeal irritation become apparent and vomiting is usual. Papilloedema is sometimes seen immediately or within a few days or weeks, but a more typical, if uncommon sign observed on ophthalmoscopy is a brick-red subhyaloid haemorrhage, spreading outwards from the edge of one or both optic disks. In many cases there is evidence of damage to cranial nerves or to the brain itself. Unilateral or bilateral sixth-nerve palsies are common, or alternatively one third cranial nerve may be paralysed. Depending upon the situation and severity of any intracerebral extension of the haemorrhage, aphasia, a monoparesis, hemiparesis or hemiplegia may be found. Similar signs are sometimes the result of coexistent cerebral infarction which is a common complication of subarachnoid haemorrhage and which results from arterial spasm or from tearing or compression of sulcal arteries by the force of the effused blood in the subarachnoid space. Rarely, bleeding breaches the arachnoid and produces a subdural haematoma. When the patient is comatose with a dense hemiplegia, clinical diagnosis from primary intracerebral haemorrhage with rupture into the subarachnoid space can be difficult or impossible and will depend usually upon the patient's age and upon the presence or absence of evidence of severe hypertension and atherosclerosis. It should be noted, however, that in the initial stages of the illness, transient arterial hypertension is common, resulting probably from hypothalamic compression, and temporary albuminuria and glycosuria can also result from this cause.

Although in many cases the diagnosis is self-evident, a lumbar puncture is generally necessary for confirmation, and also in order to distinguish the condition from disorders such as meningitis or cerebral abscess, with which it may occasionally be confused, particularly if the onset is less abrupt than usual. This investigation should be performed with care, removing only enough fluid to establish the diagnosis and may even be contraindicated if there are signs indicating intracerebral haemorrhage, in view of the risks of tentorial herniation. Indeed, whenever possible, a CAT scan should be performed to exclude the presence of an intracranial haematoma before a diagnostic lumbar puncture is carried out. The CSF is found to be deeply and uniformly bloodstained, unlike the early tingeing with blood, disappearing as the fluid flows, which can result from damage to vertebral veins caused by the exploring needle. Furthermore, on centrifuging, the supernatant fluid is found to have a faint orange tinge (due to oxyhaemoglobin) within four to six hours of the onset, and becomes deeply yellow or xanthochromic (due to bilirubin) within 36 to 48 hours.

With conservative treatment, including bed rest, sedation and relief of headache by appropriate drugs, along with prophylactic antibiotics given to avoid respiratory and urinary infection, between 40 and 50 per cent of patients die within eight weeks of the ictus. Of these, some two-thirds die from the effects of the first bleed, often within 24 hours, but the remaining one-third succumb to a second, more catastrophic haemorrhage, which is particularly liable to occur within the second week after the first attack. About 10 per cent of those patients who are still alive eight weeks after the onset will die of recurrent bleeding before six months have elapsed and another 10 per cent in the subsequent months or years. Of the long-term survivors, only one-third are symptom-free, while another third have severe and disabling sequelae, including hemiparesis, headache, epilepsy and psychoneurosis, and the remainder have less severe residual symptoms.

Although the indications are not yet final and definitive, it is now clear that the prognosis of the condition can be radically improved by the judicious application of surgical methods of treatment. Nothing can at present be done to save those patients who die within the first two or three days, as surgical procedures carried out on the unconscious patient at this time carry almost a 100 per cent mortality. And there are also some patients who for reasons of age and general conditions are unsuitable candidates for surgery. But most patients who survive beyond the first few days should be considered with the possibility of operative procedures in mind. First, however, the surgeon must have full information about the situation and nature of the lesion responsible for the haemorrhage. He must also know whether there are complications such as cerebral infarction or intracerebral or subdural haemorrhage. Unfortunately clinical examination is of little help; for although it is reasonable to conclude in a hemiplegic patient that the bleeding point is on the opposite side, it is usually impossible to localise a bleeding aneurysm or angioma, or to distinguish between the clinical effects of intracerebral haemorrhage and of cerebral infarction in such cases. Thus everything depends upon the results of the CAT scan and cerebral angiography, which should ideally be performed within a few days after the first bleed. Both carotid and both vertebral arteries should be injected because of the possibility that multiple aneurysms may be present and also in an attempt to study the collateral circulation. If vertebral arteriography gives negative results, as it does in up to 20 per cent of cases, this may mean that the causal aneurysm has clotted. There is some evidence that in cases with negative arteriograms the prognosis is considerably better than the average. If, however, an aneurysm or angioma, or some other causal lesion is demonstrated, the surgeon can decide whether the lesion is surgically accessible and will then choose his time to operate depending upon the size and situation of the lesion and the age and condition of the patient. The most appropriate time is often at about seven days after the haemorrhage, when there is a chance of preventing those fatal recurrent haemorrhages which are particularly common in the second week and when arterial spasm, which greatly increases the risks of surgical treatment because of the danger of infarction, has usually passed off. The CAT scan or angiogram may also demonstrate complications of aneurysmal rupture such as intracerebral or subdural haematoma which require surgical treatment in their own right. The use of hypothermia as an aid to anaesthesia has been a valuable aid in such cases as it reduces cerebral metabolism. With further improvements in surgical and anaesthetic techniques it is reasonable to predict an increasing reduction in the mortality and morbidity of this condition.

Cerebral Infarction

A cerebral infarct can be caused by the sudden embolic occlusion of a cerebral artery, by the gradual thrombosis of an artery, or by a combination of arterial narrowing with other factors which cause the blood supply of a part of the brain to be reduced below a critical level. Atherosclerosis, hypertension, heart disease (including cardiac dysrhythmia), single or multiple episodes of profound hypotension, and less often increased coagulability of the blood (as in pregnancy or in patients taking oral contraceptive drugs which contain oestrogen), haemoconcentration (due to dehydration) and an increase in circulating red cells (as in polycythaemia vera) are some of the principal aetiological factors.

Cerebral Embolism
In cerebral embolism the onset is usually abrupt and if the artery blocked is a major one, loss of consciousness or even sudden death may occur. In less severe cases, consciousness is retained but the patient develops a hemiplegia or other evidence of a rapidly developing focal cerebral lesion. Headache is not usually a feature. When a minor artery is blocked there may simply be transient confusion, speech disturbance or monoparesis, a 'little stroke', which clears up rapidly owing to establishment of the collateral circulation. Indeed in many cases of cerebral embolism, even those with a complete hemiplegia, there is rapid improvement, leading

sometimes to complete recovery within a few days or weeks, though some patients do remain seriously disabled. For every embolus there must be a source, generally in the heart or great vessels. Cerebral embolism in subacute bacterial endocarditis and in mitral stenosis is a well-recognised complication, but the frequency of its occurrence following mural thrombosis in the chambers of the heart after cardiac infarction, as well as embolism from thrombi forming on atheromatous plaques in the aorta and carotid arteries, were less well appreciated until comparatively recently. Less common causes include the prolapsing mitral valve (which may give vegetations on the valve leaflets which can cause cerebral embolism in young adults) and atrial myxoma (a rare condition largely limited to females). Recent evidence indicates that attacks of recurrent cerebral ischaemia (*see below*) are usually due to repeated micro-embolism either of platelet thrombi or of cholesterol derived from breakdown of an atheromatous plaque. The presence of a bruit over one of the major vessels in the neck may indicate a localised stenosis due to a plaque or mural thrombus from which such emboli can arise. Hence in any patient with a sudden onset of a hemiplegia or of less striking focal signs, a careful search should be made for a source of emboli, and particularly for evidence of cardiac disease. This is of considerable importance, as cerebral embolic episodes are for obvious reasons likely to be multiple and there is now some evidence to indicate that the danger of a major stroke can sometimes be averted by cardiac or arterial surgery or by treatment with aspirin or anticoagulant drugs.

Cerebral Thrombosis
The remaining conditions which cause cerebral infarction have for long been grouped together under the broad general heading of 'cerebral thrombosis'. This title is often a misnomer, as there are many cases in which no actual arterial occlusion can be demonstrated. The condition is commonest in patients over 60 years of age but is nowadays occurring with increasing frequency in patients who are aged between 40 and 60 or even younger. Characteristically, the patient retires to bed perfectly well and wakes up next morning to find that one arm and leg are paralysed and perhaps that he cannot speak; or he may not discover the weakness until he attempts to stand and the leg gives way. Often there is no headache and no serious impairment of consciousness, though mild or moderate confusion is common. Rarely, headache is severe and has been attributed to compensatory vasodilatation in anastomotic vessels, or to cerebral oedema causing an increase in the intracranial pressure. Much depends, of course, upon the size of the infarct and its situation. If it is large, the patient may be comatose, owing to swelling of the affected hemisphere, while if the brain stem is affected, rather than the cerebral hemisphere, vertigo, vomiting and diplopia are often prominent features. A mild attack of confusion, and transient weakness or numbness of one arm may be the only evidence of a

small infarct. The differential diagnosis between a large infarct and a small intracerebral haemorrhage is difficult clinically but has become much easier with the advent of the CAT scan. When this is not available, examination of the CSF may help since the fluid usually contains frank blood or a good many red cells, in a cerebral haemorrhage. But even in cerebral infarction, red cells may be present and a slight to moderate rise in white cells and in the protein content of the fluid is not uncommon.

The size and anatomical delimitation of the infarct and hence the neurological signs depend upon many factors. In some typical cases angiography or autopsy reveals a large thrombus in, say, the internal carotid, vertebral or basilar artery or in one of their distal branches, giving an infarct in the expected distribution. In many others, however, no arterial thrombosis is demonstrated, although arterial narrowing produced by atheroma is widespread, affecting some arteries more than others, and the infarct may lie in the territory supplied by the narrowest of these vessels. There is evidence that in some such cases a fall in blood pressure may have been the final precipitating factor which produced infarction without arterial occlusion, due to a selective fall in blood flow through a particularly narrow vessel. Sometimes a cardiac infarct can present with cerebral symptoms in this way, or else the reduction in blood pressure which occurs during sleep or results from treatment with hypotensive drugs may be sufficient to tip the scales. Hypotension resulting from haemorrhage or from a prolonged or unusually severe episode of cardiac dysrhythmia may have a similar effect. On the other hand, paradoxically, similar infarcts may develop in hypertensive patients when the blood pressure is increased. Another important determining factor is the efficiency of the collateral circulation through the circle of Willis and through arterial anastomoses in the meninges. Furthermore, the importance of narrowing of, or thrombosis in, the main trunks of the carotid, vertebral and basilar arteries has been increasingly recognised as these processes may cause reduced blood flow, embolism, or a spread of thrombosis to their distal branches. Atheroma is one important aetiological factor, but both transient hypotension and hypertension clearly play a part. Hence one must guard against the over-enthusiastic use of hypotensive drugs in patients who are atherosclerotic as well as hypertensive. On the other hand, as severe hypertension precipitates spasm of small arteries and arterioles which in turn contribute to infarction in such cases a moderate reduction in the blood pressure should be achieved. Indeed there is now substantial evidence to indicate that the effective treatment of hypertension is reducing the incidence and severity of both cerebral haemorrhage and infarction.

There is also evidence to indicate that in hypertensive patients with 'small vessel disease' rather than the 'large vessel disease' due to atheroma which usually causes large areas of infarction, small spaces which may be infarcts ('lacunes') may occur in either the internal capsule or brain stem.

Such tiny lesions have been shown to be associated with certain clinical syndromes including 'unilateral ataxia and signs of pyramidal tract of dysfunction on the same side, involving the leg more than the arm', a 'pure motor hemiplegia' (without sensory dysfunction), a 'pure sensory stroke' and the so-called 'dysarthria-clumsy hand syndrome' (dysarthria with cerebellar ataxia in one arm).

Transient Ischaemic Attacks

While transient hypotension or a reduced cerebral blood flow resulting, say, from episodes of cardiac dysrhythmia, certainly account for some transient ischaemic attacks, whether these involve the cerebral hemispheres or the brain stem, most seem to be due to recurrent micro-embolism. The emboli consist either of platelets or of cholesterol and arise from mural thrombi or from atheromatous plaques in the large vessels in most cases. The consistency of the clinical pattern of the attacks is probably accounted for by laminar flow in the cerebral arteries which determines that a particle becoming free in the lumen at the same point usually reaches the same peripheral branch of the vessel. These attacks are particularly common in patients with carotid or vertebro-basilar insufficiency and were previously attributed erroneously to hypertensive encephalopathy or to vascular spasm. Patients with stenosis or even occlusion of one internal carotid artery often experience at frequent intervals over several days, weeks or months, recurrent brief attacks of weakness or paraesthesiae in the contralateral limbs, and particularly in the hand and arm. Often there are episodes of transient blindness in the homolateral eye, owing to involvement of the ophthalmic artery, a branch of the internal carotid. Micro-emboli are often seen in the retinal arteries in such cases. Pulsation in the affected internal carotid artery may be reduced on palpation in the tonsillar fossa, and the arterial pressure in the retinal arteries on the same side is also often reduced on ophthalmodynamometry. A systolic bruit over one common or internal carotid artery is a valuable sign, often indicating carotid stenosis. Patients suffering from basilar insufficiency experience similar transient attacks involving many brain-stem structures, now on one side of the body and now on the other, and including such features as vertigo, diplopia, transient hemianopia or bilateral blindness due to posterior cerebral artery insufficiency, paraesthesiae and weakness of one limb, of one arm and leg, or of all four limbs. It is important to recognise the significance of these symptoms early, since total occlusion of the artery can produce a complete hemiplegia (in carotid occlusion) or quadriplegia and death (in basilar occlusion). Doppler ultrasonography can be helpful in demonstrating reduced blood flow through a stenosed artery, but in order to demonstrate stenosis or occlusion of the major arteries in the neck, four-vessel arteriography carried out by aortic arch catheterisation is needed. The intracranial arteries must also be visualised since management may have to be modified if there are intracranial as well as extracranial stenoses or occlusions. One syndrome which has been defined by this method is the so-called 'subclavian steal syndrome'. If the subclavian artery is occluded at its origin, then blood may travel in a retrograde manner down the ipsilateral vertebral artery in order to supply the arm. In such cases the radial pulse and arterial blood pressure are usually reduced in the affected arm, there is often a bruit in the root of the neck, and exercising the arm may give rise to manifestations of vertebro-basilar insufficiency due to brain stem ischaemia.

The natural history of recurrent cerebral ischaemia is variable. Some such patients do go on to suffer major episodes of infarction but in others the attacks cease spontaneously, despite complete occlusion of the affected major vessel, due to the increased efficiency of collateral arterial channels. Thus the external carotid artery can sometimes supply intracranial structures by means of retrograde flow through the ophthalmic when the internal carotid is totally occluded. When the subclavian artery is occluded at its origin or when an arterial stenosis in the neck is demonstrated surgical thrombo-endarterectomy may abolish the ischaemic attacks and restore normal blood flow; but a totally occluded internal carotid artery can rarely be disobliterated surgically. When a stenosis or occlusion is demonstrated in a situation which is not surgically accessible (e.g. in the carotid siphon) then there may be an indication for giving aspirin or anticoagulant drugs (*see* p. 454) particularly if the emboli responsible for the ischaemic attacks seem likely to consist of platelets and not cholesterol.

The Syndromes of the Cerebral Arteries

Many eponymous clinical syndromes have been attributed to the occlusion of individual cerebral arteries. Of these, some occur consistently, and in a stereotyped manner, while others are rare. The fact that many cases of unquestionable cerebral infarction do not fulfil the diagnostic criteria of these classical syndromes demonstrates the variability in distribution of some of the cerebral arteries and of the anastomotic channels which exist in the meninges. In general, however, perforating arteries are true end-arteries and occlusion of these vessels can often be recognised clinically. A diagrammatic representation of the cortical distribution of blood from the major cerebral arteries is given in Fig. 19.

Internal Carotid Artery Thrombosis

The syndrome of transient ischaemic attacks resulting from stenosis of this vessel has already been described. When complete occlusion occurs, however, there is often a complete contralateral hemiplegia, with aphasia if the dominant hemisphere is involved. Alternatively, if the collateral circulation is satisfactory, the clinical features may resemble those of middle cerebral artery occlusion, while on occasion, symptoms are transient, and disability trivial. Occlusion of this artery has replaced meningo-vascular syphilis as the commonest cause of hemiplegia in adults in the

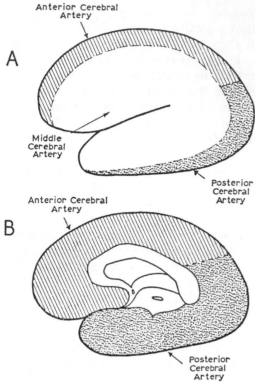

Fig. 19. A diagrammatic representation of the distribution of blood flow from the three major cerebral arteries to the cerebral hemispheres.

third and fourth decades. It may complicate pregnancy or oral contraceptive medication and can follow trauma to the neck. Rarely kinking of the vessel in the neck or fibromuscular hypoplasia of its wall appear to be contributing factors. A carotid arteritis with occlusion, sometimes due to a spread of inflammation from cervical lymph nodes, may account for some cases of acute infantile hemiplegia. Occlusion of a perforating branch of the *posterior communicating artery,* itself a branch of the internal carotid, causes infarction of the subthalamic nucleus (corpus Luysii), giving contralateral hemiballismus. Occlusion of the *anterior choroidal* branch of the internal carotid is often asymptomatic but can give contralateral hemianopia, hemiplegia and hemihypalgesia.

The Middle Cerebral Artery
Occlusion of the main trunk of the middle cerebral artery gives a contralateral hemiplegia and sensory loss of cortical type. When the obstruction lies more distally weakness involves mainly the face, arm and hand. Motor aphasia is common, sensory aphasia less so, but the latter

does occur at times, and a hemianopia is occasionally seen due to infarction of the optic radiation in the temporal lobe.

The Anterior Cerebral Artery

When the main trunk of this artery is occluded, this results in a contralateral hemiplegia with crural dominance (i.e. greater weakness of the leg than of the arm). Cortical sensory loss and aphasia are often present. When Heubner's artery, a penetrating branch which supplies the anterior limb of the internal capsule, is occluded, there is paralysis of the contralateral face and upper limb and often some sensory loss of spinothalamic type in the contralateral limbs.

The Posterior Cerebral Artery

The principal effect of thrombosis of this artery is a contralateral homonymous hemianopia. When perforating branches to the thalamus are involved, a contralateral thalamic syndrome may develop, while lesions of the visual association area in the dominant hemisphere occasionally result in visual agnosia.

The Basilar Artery

Transient ischaemic attacks attributable to vertebro-basilar insufficiency were described above. Total occlusion of the basilar artery is generally soon fatal, with loss of consciousness, a decerebrate state, or quadriplegia, but a myriad of clinical syndromes can occur as a result of occlusion of its individual perforating branches. Thus Weber's syndrome consists of a unilateral third cranial nerve palsy and a contralateral hemiplegia. The Benedikt syndrome is a third-nerve palsy with ipsilateral cerebellar ataxia. A paralysis of the sixth and seventh cranial nerves on one side with a contralateral hemiplegia constitutes the Millard–Gubler syndrome, while the Foville syndrome consists of a sixth-nerve palsy, paralysis of conjugate ocular deviation to the side of the lesion, and again, as a rule, a contralateral hemiparesis. Occlusion of the internal auditory artery may give sudden unilateral deafness and severe vertigo. Apart from these classical syndromes, many other clinical phenomena may be attributable to basilar artery insufficiency, including such features as cranial nerve palsies in various combinations, ipsilateral cerebellar signs, and contralateral hemiplegia or hemianalgesia.

The Superior Cerebellar Artery

The characteristic features of superior cerebellar artery occlusion are first, ipsilateral cerebellar ataxia often with choreiform movements; and secondly, contralateral hemianalgesia with preservation of finer sensory modalities.

The Posterior Inferior Cerebellar Artery
Occlusion of this branch of the vertebral artery gives a typical clinical picture which is one of the commonest brain-stem vascular syndromes (Wallenberg's syndrome). In fact it more often results from a thrombus in the vertebral artery itself and not in its posterior inferior cerebellar branch. The onset is usually abrupt with vertigo and vomiting, and sometimes with pain in one side of the face. There is often dysphagia at the onset and the palate is paralysed on the side of the lesion, while there are also 'cerebellar' signs in the limbs on this side. An ipsilateral Horner's syndrome is often present, and there is usually dissociated anaesthesia to pain and temperature on the same side of the face and over the opposite half of the body below the neck. This sensory loss is, however, variable and a complete contralateral hemianalgesia is not uncommon.

Although many other syndromes of the cerebral arteries have been described, these are the commonest. It is particularly important to recognise the nature of transient ischaemic attacks as these can often be treated effectively.

Prognosis
Cerebral infarction is fatal in up to 20 per cent of cases. When the infarct is small or the causal ischaemia relatively transient, complete recovery can take place within a few days and this occurs in about 20 per cent of patients. In the remaining 60 per cent some degree of disability persists. For instance, up to 20 per cent later develop focal or generalised seizures as a sequel of the illness. Indeed it seems likely that some cases of 'epilepsy of late onset' are due to pre-existing, symptomless or unrecognised, cerebral infarction. Even after a complete hemiplegia has developed, remarkable degrees of recovery may be seen and most patients are eventually able to walk after some weeks or months, although in cases of middle cerebral or carotid occlusion there is often little recovery of function in the affected hand. Aphasia, too, can recover to a surprising extent, either spontaneously or with appropriate speech training which may have to be continued in selected cases for many months. Recovery from brain-stem vascular syndromes is also virtually complete in some cases. The prognosis is particularly favourable in 'posterior inferior cerebellar artery thrombosis' in which after a few months the only residual signs may be a Horner's syndrome on one side and a contralateral hemianalgesia; occasionally persistent dysphagia is troublesome. Recurrent infarction occurs after a greater or lesser period in about half the survivors, but the remainder remain free from such episodes, often for several years.

Moya-Moya Disease

This rare condition, originally described in the Japanese, but subsequently recognised in Western countries, is one in which there is spontaneous occlusion of the major vessels of the circle of Willis so that the cerebral hemispheres are supplied with blood through a network of small vessels resembling the rete mirabile of lower mammals. The cause is unknown; the clinical manifestations include variable focal neurological deficits, convulsions and subarachnoid haemorrhage. The condition is seen especially in children and young adults, and is commoner in females.

Hypertensive Encephalopathy

This term identifies a disorder of acute onset in which severe arterial hypertension is associated with headache, nausea, vomiting, confusion, convulsions and stupor or coma. Usually the condition occurs only in patients with malignant hypertension or in the terminal stages of chronic nephritis; papilloedema and advanced retinopathy are invariably present. Focal neurological symptoms and signs are not a part of this syndrome as a rule but imply the presence of complicating factors such as 'thrombosis', embolism, or haemorrhage.

Cerebral Atherosclerosis

This term is used to describe the progressive degenerative disorder which results from widespread atheroma of the cerebral vasculature with consequent intermittently-progressive ischaemia of the brain. It ultimately gives an irreversible dementia (multi-infarct dementia), but the progress of the disorder is invariably step-like, and it is unwise to accept this diagnosis as a cause of dementia arising in the presenium or in the elderly unless there have been transient episodes of confusion, paraesthesiae, aphasia or paresis, to indicate that one or more 'little stroke' has occurred. In the late stages dementia is severe, the patient is doubly incontinent, but often has a voracious appetite, and may have few signs of neurological abnormality save for brisk tendon reflexes and extensor plantar responses.

A clinical picture which develops in some such cases is that of **pseudobulbar palsy**. This syndrome is characterised by over-emotionalism, often with pathological laughing and crying and gross lability of the affect, along with spasticity of the muscles of speech and swallowing, due to bilateral pyramidal tract lesions in the upper mid-brain or cerebral hemispheres. Some dysarthria and dysphagia and pathological over-emotionalism are often seen too in the syndrome of so-called **atherosclerotic Parkinsonism** in which hypertensive and atherosclerotic patients show little if any facial masking, but commonly demonstrate a shuffling gait, similar to that of paralysis agitans, and progressive rigidity of the limbs; usually, however, they also show evidence of dementia, the deep tendon reflexes are greatly exaggerated, and the plantar responses extensor. Pathologically and clinically pseudobulbar palsy and atherosclerotic Parkinsonism are closely related.

Cerebral Venous Sinus Thrombosis

The effects of suppurative thrombosis of intracranial venous sinuses have already been described (p. 280). Aseptic thrombosis of the cavernous sinus is rare but this pathological process can occur, apparently spontaneously, in the lateral or sagittal sinuses, causing the syndrome of benign intracranial hypertension, or pseudotumour cerebri. The characteristic features are headache and papilloedema in a patient whose consciousness is often unimpaired, who looks well, who may have no localising neurological signs, and is found to have normal cerebral ventricles on CAT scan or ventriculography. The condition can complicate otitis media or malignant disease, it may develop during pregnancy or after head injury, and sometimes occurs spontaneously, particularly in young and rather obese women. Cortical thrombophlebitis in childhood or in pregnancy is sometimes different in its presentation and may give focal fits and neurological signs (e.g. hemiplegia) which resolve unusually rapidly. Occasionally, when thrombosis of the sagittal sinus is extensive, the patient is semicomatose and has fits and focal neurological signs (hemiparesis or paraplegia) due to venous infarction of the superior aspect of the cerebral cortex; subarachnoid haemorrhage sometimes occurs as a result.

Temporal, Giant-cell or Cranial Arteritis

This condition, which is commonest in patients over 65 years of age, is related to the other diseases of the 'collagen' or connective tissue group. Characteristically the patient suffers general malaise with vague aches and pains in the limbs and joints, fever and loss of appetite. There is also temporal headache and tenderness of the neck and scalp. The temporal and occipital arteries are nodular, tender and sometimes thrombosed. Sometimes there is little clinical evidence of disease in the temporal arteries and the presenting features are those of polymyalgia rheumatica (*see* p. 385). The most important complication is occlusion of the central retinal artery; this condition is the commonest cause of sudden unilateral blindness in the elderly. If the disease is not treated the second eye can be involved soon afterwards. Rarely, the arotid, cerebral and coronary arteries are affected to give cerebral or cardiac infarction. The erythrocyte sedimentation rate is invariably raised and the condition responds rapidly to steroid therapy.

Other 'Collagen' or 'Connective-tissue' Diseases

Occasionally polyarteritis nodosa and systemic lupus erythematosus give rise to neurological symptoms due to involvement of the small arteries of the brain or spinal cord (*see* p. 303). There is also a rare form of diffuse granulomatous angiitis of the cerebral vessels of unknown cause which affects young people and usually progresses to a fatal termination in about two years. Thrombotic microangiopathy (thrombotic thrombocytopenic purpura) is a rare condition in which fever, haemolytic anaemia, convulsions, confusion and variable pareses of the limbs may occur due to blockage of capillaries in the brain and elsewhere by platelet thrombi. The condition runs a fulminant course, there is thrombocytopenia and a high erythrocyte sedimentation rate, and treatment with steroid drugs is usually ineffective.

Buerger's Disease

Thromboangiitis obliterans has been thought to involve the cerebral vasculature to give a clinical picture which is dominated by fits, progressive dementia and variable palsies of the limbs but most cases so diagnosed have proved to be suffering from atherosclerosis.

Pulseless Disease *(Takayasu's Disease)*

This is a condition, first described in Japan, in which non-specific arteritis of the aortic arch occurs in young people and results in slow progressive occlusion of medium-sized arteries. No limb pulses may be palpable. As the carotid and vertebral arteries are involved, symptoms and signs of progressive or repeated cerebral infarction commonly appear in such cases. True pulseless disease is rare in Great Britain and the United States, but a similar syndrome may occur in middle-aged or elderly patients due to atherosclerosis.

Unruptured Saccular Aneurysms

Unruptured aneurysms of the cerebral vessels often give no symptoms, but they can simulate basally-situated space-occupying lesions if they become large enough to compress cranial-nerve trunks or other important structures. A supraclinoid aneurysm of the internal carotid artery is a common cause of an isolated third nerve palsy, while a suprasellar aneurysm can be responsible for chiasmal compression and hence for appropriate visual-field defects. An aneurysm within the cavernous sinus may give paralysis of the third, fourth and sixth cranial nerves on the affected side, along with sensory loss in the distribution of the first and second divisions of the ipsilateral fifth nerve. If an aneurysm in this situation ruptures, pulsating exophthalmos develops and a loud bruit can be heard over the affected eye. A similar carotico-cavernous fistula rarely follows head injury in the absence of an aneurysm.

Arteriovenous Angioma

Small angiomas in the substance of the cerebrum may produce no symptoms until they bleed, resulting in subarachnoid haemorrhage. Others are associated with headaches closely resembling migraine, often strictly limited to the side of the head upon which the angioma lies, while yet others give rise to focal fits and neurological signs (aphasia, hemiparesis), as they expand in size. Large angiomas are occasionally big enough to starve the surrounding brain of blood, resulting in dementia. A cranial bruit is often heard on the scalp overlying the intracranial lesion or over the appropriate internal carotid artery in the neck. Similar angiomas of the brain stem and posterior fossa are comparatively rare, but can be responsible for repeated episodes of brain-stem dysfunction occurring over a period of several years, resembling in some respects attacks of vertebro-basilar insufficiency and in others, repeated brain-stem episodes of multiple sclerosis.

Sturge–Weber Syndrome

This is a congenital malformation of precapillaries in the cerebral cortex, involving as a rule one parietal and occipital lobe and giving a characteristic radiological pattern of subcortical calcification outlining the cerebral gyri. Usually such patients have frequent fits and a contralateral hemiplegia. An invariable feature of the syndrome is a 'port-wine' naevus of the face on the affected side, often with a unilateral congenital ox-eye (buphthalmos).

Vascular Disorders of the Spinal Cord

By comparison with cerebral vascular disease, disorders of the spinal vasculature are relatively uncommon.

Spinal Subarachnoid Haemorrhage

This rare variety of subarachnoid haemorrhage causes sudden and severe pain in the back. This spreads into the arms and legs, depending upon which spinal roots are principally affected through being in close proximity to the bleeding point. Headache and neck stiffness often develop subsequently if the haemorrhage is sufficiently extensive and extends to the cranial subarachnoid space. There may be neurological signs of variable extent in the limbs, depending upon the aetiology of the bleeding and the amount of damage to the spinal cord and/or nerve roots which has taken place. The commonest cause is an arteriovenous angioma of the spinal cord but it can also be symptomatic of a cauda equina tumour, such as an ependymoma of the filum terminale or even a neurofibroma.

Intramedullary spinal haemorrhage is an extremely rare event; this spontaneous variety of haematomyelia gives a clinical picture resembling that of the traumatic condition (*see* p. 265). It is usually the result of bleeding from small vascular anomalies (angiomas, telangiectases) within the cord.

Anterior Spinal Artery Thrombosis

The anterior spinal artery, formed by the fusion of branches from each vertebral artery at the level of the foramen magnum, descends in the anterior median fissure of the spinal cord and supplies, by means of its perforating branches, the greater part of the spinal cord apart from the posterior columns. The latter area receives its blood supply from two posterior spinal arteries which are also branches of the vertebral arteries and descend on the posterolateral aspect of the cord but which are smaller and less constant. Throughout the dorsal region the anterior spinal artery receives contributions from radicular arteries which are derived from the intercostals and in the lumbar region lumbar arteries also contribute. Indeed the most important artery supplying the cord below the D10 segment is the great anterior medullary artery of Adamkiewicz which arises from the lumbar aorta. Thrombosis of the anterior spinal artery gives massive infarction of the spinal cord with a complete flaccid paraplegia, retention of urine and sensory loss to pain and temperature below the level of the lesion. Only some light touch and position and joint sense may be retained. The condition is generally due to atherosclerosis and hence occurs in the elderly. When it develops in the upper cervical region there is a complete quadriplegia with respiratory paralysis, and death follows rapidly. More often the upper level of the paralysis and sensory loss is at about the D10 dermatome and in such a case occlusion of the artery of Adamkiewicz may be responsible. The latter syndrome is an important immediate complication of a dissecting aneurysm of the aorta which occludes the mouths of its branches. The paraplegia is irreversible and many patients so afflicted soon die from urinary or respiratory infection.

It is, however, becoming increasingly clear that a syndrome of incomplete infarction due to embolism or occlusion of radicals of the anterior spinal artery is not as uncommon as was once believed, and in such a case there is paresis rather than paralysis and partial recovery often occurs. Indeed a syndrome of combined but asymmetrical lower and upper motor neurone weakness confined to the lower limbs with variable sensory loss, in which myelography gives normal findings, is often due to an **ischaemic myelopathy**. Other patients prove to have episodes of transient spinal cord dysfunction comparable to transient cerebral ischaemic attacks, often following exertion ('intermittent claudication of the spinal cord'). Intermittent ischaemia or 'claudication' of the cauda equina is even more common. Such patients usually complain of pain or paraesthesiae in one or both legs occurring on exertion and relieved by rest but have normal peripheral pulses. Examination after exercise may demonstrate motor weakness, loss of reflexes and/or sensory loss which disappear with rest. Radiography and myelography in such cases usually demonstrate either a bony stenosis of the lumbar canal or a central disc protrusion and the condition can be cured by surgical laminectomy and decompression.

Spinal Venous Thrombosis

A form of subacute necrotising myelopathy, giving a slowly ascending paraplegia, has been attributed to widespread thrombosis of vertebral veins, but is rare. It is particularly liable to occur in patients with chronic cor pulmonale and myelography may demonstrate dilated veins on the surface of the cord. Some authors believe that this syndrome is due to a venous angioma rather than to venous thrombosis.

References

Adams, R. D. and Victor, M., *Principles of Neurology*, 2nd ed. (New York, McGraw-Hill, 1981).

Greenhalgh, R. M. and Rose, F. C. (Eds.), *Progress in Stroke Research, 1.* (London, Pitman Books, 1979).

Hughes, J. T., *The Pathology of the Spinal Cord* 2nd ed. (London, Lloyd-Luke, 1978).

Hutchinson, E. C. and Acheson, J. *The Natural History of Cerebral Vascular Disease,* Major Problems in Neurology, No. 4 (London, Saunders, 1975).

Marshall, J., *The Management of Cerebrovascular Disease,* 3rd ed. (London, Churchill, 1976).

Ross Russell, R. W. (Ed.), *Cerebral Arterial Disease* (Edinburgh and London, Churchill Livingstone, 1976).

Toole, J. F. and Patel, A. N., *Cerebrovascular Disorders,* 2nd ed. (New York, McGraw-Hill, 1974).

Walton, J. N., *Subarachnoid Haemorrhage* (Edinburgh, Livingstone, 1956).

18 Disorders of the Lower Motor Neurone and Voluntary Muscles

There is a large and important group of diseases and symptom-complexes, often referred to as the neuromuscular disorders. These are characterised by weakness and/or wasting of the voluntary muscles, due to disordered function of the lower motor neurones or of the muscles themselves. Many of these conditions are chronic, progressive, and relatively uninfluenced by treatment, but others, which are superficially similar, can be treated effectively. Hence differential diagnosis of the disease entities falling into this group is very important, and apart from the clinical criteria which are of value in this connexion, and which will be outlined below, certain special investigations, including techniques of electrodiagnosis and muscle biopsy (*see* pp. 58 and 39) have an important place. The first step in diagnosis must be to identify the site of the pathological change; the lesion may lie in the motor nuclei of the cranial nerves, in the anterior horn cells of the spinal cord, in the spinal roots or nerves, in the peripheral nerves or plexuses, in the neuromuscular junction, or in the skeletal muscles themselves. The coexistence of abnormalities of sensation can be of considerable assistance in this process of identification. Next it is necessary to determine if possible the nature and aetiology of the pathological process. Unfortunately there are still many diseases in this group whose aetiology and pathogenesis remain obscure. Several of those of known cause have been considered in previous chapters. Thus muscular weakness and/or atrophy is a striking feature of many cases of acute anterior poliomyelitis, of postinfective polyradiculitis, and of 'collagen' disease affecting the peripheral nerves (*see* pp. 285, 302 and 303). Involvement of the anterior horn cells of the spinal cord, with resulting muscular atrophy, is often found in disorders such as syringomyelia, and amyotrophy due to lesions in the cord or peripheral nerves is seen in some of the hereditary ataxias (*see* p. 245). Furthermore, intra- and extra-medullary spinal neoplasms (*see* p. 336) or traumatic disorders of the spinal cord, roots, plexuses or peripheral nerves (*see* pp. 264–276) may have a similar effect. This chapter will consider those conditions not previously mentioned.

The Spinal Muscular Atrophies

Four principal conditions can provisionally be classified in this group. The first is a progressive genetically-determined disorder of the anterior horn cells, occurring either in infancy, childhood or adolescence, or in adult life. The second is adult motor neurone (or motor system) disease, the third the neuronal sub-variety of peroneal muscular atrophy and the fourth is scapuloperoneal muscular atrophy.

Progressive Spinal Muscular Atrophy (SMA)

The most severe form of this condition **(Werdnig–Hoffman disease**, also known as acute infantile spinal muscular atrophy or SMA Type I), which typically begins in the first six months of life, but can also be present at birth, affects babies of either sex. It is inherited as an autosomal recessive trait, so that it often affects more than one member of a sibship. Indeed the number of affected children in any one family often exceeds the expected one in four incidence. Usually the parents observe that the child is not moving his limbs normally, that he is unable to hold up his head or to sit, that he is generally limp and 'floppy' and when picked up he tends to slip through the hands. Gradually muscular weakness and generalised hypotonia increase, affecting first the muscles around the shoulder girdle and pelvis and later those of the chest wall, so that there is a characteristic indrawing of the lower ribs at the diaphragmatic attachment on inspiration. The infant, who is at first sight healthy and well-nourished, is seen to lie in a typical posture with the arms abducted on either side of the head, and with the legs abducted and externally rotated at the hips. Later there is weakness of the muscles of deglutition, and fasciculation in the tongue is seen. Most affected children die from respiratory infection before the end of the first or second year of life. Unfortunately there is no specific treatment.

In some other patients and families also demonstrating autosomal recessive inheritance the condition presents with muscular weakness and hypotonia resembling that seen in Werdnig-Hoffmann disease in the second six months of life or in the second year. The paralysis is less severe than in the acute variety and often the disease process appears to arrest leaving the child severely crippled by muscular weakness, contractures and secondary skeletal deformity. These children, who may never be able to walk or even sit unsupported, often survive into the second or third decade; in them orthopaedic measures and appliances designed to reduce contractures and deformity are particularly important and must be started early. Some authorities regard this as a separate sub-variety of SMA (SMA Type II) and classify it separately from juvenile SMA (SMA Type III), while others suggest that this condition represents only the most severe end of a spectrum of varying severity in the subacute or chronic variety of SMA which may begin in childhood or adolescence. The latter view is based upon the observation of severe late infantile and benign juvenile cases within the same sibship. In the juvenile cases weakness may first appear in the proximal limb muscles later in the first decade or even in the second or third, when the picture is easily mistaken for that of muscular dystrophy (these are cases of 'pseudo-myopathic' spinal muscular atrophy, the so-called **Kugelberg-Welander syndrome**). In such cases the weakness involves proximal muscles of the lower and upper limbs giving postural changes, a waddling gait, and other features like those of muscular dystrophy. However, some muscles (e.g. deltoid) which are often spared in the early stages of a dystrophic process are commonly involved early and fasciculation may be seen in the tongue or elsewhere. Many such cases have undoubtedly been regarded in the past as examples of muscular dystrophy and the true diagnosis has only become apparent when modern methods of investigation (e.g. electromyography and muscle biopsy) have been employed. The distinction is not academic, as benign spinal muscular atrophy of childhood, adolescence, and early adult life often arrests or runs a more benign course than does muscular dystrophy, and the patients can sometimes be improved by vigorous physiotherapy. It is now evident that many patients thought to have developed limb-girdle muscular dystrophy in later adult life are in fact suffering from a similar autosomal recessive benign spinal muscular atrophy. In such cases diagnosis from motor neurone disease (*see below*) rests upon the family history, the absence of signs of upper motor neurone dysfunction, the relative symmetry of the muscular weakness and wasting and its onset usually in proximal rather than distal limb muscles.

Motor Neurone Disease

This is a disease of adult life which usually begins after the age of 40, though it appears occasionally in younger individuals. In Britain, the USA and most Western countries it is usually sporadic, occurring equally in the two sexes. However, a form of the disease which is inherited by an autosomal dominant mechanism has been described, but in such families the condition is often clinically atypical and it may run an unusually benign course. In the Chamorro people on the island of Guam and in other parts of the Western Pacific, a severe form of the disease is very common and is often associated with features of Parkinsonism and dementia (the Parkinsonism-dementia complex) in affected individuals. It is still uncertain as to whether this Western Pacific form is genetically determined or due to an unidentified environmental factor.

The pathogenesis of the condition is obscure; cases have been described as developing many years after an attack of paralytic poliomyelitis and occasionally after encephalitis lethargica, while trauma has been implicated as a contributory factor in isolated instances, but the significance of these observations remains doubtful. A 'slow virus' infection has been postulated but all attempts to isolate a virus from such cases have been unsuccessful so that the progressive degenerative changes which occur in the motor nuclei of the cranial nerves, in the anterior horn cells of the spinal cord, and in the pyramidal tracts remain unexplained. Even though minor pathological changes have been discovered in sensory pathways in certain cases it is a diagnostic axiom that clinically-recognisable sensory disturbances are absent. Although they merge with one another, three distinctive clinical syndromes, namely progressive bulbar palsy, amyotrophic lateral sclerosis and progressive muscular atrophy, have been described as typifying the variable clinical presentation of the disease. In progressive bulbar palsy the motor cranial nerve nuclei are predominantly affected, in amyotrophic lateral sclerosis the pyramidal tracts, and in progressive muscular atrophy the anterior horn cells of the cord, but in almost all cases there is eventually evidence of lesions in all three sites.

Progressive Bulbar Palsy

The first symptom of this condition is often dysphagia, and dysarthria soon follows, though difficulty in speaking may come first. Indeed isolated dysarthria of gradual onset in the absence of other symptoms and signs should always suggest the diagnosis when appearing in middle or late life. Food, particularly solid particles, sticks in the back of the throat, choking is frequent and later there is often regurgitation of fluid down the nose owing to palatal paralysis; the voice, as well as being slurred, acquires a nasal quality. On examination there is paresis of palatal, pharyngeal and tongue muscles; profuse fasciculation of the tongue is evident, and the jaw jerk is exaggerated. Fasciculation is also observed as a rule in shoulder girdle muscles and there are usually signs of pyramidal tract dysfunction in the limbs. Often features of pseudobulbar palsy (*see* p. 353) due to bilateral pyramidal tract involvement accompany those of true bulbar palsy due to lower motor neurone lesions. The disease is progressive, leading to complete bulbar paralysis with the serious nursing problems which this entails, along with weakness and spasticity of the limbs. Tracheostomy and tube-feeding may be necessary. Most patients die from respiratory infection within one or two years.

Amyotrophic Lateral Sclerosis

The usual presenting symptom in this disorder is difficulty in walking due to stiffness of the legs, or else dragging of one leg with subsequent involvement of the other. Physical examination reveals a spastic quadriparesis with strikingly increased tendon reflexes in all four limbs and extensor plantar responses. There is no abnormality of sensation and the abdominal reflexes are often retained until late in the course. In the early stages there are few indications of lower motor neurone dysfunction but there is generally some fasciculation in the shoulder girdle and thigh muscles and subsequently muscular atrophy appears. However, the clinical picture is sometimes one of bilateral pyramidal tract disease for some years before signs of lower motor neurone lesions develop. Symptoms and signs of bulbar paralysis appear late; in these cases it is spasticity and weakness due to the upper motor neurone lesions which are the principal cause of disability. Nevertheless weakness of the bulbar muscles ultimately causes death in most cases, usually in two to five years from the onset.

Progressive Muscular Atrophy

In this, the most benign presentation of motor neurone disease, the first symptom is usually weakness of muscles in one hand or forearm; less commonly leg muscles are first affected, when a progressive foot drop is the usual manifestation. The weakness progresses insidiously; at first the only symptom may be clumsiness of fine movements of the fingers (inability to fasten buttons, to sew or to write) but subsequently the grip is affected or wrist drop develops, and the weakness spreads up the arm. In the early stages, fasciculation is often scanty, but later it becomes prominent. There may be considerable difficulty in distinguishing the early manifestations of this disease from those due to cervical root, peripheral nerve or plexus lesions, but subsequently it becomes clear that the distribution of muscular weakness and wasting is more extensive than could be accounted for by involvement of a single peripheral nerve or of one or two motor roots. Eventually there is extensive involvement of the muscles of the limbs and trunk, but the signs are usually asymmetrical at first. Because of extensive muscular atrophy, the tendon reflexes sub-served by the affected muscles are commonly lost, and evidence of pyramidal tract involvement is often lacking for some time, but in the end the plantar responses usually become extensor and bulbar palsy develops. The absence of sensory loss generally serves to distinguish this condition from peripheral neuropathy, but when fasciculation is scanty, diagnosis from a predominantly motor polyneuropathy can be difficult if not impossible, though electromyography and motor nerve conduction velocity measurements, usually normal in motor neurone disease and often reduced in polyneuropathy, may be helpful. The natural history of this condition is variable; the average duration of the illness before it ends fatally, again as a rule from respiratory infection, is between 18 months and five years, but in some proven cases the total duration has been as long as 10 or 15 years or even longer.

Peroneal Muscular Atrophy (Charcot-Marie-Tooth Disease)

This condition, previously mentioned in Chapter 12, is related to the other conditions of the hereditary ataxia group, and is often in many respects the most benign of all the chronic progressive neurological diseases. It is usually inherited as either an autosomal dominant or autosomal recessive trait, affects either sex, and begins usually in adolescence or early adult life. Very occasional families have shown X-linked inheritance. Recent pathological evidence suggests that this syndrome results from two or possibly three distinct pathological processes but that the nature of the process is consistent in the affected members of a single family. In one form of the disease the neuropathy is due to axonal degeneration and the lesion may lie either in the anterior horn cell or in the peripheral axons; in the other it is demyelinating, with slowing of nerve conduction and there may be hypertrophy of peripheral nerves. Of these sub-varieties the hypertrophic demyelinating form is the commonest and usually the most benign with total restriction of weakness to distal limb muscles. The axonal variety is much less common and it, like the neuronal (distal spinal muscular atrophy) type, ultimately spreads to involve proximal muscles. The first symptoms are usually those of unilateral or bilateral foot drop. Subsequently the calf muscles are involved so that there is severe weakness of dorsiflexion, plantar-flexion, inversion and eversion of the feet and there is a striking atrophy of all muscles below the knee. The picture of an 'inverted champagne bottle' limb, with bilateral pes cavus, in which the thin legs contrast strikingly with the normal thighs, is characteristic. In most cases the intrinsic muscles of the hands are also affected to give a bilateral 'claw hand', but the muscular involvement does not often spread to involve the upper arms. Except in the neuronal type there is often loss of vibration sense in the lower limbs, but impairment of cutaneous sensibility is uncommon. Despite their disability, many patients remain active and survive to a normal age. Appliances to control foot-drop are usually required and greatly improve walking.

Scapuloperoneal Muscular Atrophy

This rare disorder, of dominant inheritance, is usually due to anterior horn cell disease, less often myopathic. In the legs the changes resemble those of peroneal muscular atrophy, while in the upper limbs there is winging of the scapulae. It is much more benign than progressive muscular atrophy, with which it is often confused.

Lesions of Motor Cranial Nerves, of Spinal Roots and of Peripheral Nerves

Many disorders which could reasonably be considered under this heading have already been described. Thus dysfunction of the nerves to the extrinsic ocular muscles was discussed in Chapter 8 (pp. 165–175). Infective and allergic conditions involving spinal roots were described in Chapter 14 (pp. 302–304), while trauma to roots, plexuses and peripheral nerves was considered in Chapter 13 (pp. 269–276). There remain to be considered some abnormalities of the facial nerve and of other motor cranial nerves, the clinical effects of intervertebral disk prolapse, of cervical spondylosis, and the differential diagnosis of disorders causing pain in the arm or wasting of the small hand muscles.

Facial Paralysis

A lower motor neurone lesion of the facial nerve can be distinguished from an upper motor neurone type of facial palsy by the fact that in the former all the facial muscles on one side are equally affected, while in the latter the weakness involves principally the muscles of the lower face, and movement of those around the eye is comparatively unimpaired. A complete unilateral facial palsy can be due to a nuclear lesion, as in poliomyelitis, multiple sclerosis, pontine infarction or tumour, or rarely, motor neurone disease. It can also result from lesions of the nerve trunk in its intracranial course, when it is involved in a cranial polyneuropathy, constricted by granulomatous inflammation in the subarachnoid space (meningitis, sarcoidosis, meningovascular syphilis) or compressed by a tumour (e.g. acoustic neuroma) or deposits of a reticulosis. The commonest conditions giving facial palsy due to damage to the nerve in its course through the temporal bone are otitis media and herpes zoster of the geniculate ganglion (the Ramsay Hunt syndrome). In its extracranial course the nerve may be damaged by disease of the parotid glands; bilateral facial palsy is a rare presenting feature of acute leukaemia or sarcoidosis.

The commonest variety of unilateral facial palsy is, however, **Bell's palsy** which can occur at any age and in either sex and is of unknown aetiology, although a swelling of the nerve in the narrow bony canal above the stylomastoid foramen has been postulated as its cause. It may follow exposure to cold or a draught but often arises without apparent precipitating cause. A viral cause has been proposed but remains unconfirmed. Often the patient awakens to find that he is unable to close the eye on the affected side, that the furrows on this side of the forehead are lost, and that the mouth is drawn over to the sound side. Occasionally there is hyperacusis in the ipsilateral ear due to involvement of the nerve to the stapedius. In some cases the paralysis is incomplete; when this is so, if there is no progression over the course of the first two or three days, complete recovery generally occurs within one to two weeks. More often the paralysis remains complete for two or three weeks and then begins to recover; and recovery then is complete as a rule within two or three months. In a comparatively small number of cases there is actual division of certain nerve fibres (neuronotmesis) and regeneration is necessary. In such a case recovery may take several months and even then is generally incomplete, as some of the regenerating nerve fibres go astray. Commonly in such a case a degree of permanent facial contracture develops, a factor which improves the appearance of the face while at rest, though paralysis is still evident on movement (e.g. smiling). Occasionally, too, clonic facial spasm (*see below*) is a sequel. Another rare complication is involuntary lacrimation during eating (the syndrome of 'crocodile tears') due to the fact that regenerating autonomic fibres intended for the salivary glands reach the lacrimal glands instead. During the acute stage, it may be necessary to protect the cornea of the eye which cannot be closed. The cosmetic appearance can be improved by the use of strips of transparent adhesive tape (e.g. 'Sellotape'). Treatment with steroid drugs or ACTH has been advocated but is only of value if given immediately after the onset, and surgical decompression of the facial canal is usually performed too late to help, as it is only done when it is evident that spontaneous recovery is not taking place. Unfortunately, electromyography gives relatively little information of prognostic value until about three weeks after the onset. However, if electrical conduction in the facial nerve can be demonstrated one week after the onset of paralysis this is a good prognostic sign. Electrical stimulation of the paralysed muscles has often been used but is of dubious value and may increase contracture. In long-standing facial paralysis, cosmetic plastic surgery has a limited but definite place. Some patients suffer repeated attacks of Bell's palsy, now on one side of the face and now on the other, but this is relatively uncommon. Recurrent familial facial palsy associated with congenital fissuring of the tongue is called Melkersson's syndrome.

Hemifacial Spasm

This condition, also called clonic facial spasm, is commonest in middle-aged or elderly women. It is thought to be due to a benign irritative lesion of unknown aetiology involving the nerve in its bony canal. It gives intermittent fine twitching in one orbicularis oculi which later spreads to involve the remaining facial muscles on the same side. The spasms can eventually be quite powerful, and rapidly though irregularly repetitive. In the early stages it may resemble a tic and is certainly accentuated by emotional stress, but tics are usually bilateral so that the strictly unilateral movements of hemifacial spasm are diagnostic. The condition differs from the slow rippling movements of facial myokymia which may be a rare manifestation of multiple sclerosis. The EMG is often helpful in demonstrating 'grouped' motor unit discharges (each consisting of two or three motor unit action potentials) which repeat rhythmically. Eventually progressive facial paralysis often develops on the affected side and the movements cease. The condition is embarrassing and inconvenient and little influenced by drugs although diazepam may damp down the movements. Decompression of the facial canal has been advocated but is rarely successful; alcohol injection or operative division of certain fibres of the nerve has been tried but the spasm is then exchanged for a partial facial paralysis. Exploration of the nerve in the posterior fossa has revealed compression of its trunk by an artery in some cases.

Lesions of Other Motor Cranial Nerves

Isolated lesions of other motor cranial nerves are rare, but their nuclei can be damaged by brain stem lesions, while the nerves themselves may be compressed by space-occupying lesions or involved in inflammatory exudate either intracranially or extracranially. A lesion of the motor root of one **trigeminal nerve** gives atrophy and weakness of the masseter, temporalis and pterygoids on the affected side with consequent asymmetrical jaw movement. The **glossopharyngeal** nerve supplies only the stylopharyngeus muscle, so that its motor function cannot be tested. The **vagus** nerve, however, supplies the muscles of the soft palate and pharynx, so that a unilateral lesion of this nerve paralyses these structures on the affected side. When such a lesion is present, the soft palate and uvula deviate to the side away from the lesion, and there is a 'curtain' movement of the posterior pharyngeal wall, again to the opposite side; often this is seen when the patient says 'Ah'. Unilateral paralysis of laryngeal muscles, which can also result from lesions of the recurrent laryngeal branch of the vagus (due to secondary neoplasm or reticulosis in mediastinal lymph nodes, to an aortic aneurysm, or thyroid carcinoma) gives hoarseness of the voice and paralysis of the ipsilateral vocal cord which can be seen on laryngoscopy. A lesion of the **spinal accessory** nerve gives atrophy and weakness of trapezius and sternomastoid on the affected side, while a unilateral **hypoglossal** palsy results in atrophy and fasciculation of one half of the tongue, which, when protruded, deviates to the affected side.

Prolapsed Intervertebral Disk

The intervertebral disk consists of an outer fibrocartilaginous ring, the annulus fibrosus, and a central semifluid portion, the nucleus pulposus. As a result of a degenerative process of unknown aetiology, the annulus fibrosus may be breached, allowing the nucleus pulposus to herniate through the gap so formed. If this gap lies posteriorly in the annulus, as is usual, the prolapsed disk may encroach either upon the spinal canal (a central protrusion) or upon an intervertebral foramen (a lateral protrusion). An acute lateral prolapse of a cervical disk will usually compress a spinal root or nerve, giving the clinical syndrome of brachial neuralgia, while a similar lateral protrusion of a lumbar disk is the commonest cause of sciatica. An acute central protrusion in the cervical region causes sudden compression of the cervical cord, with symptoms and signs of partial, or even complete, paraplegia or quadriplegia depending upon the size of the protrusion and the level of the lesion, while in the lumbar region a similar acute prolapse may give a cauda equina syndrome of acute onset. Dorsal disk protrusions are comparatively rare, but when they do occur, the spinal canal is so narrow in this situation that there is generally evidence of spinal cord compression.

The clinical syndromes resulting from disk prolapse can occur in either sex, but are more common in men; they are most often observed in middle and late life, as increasing age contributes to disk degeneration, but may occur in early adult life. Trauma plays an important role, as symptoms may develop first after sudden exertion (a twisting movement, hyperextension of the neck, straining to lift a heavy object). Almost certainly such traumatic incidents do no more than to precipitate prolapse of a degenerating disk which would eventually have ruptured spontaneously.

The first symptom is generally pain in the neck or back, with tenderness over the spinous processes of the affected vertebrae and with pain and tenderness in the spinal muscles (owing to protective spasm). This is why the first symptoms of an acute intervertebral disk prolapse are commonly attributed to 'stiff neck', 'fibrositis' or 'lumbago'. Movements of the affected area of the spine may be intensely painful. When the protrusion is central, weakness and paraesthesiae in the lower limbs and retention of urine are often seen immediately. If the lesion is cervical there will be signs of a symmetrical paraparesis, while if it is lumbar, there are usually lower motor neurone and sensory signs in the lower limbs indicating involvement of multiple roots of the cauda equina. In a laterally-situated prolapse in the cervical region, pain of an intense burning character spreads over the shoulder and down the arm, along the dermatome innervated by the affected root. In the lumbar region the pain travels down the back of the thigh and leg and often into the foot, although occasionally in a case of high lumbar disk protrusion it radiates down the front of the thigh. Typically the pain is made worse by movement, and by coughing or by straining, which temporarily increase the pressure in the spinal canal. Often, too, it is worse when the patient is warm in bed at night. Peripheral nerves (e.g. the sciatic) which receive contributions from the affected root, are tender and painful when stretched. When the lesion is cervical, lateral flexion of the head towards the side of the prolapse is painful (Spurling's sign) while in sciatica, straight-leg raising on the affected side is restricted and painful (Lasègue's sign).

Compression of a motor root by the prolapsed disk often produces in due course muscular weakness, fasciculation, atrophy and reflex changes, depending upon which root is involved; affection of the sensory root gives subjective numbness and paraesthesiae and objective sensory loss in the appropriate dermatome. In the cervical region, the commonest levels of disk prolapse are at C5–6, in which case the fifth cervical root is involved and at C6–7, giving compression of the C6 root. In either case, the deltoid, biceps and brachioradialis muscles may be weak or atrophic and the biceps and radial jerks are commonly depressed. In the lumbar region the sites of election are L4–5 (L5 root) and L5–S1 (S1 root). In either event a partial foot drop may result, but when the disk protrudes at the higher level the pain usually radiates down into the dorsum of the foot and the reflexes are intact, while compression of the S1 root gives pain along the outer border and sole of the foot and an absent ankle jerk. In a case of acute disk prolapse, spinal radiographs are often normal, but sometimes the affected disk space is narrowed. A moderate rise in the CSF protein (up to 1.0 g/l, or more if there is a complete block) is not uncommon.

Commonly with rest and analgesics alone the symptoms of an acute disk prolapse resolve within a few days or weeks, but exertion may cause a recurrence of symptoms, often after months or years. When bed rest fails, immobilisation in plaster or in a plastic cervical collar or lumbar support may be needed; alternatively, either intermittent or continuous spinal traction may be tried. Manipulation has many advocates, and is occasionally very successful, though in the cervical region particularly, it carries considerable risks of damage to the spinal cord. Myelography (which is less successful in demonstrating lateral rather than central protrusions) followed by surgical decompression of the spinal cord, affected root(s) or spinal nerve(s) and removal of the prolapsed fragment of nucleus pulposus, are usually indicated if there is evidence of severe muscular weakness, extensive sensory loss or impairment of sphincter control, or in cases of prolapsed lumbar disk in which all other measures have failed to relieve pain.

Cervical Spondylosis

This term is utilised to describe the chronic changes which occur in the cervical spine as a result of long-standing multiple or single intervertebral disk lesions, and which can cause a variety of symptoms and physical signs due to compression of cervical nerve roots and of the spinal cord (cervical myelopathy). This name should not be given to the syndrome of acute cervical disk prolapse, either central or lateral. When part of an intervertebral disk has been prolapsed for some time the protruding portion becomes at first fibrotic but later is calcified and bony-hard. A firm bar of tissue is thus created along the posterior aspect of the disk (and often on its anterior aspect as well); this is usually associated with overgrowth of the margins of the contiguous vertebrae to give bony spurs or osteophytes (so-called lipping). Commonly these bars and lips also encroach upon the intervertebral foramina, and this encroachment is shown in oblique radiographs of the spine. These changes are usually observed at several levels. The resulting changes in spinal radiographs are often referred to as indicating 'osteoarthritis'. Such appearances are found in many manual workers and in fewer sedentary workers after middle-age; some have no neurological symptoms and signs. Hence, it follows that these radiological changes are often found coincidentally in patients with other neurological diseases, including multiple sclerosis, syringomyelia, motor neurone disease, and even spinal tumour; therefore it is unwise to assume that spondylosis necessarily accounts for the patient's symptoms even though this may ultimately prove to be the case.

The syndrome of **cervical myelopathy** resulting from spondylosis is a disorder of middle- and late-life and is much commoner in men than in women. There may have been symptoms in the past (episodes of stiff neck, or 'neuritis' in the arms) to indicate previous acute incidents of disk prolapse, while even in the chronic stage the patient sometimes complains of intermittent pain or stiffness in the neck, or of pain down one or both arms. Variable degrees of wasting and weakness of upper limb muscles, sometimes with fasciculation, may be observed on one or both sides, but these changes are not invariable and often unobtrusive; most symptoms are referable to the lower limbs. The muscles usually involved in the arms are the spinati, deltoid, biceps and triceps, as the roots which are most often compressed are those of the C5, 6 and 7 segments; involvement of intrinsic hand muscles is very rare but can result from ischaemia of anterior horn cells due to cord compression above the D1 segment. A common and valuable sign is inversion of the biceps or radial reflexes. The biceps jerk is said to be inverted if tapping the biceps tendon produces contraction of the triceps; while the radial jerk is inverted if a tap on the brachioradialis tendon produces no contraction of this muscle, but finger flexion. These signs, if present, imply that there is a lesion of the C5 or C6 segment of the cord, breaking the reflex arc for reflexes which utilise these cord segments, but at the same time compressing the pyramidal tract to give exaggeration of those reflexes whose pathways pass through lower segments. The usual symptoms and signs in the lower limbs are those of progressive spastic paraparesis, which is often, but not always, asymmetrical at first.

This syndrome is probably the commonest cause of a spastic paraparesis developing in late middle-life. Usually the patient describes a gradual onset with dragging and stiffness of one leg or with some aching pain in the limb after walking any distance. Paraesthesiae are relatively uncommon, but occasionally 'electric shocks' in the trunk and legs on flexion of the neck (Lhermitte's sign) are experienced. On examination there are signs of a spastic paraparesis with exaggerated tendon reflexes and extensor plantar responses. Absence of vibration sense in the lower limbs is common, due to posterior column involvement, but sensory loss of spinothalamic type is seen less often. In other words, the syndrome can mimic cervical cord compression due to a tumour or a focal cord lesion resulting from any cause. The symptoms are usually slowly progressive, but less rapidly than in a case of cord tumour, while the absence of remissions is helpful in distinguishing the condition from multiple sclerosis. Prolonged clinical arrest is, however, seen in some patients. Diagnosis in the end depends upon myelography, which reveals in such cases one or, more often, several indentations of the column of myodil opposite the affected disk spaces. The cord is often compressed between the disk protrusion anteriorly and an infolded ligamentum subflavum posteriorly. An ever-present danger in cases of this type is complete quadriplegia due to cervical cord contusion, which, as a result of narrowing of the cervical canal, may follow a relatively mild hyperextension injury of the neck. In the average case, although disability slowly increases, the patient is not totally disabled and often the symptoms of cord compression seem after a time to become no worse. Although often used a cervical collar is of little value except in relieving pain; surgical decompression of the cervical canal may be indicated when deterioration is comparatively rapid and when there is myelographic evidence of a large central disk protrusion at one or two levels. Removal of the affected disks and fusion of the cervical spine using an anterior approach (the Cloward operation) also has its advocates.

The Causes of Pain in the Arm

It is convenient at this point to mention briefly some important causes of the syndrome of brachial neuralgia or pain in the arm. The anatomical situation of the cause of the pain must first be considered; the conditions mentioned have all been discussed previously. Among the spinal disorders which may cause pain of root distribution in the upper limb are poliomyelitis, syringomyelia, multiple sclerosis and intramedullary tumour (intramedullary lesions); shoulder girdle neuritis (neuralgic amyotrophy), arachnoiditis and extramedullary tumours (extramedullary lesions); acute cervical disk prolapse, cervical spondylosis, and neoplasia in a vertebral body (lesions of the spinal column). Outside the spinal column, the commonest causes are cervical rib (pain down the inner side of the arm), the ill-defined costoclavicular outlet syndrome, tumours (i.e. neurofibroma or metastases in the root of the neck) of the brachial plexus or peripheral nerves, and, at the wrist, compression of the median nerve in the carpal tunnel. A bronchogenic carcinoma at the apex of the lung (Pancoast's superior pulmonary sulcus tumour) is a not infrequent cause of pain in the arm associated with an ipsilateral Horner's syndrome due to involvement of the stellate ganglion. Pericapsulitis of the shoulder joint, giving an immobile painful joint or one with only slight restriction of movement but with a tender capsule, is often associated with pain at the insertion of the deltoid and occasionally with painful brawny swelling of the hand (the shoulder-hand syndrome); the latter, if long-standing, may lead to atrophy and decalcification of bones (Sudeck's atrophy). Often, too, patients referred to neurological clinics with pain in the forearm, spreading down the dorsum into the fingers, prove to be suffering from a 'tennis-elbow' syndrome with local tenderness over the common extensor origin at the lateral epicondyle of the humerus or at the neck of the radius.

The Causes of Wasting of Small Hand Muscles

The conditions which cause wasting of the small muscles of the hands can be similarly classified. The commonest spinal cord lesions to have this effect are haematomyelia, poliomyelitis, motor neurone disease, syringomyelia, spinal muscular atrophy and peroneal muscular atrophy. A similar effect may result from an extramedullary tumour at the D1 level, or from arachnoiditis, but is rare in cervical spondylosis or acute disk lesions as the D1 root is not commonly compressed. Wasting of all the small hand muscles can be the result of any lesion of the inner cord of the brachial plexus; common lesions at this site include birth injury (Klumpke's paralysis), a hyperabduction injury during anaesthesia, compression by the head of the humerus following shoulder dislocation, tumours of the brachial plexus, and compression by a cervical rib or in the thoracic outlet. All the small hand muscles become atrophic as a rule in cases of motor polyneuropathy, but when there is an ulnar nerve lesion, those of the lateral half of the thenar eminence are spared, while the latter muscles are selectively involved when there is a lesion of the median nerve (as in the carpal tunnel). Hence atrophy of all the small hand muscles usually indicates disease of the D1 segment of the cord, of the D1 root, of the inner cord of the brachial plexus, or a diffuse disorder of peripheral nerves or anterior horn cells; atrophy of the lateral half of the thenar eminence generally indicates a median nerve lesion, while sparing of these muscles but atrophy of the others, giving a 'claw hand,' indicates an ulnar nerve lesion. The presence or absence of sensory signs, and their distribution, are of additional value in differential diagnosis. Wasting and weakness of these muscles is rare in myopathies but may occur late in limb-girdle muscular dystrophy; it is, however, an early sign of the rare distal form.

Peripheral Neuropathy (Polyneuropathy)

This condition, often entitled peripheral neuritis or polyneuritis, is more properly called peripheral neuropathy or polyneuropathy as inflammatory changes are rarely discovered in the affected nerves except in post-infective cases. Pathologically there are two principal varieties. In one the process is one of axonal degeneration; surviving nerve fibres conduct at a normal rate but the muscle action potential evoked by stimulation of a motor nerve, or the sensory nerve action potential evoked on stimulating a sensory nerve, is reduced in amplitude. In the second type the neuropathy is demyelinating and conduction velocity is slowed. Any process of recurrent demyelination and remyelination may result eventually in Schwann cell proliferation and nerve hypertrophy. In severe axonal neuropathy there is often secondary demyelination, while primary demyelination ultimately causes axonal damage as a rule, so that in many cases there is evidence of both types of process. Nevertheless, nerve conduction studies, and sometimes sural nerve biopsy, may help to determine the nature of the predominant pathological process thus giving a clue to aetiology. The neuropathies are a group of clinical syndromes of multiple aetiology in which there are features indicating simultaneous involvement of many peripheral nerves. The clinical picture of sensorimotor neuropathy is therefore one of weakness of lower motor neurone type with eventual atrophy, in the peripheral limb muscles; there is usually symmetrical sensory impairment in 'glove and stocking' distribution, and the tendon reflexes are absent. In contradistinction to 'glove and stocking' sensory loss of hysterical origin, that due to polyneuropathy does not usually show a sharp margin between the area of sensory impairment and that of normal sensation, but the change is gradual. Furthermore, a 'flare' response following a scratch is absent in polyneuropathy if sensory fibres are severely involved, but is present in hysteria. Sometimes motor fibres are predominantly affected (motor neuropathy) and sometimes sensory (sensory neuropathy). Often the affected skeletal muscles, particularly those of the calves, are tender. While distal weakness in the upper and lower limbs is the rule, paradoxically postinfective polyneuropathy (the Guillain–Barré syndrome—*see* p. 302) often affects proximal upper and lower limb muscles first and the neuropathy is predominantly motor, so that in subacute cases the clinical picture may superficially resemble that of a myopathy such as polymyositis. Many variations in the clinical picture occur from case to case and depend in part upon the aetiology of the illness. It is therefore essential initially to classify and define the known causes of this syndrome according to present knowledge. A provisional classification, which is not intended to embrace all types but simply the more important, is given below.

Classification

1. *Infective*: leprosy, infective mononucleosis.

2. *Postinfective*: (*a*) due to specific exotoxins—diphtheria; (*b*) postinfective (probably allergic)—the Guillain–Barré syndrome, serum neuropathy; (*c*) complicating specific infections—typhoid fever, dysentery, etc.

3. *Metabolic*: (*a*) nutritional—vitamin B_1, B_6 or B_{12} deficiency, alcoholism, pregnancy, etc.; (*b*) heavy metal poisoning—arsenic, mercury, gold, copper, etc.; (*c*) other poisons—triorthocresyl phosphate, isoniazid, acrylamide, vincristine, thalidomide, nitrofurantoin, chloroquine, clioquinol, disulfiram, *n*-hexane, phenytoin, organic poisons; (*d*) diabetes mellitus; (*e*) hyperinsulinism; (*f*) myxoedema; (*g*) acromegaly; (*h*) uraemia.

4. *Vascular:* polyarteritis nodosa; systemic lupus erythematosus; other 'collagen' or 'connective-tissue' diseases; leukaemia and dysproteinaemas.

5. *Genetically-determined*: peroneal muscular atrophy (neuropathic form); familial interstitial hypertrophic polyneuropathy (Dejerine–Sottas); hereditary sensory neuropathy; heredopathia atactica polyneuritiformis (Refsum's syndrome); neuropathy in metachromatic leucodystrophy and Krabbe's disease; neuropathy in primary amyloidosis; acute porphyria.

6. *Unknown Aetiology*: carcinomatous neuropathy; chronic progressive polyneuropathy.

The infective and postinfective varieties of polyneuropathy have already been described (*see* pp. 283–303). They are mainly demyelinating in type. In **leprosy** the clinical picture is one of progressive involvement of individual peripheral nerves with thickening of the nerve trunks and patchy cutaneous anaesthesia. Isolated palsies of single peripheral nerves (the facial or, say, the median or ulnar) or a symmetrical sensorimotor neuropathy are occasional complications of infective mononucleosis. The polyneuropathy due to **diphtheria** exotoxin usually begins within 10 days of the acute infection and first involves muscles near to the infected area, so that dysphagia and palatal palsy are often the first manifestation; in more severe cases, a symmetrical polyneuropathy of all four limbs develops in about four to six weeks. The **Guillain–Barré syndrome** is the commonest cause of acute ascending paralysis, but more often gives a subacute, predominantly motor, symmetrical neuropathy beginning in peripheral limb muscles and associated with a raised CSF protein. Indeed, a rise in the protein content of the fluid is a feature common to many varieties of polyneuropathy especially when demyelinating, but the values recorded in the postinfective cases are generally the highest of all. A polyneuropathy of non-specific type can also complicate many specific infective disorders. In most of these the neuropathy should probably be regarded as postinfective and autoimmune in character.

In the metabolic group of cases, the predominantly axonal polyneuropathy resulting from a **deficiency of vitamin B$_1$** (thiamine) is well recognised. Sensory symptoms generally predominate, and the condition begins with paraesthesiae in the hands and feet; these are followed by pain and tenderness of calf muscles and by bilateral foot drop, weakness of the grip and later wrist drop. There is peripheral blunting of all forms of sensation and often excessive sensitivity of the skin of the feet. This syndrome can be the result of a primary dietary deficiency of vitamin B$_1$; in such a case there may also be tachycardia, enlargement of the heart and peripheral oedema, giving the fully-developed syndrome of beri-beri. In less severe cases the polyneuropathy develops alone. The condition sometimes begins during pregnancy, following hyperemesis gravidarum, or may result from the anorexia which occasionally accompanies depression or chronic anxiety or is the predominant symptom of anorexia nervosa. The neuropathies of **pellagra** and of pyridoxine deficiency are similar; sensory neuropathy of **vitamin B$_{12}$ deficiency** (*see* Chapter 19) is usually relatively minor in relation to the evidence of spinal cord dysfunction. The polyneuropathy which frequently complicates **chronic alcoholism** is due to thiamine deficiency and not to the alcohol itself; it only develops as a rule when the consumption of alcohol has increased to such an extent that is interferes with the intake of food. Pain and cutaneous hyperaesthesia are particularly severe in alcoholic neuropathy. Wernicke's encephalopathy (*see* p. 392) and the Korsakoff syndrome (*see* p. 120) may also be present. The polyneuropathies resulting from **heavy-metal poisoning** are similar. Thiamine, as coenzyme A, is important in pyruvate metabolism; heavy metals, by competing with thiamine for certain essential SH groups, interfere with this activity and hence produce polyneuropathy through conditioned thiamine deficiency. Lead poisoning in adults (*see* p. 406) commonly gives a neuropathy which begins with localised weakness of one muscle group (e.g. wrist drop) but polyneuropathy due to other heavy metals such as arsenic is more often generalised. A variety of polyneuropathy due to mercury poisoning (from the use of teething powders) which has virtually disappeared since these powders were abandoned, is pink disease (acrodynia). This condition produced in infants profound irritability, hypotonia of the limbs, weight loss and a reddened, scaly condition of the hands and feet.

Triorthocresylphosphate, a cholinesterase poison, which was an occasional contaminant of illicit alcoholic liquors in America in the 1930s, produced many cases of severe axonal polyneuropathy, in which paralysis and sensory impairment were often permanent (Jamaica ginger paralysis). It caused a more recent 'epidemic' of polyneuropathy in Morocco, due to the use of lubricating oil for cooking purposes. A similar syndrome may follow the use of **apiol**, taken to procure abortion. In recent years, many drugs have been found to cause polyneuropathy; **isoniazid** is one example. Usually in such cases the neuropathy recovers in a few weeks or months after the offending drug has been withdrawn. Isoniazid produces its effect through conditioned pyridoxine deficiency and sensitivity to the drug in this respect is genetically-determined, as some people excrete it quickly, others slowly. The exact mechanism by which other drugs and certain **industrial organic poisons** such as acrylamide produce polyneuropathy is unknown. The neuropathy following **sulphonamide therapy** is probably due to hypersensitivity and is in many cases related to that which may complicate polyarteritis nodosa or systemic lupus (*see below*). **Thalidomide**, now withdrawn from the market, gave a peculiarly painful distal sensory neuropathy, while **vincristine** (used for the treatment of malignant disease) and **chloroquine** give a mixed sensorimotor neuropathy with axonal degeneration, as does **nitrofurantoin,** particularly if given to patients with a high blood urea. **Clioquinol,** often used to treat traveller's diarrhoea, has also been shown after prolonged usage to produce a severe polyneuropathy with optic nerve damage, especially in Japan, and a similar syndrome believed to be due to dietary cyanide in cassava root is the cause of the **tropical ataxic neuropathy** seen in Nigeria and other parts of Africa. Sensorimotor axonal neuropathy can also be caused by **disulfiram** ('antabuse', used in the management of alcoholism), ***n*-hexane** which is used in the leather industry and in certain plastic glues ('glue-sniffers' neuropathy) and even rarely after the prolonged ingestion of phenytoin given as an anticonvulsant.

Peripheral neuropathy is a common and important complication of **diabetes mellitus**. Two principal clinical varieties exist. One, which is particularly common in the elderly, produces pain and cramp in the calves, symptoms which are particularly troublesome at night. The ankle and/or knee jerks are absent and there is some impairment of the appreciation of vibration at the ankles. The second form, which usually occurs in younger patients, is a more severe and generalised form of mixed axonal and demyelinating polyneuropathy, affecting power and sensation in all four limbs. It has been suggested that the first type is due to atherosclerosis of the vasa nervorum, the second to some as yet unidentified metabolic disorder associated with diabetes. Whether this is so remains to be proved; however, most cases of both clinical types improve when the diabetic condition is controlled. In the syndrome of **diabetic amyotrophy** wasting and weakness develop most often in one or both quadriceps muscles and rarely in other muscle groups; there may also be pain in the affected muscles. It is usually due to a localised ischaemic femoral neuropathy and also tends to improve when the diabetes is controlled. A rare diabetic autonomic neuropathy with diarrhoea, impotence and dysuria has also been described. Another rare variety of polyneuropathy, which is, however, predominantly motor in type and may therefore mimic motor neurone disease, is an occasional complication of **hyperinsulinism** due to an adenoma of the islets of Langerhans.

Amyloid neuropathy occurs in three distinctive inherited varieties, usually in genetic isolates in various parts of the world. The Portuguese variety produces progressive weakness and sensory loss in the limbs, and is often associated with autonomic dysfunction and trophic ulceration of the feet. The Rukavina and van Allan varieties are very rare; the former usually presents with a bilateral carpal tunnel syndrome due to thickening of the median nerves, the latter with sensorimotor neuropathy, nephropathy and peptic ulcer. Occasionally a neuropathy with deposits resembling amyloid in the peripheral nerves may complicate **multiple myelomatosis**. An association between peripheral neuropathy and episodes of abdominal pain and mental confusion, during which port-wine coloured urine is passed, favours a diagnosis of **acute porphyria**, which will be considered further in Chapter 19 (p. 410). Now that patients with chronic renal disease survive longer than they once did, a specific sensorimotor axonal neuropathy due to **uraemia** is increasingly common; the condition is improved by effective dialysis but may relapse as the blood urea rises.

The varieties of peripheral neuropathy which complicate cases of 'collagen' disease depend in part upon pathological changes in the vasa nervorum; they are predominantly demyelinating in type. Asymmetrical involvement of multiple peripheral nerves (mononeuritis multiplex) is a common feature of **polyarteritis nodosa**, while a symmetrical polyneuropathy develops in some cases of **rheumatoid arthritis** and **systemic lupus erythematosus** (*see* p. 304). Steroid therapy may then not only control the primary illness but also the neuropathic syndrome. Polyneuropathy is also an occasional complication of leukaemia, reticulosis and of the dysglobulinaemias.

As previously mentioned (*see* p. 248) a progressive peripheral neuropathy can be inherited. This is the case in the neuropathic form of peroneal muscular atrophy and the closely related **Dejerine–Sottas disease**. Polyneuropathy associated with nerve deafness and cerebellar ataxia occurs in **Refsum's syndrome** in which an abnormal lipid (phytanic acid) accumulates in the peripheral nerves. Similar abnormal collections of lipid may impair peripheral nerve function in metachromatic leucodystrophy and in Krabbe's disease (*see* p. 243). Polyneuropathy is also one feature of a-α-lipoproteinaemia (Tangier disease) and of a-β-lipoproteinaemia (the Bassen–Kornzweig syndrome). In **hereditary sensory neuropathy** a progressive degeneration of posterior root ganglia gives progressive peripheral sensory loss, often accompanied by perforating ulcers of the feet and necrosis of phalanges (often called acrodystrophic neuropathy or Morvan's syndrome).

Finally there are certain varieties of peripheral neuropathy of unknown aetiology. A progressive polyneuropathy of demyelinating type is a common complication of **bronchogenic carcinoma** and less commonly of malignant disease in other sites. Sometimes the symptoms and signs of the peripheral nerve disorder precede those of the primary neoplasm by months or even years. Although some of the earliest cases described were examples of pure sensory neuropathy, in most cases the affection is predominantly motor, though variable peripheral sensory loss is often found. Numerous clinical variations occur, but a common story is one of vague pain in the legs on exertion, followed by gradual diminution and eventually loss of the lower limb reflexes and then by foot drop and sensory changes. Myopathic changes are sometimes present in addition, thus giving a neuromyopathy. A negative chest X-ray is never sufficient to exclude the diagnosis of bronchogenic carcinoma, and the primary neoplasm may appear in subsequent radiographs. In rare cases, the neuropathy remits after successful removal of the primary growth, but the nature of the relationship between the malignant disease and the neuropathy remains unexplained. The final category included in our provisional classification is **chronic progressive polyneuropathy**. Many cases exist in which a progressive polyneuropathy develops without obvious cause. The number of cases so classified is steadily diminishing and there is evidence to suggest that some of these, and particularly certain cases of recurrent demyelinating polyneuropathy (in which 'onion-skin' concentric Schwann cell proliferation ultimately causes enlargement of nerve trunks), are due to a hypersensitivity reaction involving peripheral nerves and that steroid therapy may sometimes be beneficial. Certainly when there is slowing of nerve conduction indicating demyelination, when the CSF protein content is raised and when no cause for the neuropathy is evident, steroids deserve a trial. Probably, however, many causes of polyneuropathy are yet to be identified. Now that new drugs are continually being introduced into medicine and new toxins (e.g. insecticides) are to be found in man's environment the possibility of a toxic or metabolic cause should always be considered in cases for which no valid explanation can be found.

Myasthenia Gravis

The phenomenon of myasthenia consists of an abnormal degree of fatigability of skeletal muscle. If repeated contractions of an affected muscle are induced, either voluntarily or electrically, the power of these contractions becomes progressively less powerful. Hence patients with myasthenia usually find that they become weaker as the day wears on, or after exceptional effort, and improve with rest. For some time it has been known in this disease that there is a defect of neuromuscular transmission which can be partially reversed by cholinesterase inhibitors such as edrophonium or neostigmine and its analogues. However, the discovery that the condition is auto-immune and that it is due to the presence of circulating antibodies against the acetylcholine receptor (AChR) of the muscle fibre, antibodies which coat the receptors and thus interfere with neuromuscular transmission, is comparatively recent. The exact part played by thymic lymphocytes (T cells) and by humoral factors in the elaboration of these antibodies and the nature of the primary process which stimulates their elaboration remains to be determined. Methods for measuring circulating AChR antibodies are now available and are invaluable in diagnosis.

A myasthenic syndrome has been described in association with bronchogenic and, less often, other types of carcinoma but differs from true myasthenia (*see below* and p. 339). Myasthenic fatigability is occasionally observed in polymyositis or muscular dystrophy, but it is much more common for myasthenia to occur alone without other evidence of disease in the skeletal muscles or elsewhere; this syndrome is referred to as myasthenia gravis, though the benign course of many cases belies the name. It occurs in association with thyrotoxicosis much more often than could be accounted for by chance. It is seen in either sex but is much more common in females. Only rarely does it affect more than one member of a family. It can begin at any age, in childhood, in adolescence, early adult life, or even in old age. An infant born of a myasthenic mother may suffer from neonatal myasthenia for the first few days of life, but then recovers; this suggests that AChR antibodies are conveyed across the placenta from mother to child.

This disease usually affects first the external ocular, pharyngeal or jaw muscles. In about 10 per cent of cases the condition remains limited to the extraocular muscles indefinitely and in such individuals the condition is benign. A common first symptom is ptosis, either unilateral or bilateral, and/or diplopia, which become worse towards the end of the day. Difficulty in swallowing or in chewing often follow, and sometimes the jaw becomes so fatigued after a meal that it hangs open. In other severe cases, there is similar fatigability of the neck, limb and trunk muscles, and respiratory paralysis is an important and sometimes fatal complication. After months or years permanent muscular weakness and wasting, uninfluenced by treatment, develop in some cases and the affected muscles show degenerative changes on histological examination. The triceps muscle is often selectively involved in this way. The tendon reflexes usually remain brisk in true myasthenia, while in the myasthenic syndrome accompanying carcinoma they are usually lost; in the latter condition, too, the initial fatigability of an affected muscle during exercise is usually followed by a marked increase in strength.

The prognosis is very variable; in the ocular cases the disease is benign, but acute generalised cases sometimes occur which despite treatment are fatal within a few months. In cases of moderate severity, maintenance therapy with neostigmine and its analogues may achieve adequate control of the muscular weakness and allow a reasonably active existence. But anti-cholinesterase drugs are not invariably successful, especially since a dose sufficient to control weakness in one muscle group may produce cholinergic weakness in another. Additional measures often used, apart from thymectomy (*see below*) include steroid and immunosuppressive drugs and plasmapheresis (*see* Chapter 20). Spontaneous remission, which can be heralded by reduced prostigmine requirements, is not uncommon and may last for months or years. In relatively acute myasthenia occurring in young women, and in other selected cases which show a poor response to drug therapy, surgical removal of the thymus may be dramatically beneficial. The gland is enlarged in many patients and some are found to have a thymoma, which some believe should be treated with radiotherapy prior to surgery. A history of variable ptosis, diplopia, dysphagia, jaw or neck muscle weakness or weakness of the limbs should always raise the possibility of myasthenia and a diagnostic intravenous injection of 10 mg of edrophonium, a drug with a rapid but transient effect, should be tried to see if the weakness is influenced thereby. It is wise to inject 2 mg initially and to await side-effects, before proceeding to give the entire 10 mg. Management is considered in greater detail on p. 448.

Myotonia

The phenomenon of myotonia is one of apparent delay in relaxation of skeletal muscle, accompanied by a persistent electrical 'after-discharge', even when voluntary innervation of the muscle has ceased. The exact nature of the abnormality in such cases is still uncertain, although an abnormality of chloride conductance in the muscle fibre membrane has been demonstrated. A characteristic feature is that the patient, on taking a firm grasp of an object, is unable to let go, and typically a gradual uncurling of the clenched fingers, beginning in the index and middle fingers, is observed; the total period required for relaxation may be several seconds. The phenomenon can also be demonstrated by a firm tap upon the surface of a muscle, seen best in the tongue or thenar eminence, when a clear-cut 'dimple' or furrow appears and may persist for several seconds. The electromyogram (*see* p. 59) is diagnostic. Myotonia is accentuated by cold, and is usually reduced either by warmth or by repeated contraction of the affected muscles, which results in a 'wearing-off' of the phenomenon. It can be partially or completely relieved by drugs such as quinine, procaine amide, phenytoin and by steroids.

There are two major clinical syndromes in which myotonia is observed. Both are usually inherited as autosomal dominant traits. However, one of these conditions, **myotonia congenita**, is transmitted in some families by an autosomal recessive mechanism. In the dominant form, Thomsen's disease, myotonia is generalised throughout the skeletal musculature, and is present from birth. Affected infants often have difficulty in feeding and a peculiarly 'strangled' cry. The principal symptom is stiffness of the muscles, with difficulty in beginning muscular activity and in relaxing afterwards; these features are accentuated by cold and can be 'worked-off' by exercise. Generalised hypertrophy of the skeletal muscles usually develops during adolescence, but weakness and atrophy of muscles is not usually observed, and most patients survive and remain active to a normal age. The milder, recessively-inherited form of myotonia congenita usually first produces symptoms in early childhood but is otherwise similar. In **dystrophia myotonica** (myotonia atrophica), by contrast, myotonia is usually apparent only in the hands and tongue, and may even be absent clinically, though it is almost invariably present electromyographically. The first symptoms usually develop in adolescence or adult life, although in occasional cases the condition causes hypotonia and developmental delay in infancy and is then only recognised as a rule when the fully-developed disease is identified in the affected parent who is almost invariably the mother. In the affected adult, in addition to myotonia affecting the grip, there is progressive difficulty in walking. There are frontal baldness (in the male), impotence and testicular atrophy, cataracts, atrophy of the sterno-mastoids and of the facial and temporal muscles, and weakness and wasting of the peripheral muscles of the limbs, involving especially long flexors and extensors but sparing, at least initially, the intrinsic muscles of the hands and feet; these changes are due to an associated muscular dystrophy which is an essential part of the disease process. Bilateral ptosis, and a typically long, lugubrious facies are usually seen. Many patients are of low intellect; the skull vault is thick, the sella small, the EEG may be abnormal, growth hormone output is diminished and there is excessive catabolism of immunoglobulin G. The condition is progressive and eventually results in severe disability leading to a wheel chair existence, with death from cardiac failure (due to myocardial degeneration) or from respiratory infection, in middle-life. Whereas the myotonia can be relieved by drugs, the dystrophic process in the peripheral limb muscles, which is the principal cause of progressive disability, is uninfluenced by treatment.

Paramyotonia is an uncommon variant of myotonia congenita. In this condition the myotonia occurs only on exposure to cold and is then associated with attacks of generalised muscular weakness resembling closely those observed in cases of familial periodic paralysis but usually accompanied by a rise, rather than a fall, in the serum potassium (*see below*). **Myotonia paradoxa** is a term given to cases in which the myotonia is accentuated and not improved by exertion. Some such cases constitute merely an unusual form of myotonia congenita, but many in which muscular pain and stiffness increase after exertion are suffering from a rare myopathy, due to a defect in muscle glycogen breakdown in muscles which are congenitally deficient in the enzyme phosphorylase (McArdle's disease); certain others are suffering from myxoedema, a disorder which can occasionally present with muscular symptoms (pseudomyotonia).

Progressive Muscular Dystrophy

This condition, which causes progressive weakness and wasting of certain skeletal muscles, is the commonest form of genetically-determined primary degenerative myopathy. The pathological changes in the diseased muscles indicate a primary disorder of the muscle fibres and there is no conclusive evidence of disease in the central or peripheral nervous system. One rare variety of muscular dystrophy, **ocular myopathy**, gives progressive bilateral ptosis and eventually complete ophthalmoplegia and weakness of the orbicularis oculi, while another, **distal myopathy**, which is also very rare, except in Sweden, begins in the small muscles of the hands and feet and later spreads proximally in the limb muscles.

The commonest forms of muscular dystrophy fall into three principal groups which are clinically and genetically distinct. All are progressive, and uninfluenced by any form of drug treatment. The first, the **Duchenne type,** exclusively affects young boys, being inherited via a sex-linked (X-linked) recessive mechanism; often several boys in a sibship develop the condition; occasional girls affected by a similar disorder have been described and in these families the disease, which tends to be more benign, is inherited as an autosomal recessive character; recent work suggests that many but not all are suffering from spinal muscular atrophy resembling muscular dystrophy. The onset of Duchenne dystrophy is usually within the first three to five years of life; the child, who walked at the normal age, becomes clumsy in walking and running, has difficulty in climbing stairs, falls frequently and rises by 'climbing up his legs'. He walks with his abdomen protruding (accentuated lumbar lordosis) and with a typical waddle. There is progressive weakness of the proximal upper and lower limb muscles; often firm rubbery enlargement (pseudohypertrophy, partly due to fatty infiltration and partly to actual increase in muscle bulk) of the calves, and sometimes of other muscles, is seen. The progress of the disease is inexorable. Often the child is unable to walk by the time he is eight to 12 years old and later progressive contractures of the weakened muscles develop with secondary skeletal deformity, to give a tragic terminal state, from which the child is carried off by respiratory infection or by cardiac failure due to associated cardiomyopathy, often before the age of 20. A less common variety, the **Becker type**, which resembles the Duchenne type clinically and which is also inherited as an X-linked trait, is seen in occasional families; its onset is later (at 5 to 15 years) and its course more benign so that many affected individuals survive into middle life.

The **limb-girdle variety** (Erb–Leyden–Möbuis) occurs equally in the two sexes and may begin at any age though it usually does so in adolescence or early adult life; it is usually inherited via an autosomal recessive gene. The disease may begin rarely in the pelvic girdle, giving difficulty in climbing stairs and a typical waddling gait, or more often in the shoulder girdle, resulting in inability to lift the arms above the shoulders. Sometimes the muscular involvement remains confined to the shoulders or pelvic girdle for many years, but later spreads to the other group. In the shoulder girdles the trapezii, serrati, pectorals, biceps and brachioradiales are commonly involved and the deltoids are spared, to give a characteristic clinical picture. Pseudohypertrophy of muscles is occasionally seen. The prognosis in these cases is much less grave than in the Duchenne variety, but nevertheless the disease is progressive, though sometimes intermittently so; most patients are severely disabled, as a rule in middle-life, and few survive to a normal age. Up to half of all cases so diagnosed in the past are known to be suffering from benign spinal muscular atrophy (*see* p. 360) and some rare metabolic myopathies give a similar clinical picture so that diagnosis depends upon ancillary investigations.

The **facioscapulohumeral form** (Landouzy–Dejerine) is the most benign. It, too, may begin at any age (usually in adolescence or early adult life) and in either sex, but is generally inherited as an autosomal dominant trait. The facial muscles are first affected resulting in inability to close the eyes completely, a typical 'pout' of the lips and a 'transverse' smile. The shoulder girdle muscles are also involved, selectively as in some limb-girdle cases, and the disease may not spread to the pelvic girdle for many years, though the tibiales anterior are usually the first lower limb muscles to be involved. In some cases only a few muscles around the shoulders are involved and the disorder then arrests (abortive cases). Whereas the muscular weakness may progress unusually quickly in a few affected individuals, the advance of the disease is very slow in most, and some remain active, though with increasing disability, to a normal age. Recent evidence has shown that, as in the limb-girdle variety, this condition can be mimicked by spinal muscular atrophy. Scapuloperoneal muscular atrophy (p. 364) gives a very similar clinical picture except that the facial muscles are not involved; it is usually due to spinal muscular atrophy, less often to a dystrophic process.

The diagnosis of muscular dystrophy, in an established case, is rarely difficult, but in the early stages, particularly in a young child, the history of clumsiness in walking or of inability to run as quickly as other children of comparable age is often attributed to flat feet or to laziness, unless this diagnosis is borne in mind. Although the urinary output of creatine is increased, as is the serum aldolase, these tests are not specific. However, estimation of the serum creatine kinase activity, which may be raised three-hundredfold in affected young boys, is especially useful in the diagnosis of the Duchenne type but gives less abnormal results in the other varieties. This test can be used to identify the disease in its preclinical stage in the young male sibs of affected boys and is also useful in the diagnosis of the carrier state in their mothers and sisters. Carrier identification is particularly important for genetic counselling. Thus the sister of a dystrophic boy has approximately a 50:50 chance of being a carrier. If she is, then she is likely to have affected sons, but if not, her children will be normal. Thus if carriers are identified and do not have male children the number of dystrophic boys being born has been shown to diminish though some new cases will continue to result from genetic mutation. In known carriers who wish to have children, selective abortion of male fetuses (after identification of fetal sex by amniocentesis) is now widely practised and much research, using fetal blood sampling by fetoscopy and other methods is now being directed towards antenatal diagnosis of Duchenne dystrophy in the hope of moving towards a programme of selective abortion only of affected males. Carrier detection is less satisfactory in families with the Becker type dystrophy and is impossible at present in relatives of limb-girdle cases. In facioscapulohumeral dystrophy the condition is passed on only by affected individuals to half their children of either sex.

As so many other conditions may resemble muscular dystrophy, electromyography and muscle biopsy are also necessary for diagnosis. These procedures are of particular value in distinguishing muscular dystrophy from polymyositis (*see below*) and from spinal muscular atrophy and various metabolic myopathies with which the condition is most often confused. In the absence of any effective treatment, all that can be done is to keep the patients active with regular moderate exercise and avoidance of undue weight gain. Inactivity and bed rest are deleterious; every effort should be made to delay the development of contractures by passively stretching tendons which are shortening, but surgical lengthening of such tendons is not usually indicated unless the patient can be mobilised immediately afterwards. Attention should also be paid to the posture of the patients, particularly when confined to a wheelchair, and light spinal supports are sometimes required to prevent scoliosis.

Polymyositis

This name has been given to a clinical syndrome produced by combined degenerative and inflammatory changes in skeletal muscle. It does not

include suppurative and infective varieties of myositis which are comparatively rare, save for viral myositis (e.g. epidemic myalgia), which will be
discussed below. In fact, suppurative myositis is not uncommon in some
tropical countries (tropical myositis), and viruses other than Coxsackie B
(which causes epidemic myalgia' sometimes give a self-limiting myositis;
influenza is one example. The syndrome of polymyositis also excludes,
conventionally, parasitic disorders duch as trichinosis (due to eating pork
contaminated with the *Trichinella spiralis*), toxoplasmosis and trypanosomiasis cruzi (South American Chagas disease) which may also affect
skeletal muscle. In some instances the skin and mucous membranes are
also involved, in which case the condition is known as dermatomyositis,
but often the main brunt of the disease process falls upon the skeletal
muscles. Although the syndrome may embrace several diseases of varying
aetiology, in most instances the pathological process is clearly one of
so-called connective tissue disease. It is due to lymphocyte-mediated
delayed hypersensitivity; sensitised lymphocytes attack muscle, and sometimes skin and other tissues.

The syndrome has been observed in patients of all ages and in both
sexes. Acute forms of polymyositis and dermatomyositis most often occur
in adults and are characterised by generalised muscular pains and weakness
of comparatively rapid progression, associated often with a widespread
erythematous rash on the face, limbs and trunk. The proximal limb
muscles are more severely affected than the distal. The affected muscles
are tender and the patients are ill and febrile; the respiratory muscles may
be involved and the illness may end fatally within a few weeks or months.
Subacute polymyositis is much more common. In such cases muscular pain
and tenderness and symptoms of constitutional upset are often absent, and
the presenting features are those of progressive weakness and moderate
atrophy of the muscles of the shoulder and pelvic girdles. This clinical
picture can resemble closely that of muscular dystrophy, save for the fact
that in polymyositis all the proximal limb muscles are usually weakened,
and the deltoid, for instance, is not spared; furthermore the neck muscles
are often weak, dysphagia and a Raynaud phenomenon in the hands are
common, and the muscular weakness is often greater than the degree of
atrophy would suggest. This form of subacute polymyositis is particularly
common in middle- and late-life. When it occurs in childhood or adolescence there are often minor skin changes on the skin of the face and of the
hands and fingers, resembling those of early systemic sclerosis or acroscler-
osis. In some cases, the skin lesions resemble those of lupus erythematosus, while in others, there may be associated evidence of another 'collagen'
disease such as rheumatoid arthritis. Subcutaneous and intramuscular
calcification (calcinosis universalis) is not uncommon in childhood polymyositis. Another important point is that many cases of polymyositis and
particularly of dermatomyositis in middle- and late-life develop in association with malignant disease in the lung or in some other organ.

The prognosis of polymyositis and dermatomyositis is variable. Some of the acute cases are eventually fatal, despite modern methods of treatment. A few subacute cases in childhood have been known to remit spontaneously and even to recover completely; others enter a chronic stage with the development of fibrous contractures in the muscles and severe deformity (chronic myositis fibrosa). Most subacute cases occurring in adult life are progressive; very few if untreated arrest. Many cases remit completely or partially when treated with prednisone and immunosuppressive drugs (e.g. azathioprine, cyclophosphamide or methotrexate), but maintenance therapy may have to be continued for many years.

In diagnosis, a raised ESR may be helpful but this test is normal in more than a third of all cases. The serum aldolase, transaminases, creatine kinase and immunoglobulins are also often raised, but in most cases final diagnosis depends upon a combination of the clinical findings on the one hand with the results of electromyography and muscle biopsy on the other.

Polymyalgia Rheumatica

This is a disorder of middle-aged and elderly patients, of whom a few prove to be suffering from temporal or cranial arteritis. Typically it presents with diffuse muscle pain and aching which may restrict movement (getting out of the bath is often particularly difficult) but there is no muscular weakness or wasting. The ESR is invariably raised and the response to prednisone is dramatic. Maintenance treatment is often required for several months.

Epidemic Myalgia (Bornholm Disease)

This is a form of virus myositis, resulting from infection with Coxsackie B virus. It gives an acute febrile illness with severe pain in the upper abdomen and lower chest wall. Pain on breathing and coughing (pleurodynia) is a striking feature and the illness may simulate pleurisy or even an acute abdominal emergency. The condition is self-limiting, occurs in localised epidemics, and usually clears up without residual symptoms in three to five days.

Paroxysmal Myoglobinuria

Myoglobin may appear in the urine in any condition which produces sudden destruction of muscle, and if the quantity released into the blood stream is large, death may result from renal failure due to blockage of renal tubules. Causes of myoglobinuria include massive crush injuries of muscle (crush syndrome), necrosis of the anterior tibial muscles in their tight fascial compartment after prolonged exertion (the anterior tibial syndrome), acute polymyositis, and paroxysmal myoglobinuria or rhabdomyolysis. In the latter, a condition of unknown aetiology, patients experience intermittent febrile episodes, each lasting a few days, during which they develop generalised muscular pain and weakness and pass dark brown urine containing myoglobin. The condition is uninfluenced by treatment, but even after repeated attacks, recovery is often complete, though death in an attack is a rare event. The disorder usually appears first in childhood and after repeated attacks some permanent muscular weakness and wasting may be found. Recently it has been shown that muscle pain and myoglobinuria developing after exercise can be due to an inherited deficiency of carnitine palmityl transferase.

Familial Periodic Paralysis

This uncommon condition of dominant inheritance affects patients of either sex, usually from birth. Sufferers experience attacks of generalised muscular weakness which vary in severity but may occasionally be so severe as to paralyse them almost completely. A common story is that the patient wakens from sleep to find that he is unable to move. Although weakness of the skeletal musculature can be widespread and profound, swallowing is only occasionally disturbed, and respiratory muscle weakness is never sufficient to endanger life. The attacks vary in duration from one or two hours to as long as 48 hours. Commonly after a short period of total paralysis the patient is able to move but does so weakly and clumsily and may not be normal for several days. There are some cases in which the weakness is consistently localised to only a few muscle groups. The episodes are particularly likely to develop while the patient is resting after unusually heavy exertion, or after a heavy carbohydrate meal. Often they can be induced by the administration of insulin and glucose. Usually the serum potassium is low during the attacks and the weakness recovers slowly after the administration of 2–4 g of potassium chloride by mouth. Maintenance therapy with 4–5 g of potassium chloride daily and aldosterone antagonists have been used prophylactically but acetazolamide 250 mg three times daily has proved more effective in most patients. Similar episodes can occur in patients whose serum potassium is lowered as a result of other causes, as in cases of potassium-losing nephritis, renal tubular acidosis, or aldosteronism.

In some cases and families, attacks which are characteristic of the syndrome described above occur in association with a high, and not a low, serum potassium. This syndrome has been called **adynamia episodica hereditaria** or **hyperkalaemic periodic paralysis**. The attacks are often less severe and of shorter duration than in the hypokalaemic type and may follow immediately after exertion, while some patients also have myotonia.

The paralysis in these cases is accentuated by potassium but can be terminated by the use of diuretics such as chlorothiazide or acetazolamide which promote potassium excretion; these drugs are often effective if given prophylactically, and paradoxically they may also prevent attacks of the hypokalaemic type. Yet a third variety of periodic paralysis in which the serum potassium remains normal in the attacks and in which weakness is controlled by the administration of sodium and prevented by 9-α-fluorohydrocortisone 0.1 mg daily, has been described (**normokalaemic periodic paralysis**) but is probably a variant of the hyperkalaemic type. Clearly therefore it is essential in any individual experiencing attacks of this nature to estimate the serum potassium during an attack and to carry out other appropriate tests in order to identify the type of periodic paralysis from which he is suffering so that appropriate treatment may be given.

Endocrine Myopathies

This group of disorders will be described in Chapter 19 (pp. 408–410).

Other Metabolic Myopathies

In the last 30 years the increasing use of new diagnostic techniques, such as biochemical, electrophysiological and histological methods (including histochemistry and electron microscopy) has led to the definition of many previously unrecognised disorders of muscle, most of which were previously thought to be forms of muscular dystrophy. Some of these are the specific varieties of congenital dystrophy giving rise to hypotonia and weakness in infancy and childhood, to be described below. Others have been shown to be due to genetically determined metabolic disorders. While all are rare, the commonest are disorders of glycogen storage, lipid storage diseases and conditions associated with abnormal mitochondria.

The commoner glycogen storage diseases are first **McArdle's disease** due to myophosphorylase deficiency and the clinically similar condition of phosphofructokinase deficiency. These give muscle pain coming on after exertion, sometimes accompanied by myoglobinuria and physiological contracture and only slowly relieved by rest. No rise in blood lactate in the ante-cubital vein occurs after repeated contraction of forearm muscles with arterial occlusion by a tourniquet, and histochemical staining of a muscle biopsy is diagnostic. **Pompe's disease** due to acid maltase deficiency gives massive vacuolation of skeletal muscle sections due to glycogen deposition. It can give a severe diffuse cardiomyopathy which is rapidly fatal in infancy, or a subacute myopathy in adolescence or adult life. All of these conditions are due to an autosomal recessive gene.

Another vacuolar myopathy, usually presenting with a clinical picture of subacute muscular weakness like that of limb-girdle muscular dystrophy, but resulting from the deposition of neutral fat, especially in type I muscle fibres (as seen in frozen sections stained with Sudan Black), is due to autosomal recessive **carnitine deficiency;** clinical improvement in some cases follows the oral administration of carnitine.

Finally, a variety of disorders presenting either with hypermetabolism in the absence of hyperthyroidism, with ocular or oculopharyngeal muscular weakness or with a syndrome resembling limb-girdle or facioscapulo-humeral muscular dystrophy, has been shown to be associated with biochemical and morphological abnormalities of the muscle mitochondria **(mitochondrial myopathy)**. In some families there is also retinal pigmentation and cerebellar ataxia with abnormal mitochondria in the cerebellum as well as in the muscles (the Kearns–Sayre syndrome). In others, specific enzyme defects of the cytochrome enzymes of the electron transport chain are beginning to be recognised and in some such cases lactic acidosis is a troublesome complication.

The Amyotonia Congenita Syndrome ('The Floppy Infant')

To determine the nature of the pathological changes responsible for widespread weakness and hypotonia of the skeletal muscles in infancy is often a difficult matter. In most cases which present with these manifestations in severe form the disease process is one of infantile progressive spinal atrophy (Werdnig–Hoffman disease), whether the illness begins at birth or during the first year of life. Infantile polyneuropathy can also cause widespread weakness and hypotonia but nerve conduction velocity is usually reduced in such cases and the CSF protein is raised. Dystrophia myotonica (*see* p. 380) and infantile myasthenia are other uncommon causes of hypotonia. In many cases, however, the child's hypotonia is a symptom of various infective, metabolic and neurological disorders which do not primarily affect the lower motor neurone or muscles. Thus weakness and hypotonia of some degree is common in infants recovering from acute infection, in cases of intestinal malabsorption, hypocalcaemia, mental handicap, and even initially in some of flaccid cerebral diplegia. Congenital heart disease may also be associated with generalised hypotonia, as may Pompe's disease (*see above*). There exists, however, a third group of cases in which the weakness and hypotonia are benign, though of unknown aetiology, and in which improvement and sometimes complete recovery may be expected. This syndrome was first described by Oppenheim under the title of myatonia congenita or amyotonia congenita, but this diagnosis was subsequently utilised to include all infants who showed severe generalised hypotonia soon after birth. As many of these proved to be suffering from progressive spinal atrophy, this title has been discarded, and the term **benign congenital hypotonia** is now preferred by many for cases which carry a relatively good prognosis. This condition is not a single disease entity but a syndrome of multiple aetiology, although many cases show no specific identifying features and the cause of the muscular weakness and hypotonia remains unknown. These children, though weak and 'limp' or 'floppy' from birth, are never as severely paralysed as those with Werdnig–Hoffman disease and show gradual improvement. They sit up late and often do not stand or walk until late in the second or in the third year of life. Some recover completely but others, who are more severely affected in early life, improve up to a point, but no further, and have small, weak muscles throughout life. The latter condition has also been entitled 'congenital universal muscular hypoplasia' or 'benign congenital myopathy'. With the increasing use of electron microscopy to examine muscle biopsy sections, a specific morphological diagnosis is becoming possible in many more cases and relatively few now remain in this group, although there does appear to be a poorly defined non-progressive form of congenital muscular dystrophy which behaves in this way. In some cases of infantile hypotonia subsequently found to have generalised weakness and hypoplasia of muscles a curious defect of the centre of many muscle fibres can be demonstrated ('central-core' disease) while in yet others rod-shaped bodies derived from Z-bands are aggregated beneath the sarcolemma of many fibres ('nemaline myopathy'). A similar clinical picture occasionally results from mitochondrial myopathy (*see above*), or from congenital fibre type disproportion, in which there is a marked discrepancy in size between type I and type II fibres. Hypoplasia of the muscles is also seen in some individuals with long spidery fingers and a high arched palate (arachnodactyly). Another rare disorder identified in some weak and hypotonic infants by histology is 'myotubular or centronuclear myopathy', a condition in which external ocular as well as facial, limb and trunk muscles are involved and in which the muscle fibres show central chains of nuclei and superficially resemble fetal myotubes.

One final condition requires to be mentioned, namely **arthrogryposis multiplex congenita**. This is a condition of multiple contractures of skeletal muscle, combined with deformity of the limbs, which is present from birth. In some cases it appears to be due to a spinal muscular atrophy beginning in fetal life, in some to a severe myopathic process developing before birth (so-called congenital muscular dystrophy), but in most, in which there is no evidence of disease in the motor nerves or muscles themselves, to excessive intra-uterine pressure, with abnormal posturing of the limbs.

References

Bradley, W. G., *Disorders of Peripheral Nerves* (Oxford, London, Edinburgh, Melbourne, Blackwell, 1974).

Brandt, S., *Werdnig–Hoffman's Infantile Progressive Muscular Atrophy* (Copenhagen, Munksgaard, 1950).

Dubowitz, V., *Muscle Disorders in Childhood,* Vol. XVI in Major Problems in Clinical Paediatrics, Ed. Schaffer, A. J. and Markowitz, M. (London, Philadelphia, Toronto, W. B. Saunders, 1978).

Dubowitz, V. and Brooke, M., *Muscle Biopsy: A Modern Approach,* Major Problems in Neurology, Ed. Walton, J. N., No. 2 (London, Saunders, 1973).

Dyck, P. J., Thomas, P. K. and Lambert, E. H., *Peripheral Neuropathy* (London, Philadelphia, Toronto, W. B. Saunders, 1975).

Harper, P. S., *Myotonic Dystrophy*, Vol. 9 in Major Problems in Neurology, Ed. Walton, J. N. (London, Philadelphia, Toronto, Saunders, 1979).

Kakulas, B. A. (Ed.), *Clinical Studies in Myology* (Amsterdam, Excerpta Medica, 1973).

Norris, F. H. and Kurland, L. T. (Eds.), *Motor Neuron Diseases: Research on Amyotrophic Lateral Sclerosis and Related Disorders* (New York, Grune and Stratton, 1969).

Ossermann, K. E., *Myasthenia Gravis* (New York, Grune and Stratton, 1958).

Thomasen, E., *Myotonia* (Copenhagen, Munksgaard, 1948).

Tsubaki, T. and Toyokura, Y. (Eds.), *Amyotrophic Lateral Sclerosis* (Baltimore, University Park Press, 1979).

Walton, J. N., *Brain's Diseases of the Nervous System,* 8th Ed., Chapters 18 and 19 (London, Oxford University Press, 1977).

Walton, J. N., (Ed.), *Disorders of Voluntary Muscle*, 4th ed. (London, Churchill, 1981).

Walton, J. N. and Adams, R. D., *Polymyositis* (Edinburgh, Livingstone, 1958).

19 Metabolic Disorders and the Nervous System

Increasing interest has been taken of late in the group of diseases or symptom-complexes in which symptoms depend not so much upon recognisable structural changes occurring in the bodily tissues, but upon alterations in their chemical composition and metabolic activity. In many of these disorders physical changes in the affected organs eventually develop, but this is not always so, and the primary change is biochemical. Under this heading it is usual to consider the so-called deficiency disorders which result either from an inadequate intake of certain foods, and particularly of vitamins, or from impaired absorption of them. Several of these deficiency disorders can disturb the functioning of the nervous system, as may abnormalities in the endocrine glands and some specific inborn errors of metabolism. The more common and important of these conditions will be described in this chapter. The effect of poisons upon the nervous system as well as the influence of various forms of physical injury will also be considered, even though the latter is not metabolic in the strictest sense of the term.

Deficiency Disorders

Although many specific syndromes seen in man are ascribed to an insufficient dietary intake of certain vitamins, these syndromes are not solely dependent upon vitamin deficiency. Thus total starvation does not as a rule cause scurvy, pellagra or beri-beri, while manifestations of thiamine deficiency are greatly enhanced if the diet contains large amounts of carbohydrate. It thus appears that some food must be taken before typical clinical features of vitamin deficiency develop. Even so, the resultant clinical syndrome varies greatly in individual cases; it is not, for instance, clear why thiamine (vitamin B_1) deficiency produces Wernicke's encephalopathy in some cases, beri-beri in others, and optic neuritis or perhaps even 'burning feet' in yet others. Clearly, however, conditions like pregnancy, or infective illness, which increase the body's demands for vitamins, may accentuate symptoms attributable to deficiency which were previously minimal. It is the vitamins of the B group, and particularly thiamine, nicotinic acid, pyridoxine and vitamin B_{12}, which are of greatest importance in relation to the nervous system. Clinical syndromes resulting from vitamin C deficiency (scurvy) and from lack of the fat-soluble vitamins (A, D and K) are not as a rule attended by symptoms of nervous disease. The commoner manifestations of vitamin B_1 deficiency are Wernicke's encephalopathy and beri-beri, while nutritional amblyopia and the 'burning feet' syndrome are probably related, although the exact aetiology of these disorders is not yet fully understood. The clinical syndrome resulting from nicotinic acid deficiency is pellagra, while pyridoxine lack gives convulsions in infancy and polyneuropathy in later life. The usual neurological effect of vitamin B_{12} deficiency is subacute combined degeneration of the spinal cord, though disturbances of cerebral function and optic atrophy may also occur.

Wernicke's Encephalopathy

Wernicke's encephalopathy is characterised by mental disturbance, disorders of eye movement and ataxia, and results from thiamine deficiency. It is most often observed in chronic alcoholic patients in whom alcoholic beverages have gradually replaced other forms of food, and gastrointestinal irritation has contributed by producing anorexia. However, it can develop as a result of thiamine deficiency arising from any cause. It has been described as a consequence of repeated vomiting in pregnancy and as a sequel to gastrectomy. There is often an associated polyneuropathy. The principal pathological features are focal areas of haemorrhage and neuronal degeneration in the corpora mammillaria and upper mid-brain. Although in severe cases consciousness may be impaired, the characteristic mental symptoms are first, transient delirium and hallucinations, occurring particularly in alcoholic patients and resulting from alcoholic withdrawal; secondly, apathy, listlessness and variable confusion; and thirdly, most typical of all, the Korsakoff syndrome (*see* p. 120). The principal abnormality in this syndrome is a memory defect giving inability to record new impressions, from which spring disorientation in time and place and confabulation; events from the patient's remote past are described elaborately as if they had just happened. The principal neurological abnormalities accompanying these mental changes are coarse nystagmus, present in all directions of gaze, and ophthalmoplegia, which may consist merely of paralysis of both lateral recti or more often of disorders of conjugate ocular movement leading in some cases to total immobility of the eyes. A severe truncal ataxia is also present as a rule, even though signs of cerebellar inco-ordination in the limbs are often inconspicuous. A characteristic feature of Wernicke's disease is that the neurological abnormalities generally remit quickly with thiamine treatment, although the mental disturbances, and particularly those of the Korsakoff syndrome, may take weeks or months to resolve.

Subacute Necrotising Encephalomyelopathy (Leigh's Disease)

This uncommon disorder, which is inherited as an autosomal recessive trait, is an inborn error of metabolism mentioned here because the pathological changes in the affected infants resemble those of Wernicke's encephalopathy. The affected children show failure to thrive, hypotonia followed by spasticity and often convulsions, nystagmus, and optic atrophy. The condition usually begins in the first year of life; examination of the blood reveals an acidosis and a rise in the blood pyruvate due to a deficiency of pyruvate carboxylase which converts pyruvate to oxalacetate. The condition is usually fatal in six to 12 months but temporary improvement has followed the administration of lipoate. Rarely a more benign form of the disorder occurs in adults.

Beri-Beri

Although thiamine deficiency is clearly important in the aetiology of beri-beri, some additional factor is probably necessary in view of the rarity of the fully-developed syndrome in European or American chronic alcoholics and in view of the fact that it rarely occurs in its entirety except in populations fed upon milled rice. Polyneuropathy due to B-vitamin deficiency is, however, quite common in Western countries, not only in alcoholics, but in patients with prolonged anorexia due to mental disease and in elderly people living alone.

The principal clinical features of beri-beri are those of polyneuropathy (*see* p. 372). Apart from the distal muscular atrophy and sensory loss which are common to all varieties of peripheral neuropathy, a characteristic feature of this form is that the patients often complain of intense burning and tingling in the extremities and especially in the feet; touching the skin is often particularly unpleasant, so that walking becomes impossible, not as a result of muscular weakness, but because of sensory disturbance. In some individuals, these are the only manifestations ('dry' or 'neuritic' beri-beri) but generally there is also peripheral oedema, breathlessness, tachycardia and cardiac enlargement, indicating myocardial involvement. The administration of thiamine in large doses usually gives gradual improvement and eventually complete recovery.

The 'Burning Feet' Syndrome

A syndrome commonly observed in prisoner-of-war camps during World War II was one in which pain and intense burning developed in the feet, but signs of motor neuropathy were absent, and objective sensory changes were slight. Usually there was also intense itching of the scrotum with occasional ulceration. Clearly the syndrome was nutritional in origin and it responded to treatment with vitamins of the B group in high dosage;

probably it was a form of nutritional polyneuropathy but its exact aetiology was never clearly established.

Nutritional Amblyopia

In some individuals living on diets low in vitamin B, progressive blurring of vision develops and the visual fields show central or paracentral scotomas, at first for coloured objects and later for white. Clinical evidence of optic disk swelling is not a feature but if the condition is untreated, optic atrophy follows. This disorder resembles clinically and perhaps aetiologically the forms of amblyopia which have been attributed to alcohol and tobacco. It was once thought to be due to riboflavine deficiency and certainly responds to treatment with vitamins of the B group in high dosage, but recent work suggests that vitamin B_{12} deficiency is the principal factor. Hence the condition resembles the optic atrophy which may complicate subacute combined degeneration.

Tropical Ataxic Neuropathy

Optic atrophy, presumed in the past due to nutritional deficiency, is also a feature of the syndrome of tropical ataxic neuropathy which has been described in many parts of Africa, particularly in Nigeria. In this condition there is also progressive unsteadiness in walking with impairment of vibration and position and joint sense in the legs. It is now known to be due to the excessive ingestion of dietary cyanide which is present in cassava, the tuber of manioc.

West Indian and South Indian Spastic Paraplegia

A form of progressive spastic paraplegia of unknown origin has been observed both in the West Indies and in Southern India. Often there is associated evidence of posterior column dysfunction, and optic atrophy as well as nerve deafness are occasionally seen. There is no evidence that this condition is due to cyanide intoxication and inflammatory changes of granulomatous type have been found in the spinal cords of some patients in the West Indies but not in India. Toxic dietary factors (e.g. bush tea) and nutritional deficiencies have been postulated but the cause remains unknown. A similar clinical picture occurs in **lathyrism** due to the consumption of lathyrus peas.

Tobacco Amblyopia

This condition occurs particularly in heavy pipe-smokers who customarily smoke thick dark tobacco; slow visual deterioration occurs and paracentral or centrocaecal scotomas are usually found. There is some evidence that

B_{12} metabolism is involved, but the visual symptoms usually recover completely if the individual gives up smoking or changes to a more innocuous tobacco. It seems that cyanide in the tobacco or some form of sensitivity causes impaired utilisation of vitamin B_{12}. Sometimes improvement has followed the administration of hydroxocobalamin even if the patient continued to smoke. In the United States it is generally believed that alcohol is also a factor (tobacco–alcohol amblyopia).

Pyridoxine Deficiency

Pyridoxine (vitamin B_6) deficiency in early infancy can cause repeated convulsions. Recurrent seizures developed in many infants in the United States who were fed upon artificial milk which, through an accident of manufacture, was deficient in this vitamin. Nutritional pyridoxine lack can also cause polyneuropathy; isoniazid polyneuropathy is due to metabolic antagonism of pyridoxine and may be corrected by giving high doses of this vitamin.

Pellagra

Pellagra is generally attributed to dietary deficiency of nicotinic acid, but a secondary factor is often defective protein intake, as the amino acid tryptophan is a chemical precursor of nicotinic acid. Hence it occurs in individuals who are existing on a predominantly vegetable or cereal diet deficient in animal protein; it is not uncommon in vegans who refuse all foods derived from animal sources. Commonly the skin lesions of pellagra, which consist initially of erythema on the face, hands and other exposed surfaces, and later give rise to vesiculation, pigmentation and thickening of the skin, are produced by exposure to sunlight. The symptoms of nervous dysfunction, which are almost invariable in such cases, are predominantly mental. Sometimes the clinical picture is that of a severe confusional state, while in other cases there is memory impairment, apathy, fatigue, depression and insomnia. Evidence of polyneuropathy is often found, but is probably due to an associated deficiency of other B-vitamins. In some cases of apparently uncomplicated pellagra there are manifestations of spinal cord involvement, with spastic paraparesis and with variable evidence of posterior column dysfunction.

Vitamin B_{12} Deficiency

Although a primary dietary deficiency of vitamin B_{12} has been observed in vegans and its absorption may be impaired in various gastrointestinal disorders (especially intestinal 'blind-loop' syndromes, or previous gastrectomy), the clinical effects of vitamin B_{12} deficiency upon the nervous system are most often seen in patients with pernicious anaemia, in whom the dietary intake of the vitamin is adequate but its absorption is prevented by the absence of intrinsic factor in the gastric juice. Histamine-fast achlorhydria is invariable and usually there are changes in the blood or in the bone-marrow to indicate a diagnosis of pernicious anaemia. Rarely, however, neurological symptoms and signs antedate any recognisable change in the blood and even in the bone-marrow. Although the principal neurological symptoms and signs indicate disease of the spinal cord, there are occasional cases in which **cerebral symptoms** are predominant, at least initially. These symptoms include defects of intellect, of memory and of concentration, or episodes of confusion or paranoia; it may at times be difficult to distinguish these cerebral manifestations of vitamin B_{12} deficiency from the clinical features of early presenile dementia or from those resulting from any organic confusional state. Occasionally, too, there is progressive bilateral visual loss with central scotomas and **optic atrophy** is found.

Subacute Combined Degeneration of the Spinal Cord

Symptoms and signs of involvement of the nervous system occur in about 80 per cent of cases of pernicious anaemia. The principal sites of pathological change, in which initial loss of myelin with subsequent axonal degeneration occur, are the posterior columns and the pyramidal tracts. The disease process often also involves the posterior roots and peripheral nerves, giving clinical and pathological features of a predominantly sensory axonal polyneuropathy.

The clinical features of the illness depend upon which tracts of the spinal cord are principally affected. Since the lesions in the posterior columns usually predominate, the principal initial symptoms are generally paraesthesiae, tingling, numbness and pins and needles in the extremities. Commonly patients describe sensations as if a tight band of constriction were present around one toe, around a limb or about the waist, or say that the hands and feet feel swollen or as if encased in tight bandages; feelings suggesting that cold water is trickling down the legs may also occur. Physical signs may be slight but usually vibration sense is impaired early, Romberg's sign is positive, the appreciation of position in the toes and fingers is defective and the threshold for two-point discrimination is raised. As evidence of posterior column involvement becomes more severe, so the patient develops sensory ataxia, so that locomotion or maintenance of the upright posture are particularly difficult in the dark or when the eyes are closed. Impairment of appreciation of light touch in the periphery of the limbs is sometimes seen, together with tenderness of the calves, and it is these features, along with depression or absence of tendon reflexes (usually the ankle jerks), as well as evidence of impaired sensory nerve conduction, which have shown that peripheral nerves or posterior nerve roots are often involved. Rarely, pain and temperature sensation are impaired, due to changes in pain-conducting fibres of the peripheral nerves or in the spinothalamic tracts, and there may even be a sensory 'level' on the trunk but this is exceptional.

Disturbances of motor function result from damage to the pyramidal tracts. This gives the characteristic stiffness and slowness of the gait which develops in any case of spastic paraparesis, however caused. The abdominal reflexes are lost, and the lower limb reflexes may be exaggerated, with clonus, unless the lesions in the sensory pathways have interrupted the reflex arc; the plantar responses are usually extensor. The condition is, however, very variable in presentation. Usually sensory symptoms are predominant and the earliest signs may simply be those of a sensory neuropathy, but, on the other hand, there are some cases in which spasticity of the lower limbs is striking and signs of posterior column involvement, though present, are relatively slight. Hence this diagnosis should be seriously considered in any case of sensory neuropathy or spastic paraplegia which develops subacutely in adult life; even if examination of the blood and bone-marrow reveals no abnormality it is usually essential to estimate the level of vitamin B_{12} in the serum. A result of less than $100\,\mu\mu g$/ml of serum is virtually diagnostic of B_{12} deficiency. A Schilling test, examination of the gastric juice for histamine–fast achloryhydria and estimation of gastric parietal-cell antibodies will then be necessary to confirm that B_{12} absorption is impaired and that the diagnosis is one of pernicious anaemia. When gastric acidity is normal and intestinal malabsorption or a small bowel 'blind-loop' syndrome is suspected, appropriate radiological and other studies will be needed. It is of the greatest importance to recognise B_{12} deficiency, as if the condition is treated early the neurological manifestations can resolve completely after giving parenteral vitamin B_{12}. Sensory symptoms and signs are usually the first to improve and may be relieved completely, but if there is a spastic paraplegia of moderate severity before treatment is begun, there is usually some persistent residual disability.

Folate Deficiency

A deficiency of folate caused by malabsorption or by the use of anticonvulsant drugs has long been known to cause megaloblastic anaemia. It has been noted that some patients with polyneuropathy and/or myelopathy, and even some with dementia, have serum folate levels of less than $2\,\mu g$/ml. Treatment with folic acid (5 mg three times daily) has been recommended but the role of folate deficiency in the aetiology of these syndromes remains very uncertain.

Neurological Effects of Malabsorption

While vitamin B_{12} deficiency may occur as a result of intestinal malabsorption, myopathy, peripheral neuropathy and, more rarely, myelopathy have all been described as uncommon complications of coeliac disease in childhood and of tropical and non-tropical sprue in adult life and are as yet largely unexplained.

Nervous Disorders Due to Physical Agents

There are a number of physical agents which, though influencing the metabolic behaviour of many of the tissues of the body, have a particular tendency to impair profoundly the functioning of the central and peripheral nervous system. Among the aetiological agents which are important in this connexion are oxygen lack (anoxia, hypoxia), CO_2 intoxication, electricity, decompression sickness, and excessive heat or cold. Radiation injury, due either to excessive exposure to X-rays or to atomic explosions, has comparatively little effect upon the nervous system when compared with the severe damage which may be caused to the haematopoietic system. However, therapeutic irradiation of the neck or mediastinum is sometimes followed within six to 12 months by the development of a slowly progressive spastic paraparesis with sensory impairment in the lower limbs **(post-radiation myelopathy)**.

Anoxia

The commonest varieties of anoxia met with in clinical practice are those in which there is deficient oxygenation of the arterial blood due either to a failure of adequate quantities of oxygen to reach the lungs (high altitudes, drowning); or to diminished oxygenation resulting from pulmonary disease (emphysema); these cases are grouped together as **anoxic anoxia**. In mountain sickness (Monge's disease), fatigue, dyspnoea, finger clubbing, cyanosis and somnolence with a haematocrit of up to 70 per cent are common; pulmonary oedema is a rare complication. In anaemic anoxia there is a deficiency in circulating haemoglobin or a chemical alteration in the haemoglobin (as in carbon monoxide poisoning) which prevents it from carrying oxygen. Cardiac arrest occurring as a result of heart disease or during anaesthesia may also be followed by irreversible anoxic brain damage which is also sometimes seen as a complication of open-heart surgery. In the latter situation air or gas embolism is an additional hazard. Local anoxia of the tissues can of course be due to arterial disease producing **ischaemic anoxia**. Apart from local infarction of the brain, spinal cord or peripheral nerves, resulting from focal vascular occlusion due to atheroma, thrombosis or embolism, diffuse ischaemic anoxia can also be due to fat embolism (in severe limb fractures) or to widespread disease of small arteries and arterioles as in granulomatous arteritides and in thrombotic microangiopathy. Oxygen lack may have a profound effect upon the brain, but the spinal cord and peripheral nerves seem capable of resisting degrees of anoxia which produce irreversible cerebral damage. When the oxygen supply to the brain is moderately reduced over a long period, the most frequent symptoms are fatigue, drowsiness, apathy and failure of attention, followed later by impairment of judgement and of memory, ataxia and inco-ordination. Sudden profound anoxia produces almost instantaneous loss of the senses, and normally the brain cannot withstand more than three minutes of total anoxia, after cardiac arrest. If the period of anoxia is much more prolonged, respiration ceases and death rapidly ensues. After a period of from five to 15 minutes of cardiac arrest, even if the circulation is re-established, the patient may survive for a time in a semicomatose decerebrate state but full intellectual function is never restored. After less prolonged periods of anoxia the patient may gain full control of his limbs, and consciousness is restored after several hours or days, but there is commonly some degree of permanent intellectual deficit; epileptic seizures of temporal-lobe type are a frequent sequel, resulting from the pathological changes which anoxia produces in Ammon's horn and in contiguous areas of the hippocampus. In some cases of carbon monoxide poisoning the patient is initially unconscious but then may regain his senses at least to some extent after 24 to 48 hours. A relatively lucid interval may then be followed by progressively deepening coma and death (post-anoxic encephalopathy). Many cases showing partial recovery from an anoxic insult, however caused, show not only permanent dementia and severe behaviour disorders but also cerebellar ataxia (due to Purkinje cell damage), variable extrapyramidal features superficially resembling those of Parkinsonism, and spastic weakness of the limbs with extensor plantar responses. In occasional cases there may be a surprising degree of recovery even after prolonged unconsciousness so that the prognosis is difficult to predict in any single case.

Carbon Dioxide Intoxication

In some patients with chronic bronchitis and emphysema the respiratory centre appears to become increasingly insensitive to carbon dioxide which is retained in the circulation as bicarbonate due to chronic alveolar hypoventilation. The syndrome can also result from chronic respiratory insufficiency in neuromuscular disorders such as motor neurone disease, poliomyelitis, polyneuropathy, muscular dystrophy or myasthenia, especially when the diaphragm is involved; morphine or other sedative drugs may have a similar effect. In some cases there are headache, drowsiness and confusion persisting over many months but sometimes an acute syndrome characterised by intense headache, vomiting, convulsions, and papilloedema develops and can be precipitated by the administration of oxygen. As in chronic CO_2 retention, the respiratory centre fails to react to the raised level of CO_2 and respiration is then maintained by the receptors which respond to oxygen lack. Administering oxygen then removes the stimulus to respiration, raises the blood CO_2 still further and hence causes coma. Steroid drugs and diuretics may reduce cerebral oedema in such cases but some patients require intermittent positive pressure respiration for a few weeks in order to blow off CO_2 and to restore the sensitivity of the respiratory centre.

Electrical Injuries

Electrocution, occurring either as a result of accidental contact with an electrical supply or from being struck by lightning, can be immediately fatal due to cardiac arrest. In such cases there are extensive pathological changes in the brain, muscles and peripheral nerves as well as in other tissues. Less severe and more localised injuries commonly produce extensive burning or electrical necrosis of the tissues. It is not uncommon in such cases for a temporary flaccid paralysis of the lower limbs to occur, with sensory loss; this usually passes off in 24 hours and is believed to be due to profound vasoconstriction in the arteries of the spinal cord. Other syndromes resulting from focal injury to the brain, spinal cord or peripheral nerves also occur in some cases.

Decompression Sickness (Caisson Disease)

This condition, which is commonest in divers and in tunnel workers who work in an atmosphere of compressed air, is due to the release of bubbles of nitrogen into the blood stream during decompression. Many neurological symptoms, including hemiplegia, paraplegia, visual scotomas, vertigo and diplopia can occur in such cases, presumably as a result of gas embolism of the arteries of the brain or spinal cord. Symptoms of this type developing in a compressed-air worker demand immediate recompression in a hyperbaric chamber, a measure which almost invariably relieves the symptoms; subsequently decompression must be repeated much more slowly. Non-neurological symptoms include chest pain, dyspnoea, cough, aching in the limbs and infarction of bones, with subsequent arthropathy, particularly of the hip joints.

Heat Stroke

In an individual exposed to a consistently high environmental temperature, the typical manifestations of heat stroke are a rapidly mounting temperature and a hot dry skin with total absence of sweating. The patient is at first apathetic, later stuporose or comatose, and convulsions are common. Circulatory collapse soon follows if rapid cooling is not instituted. Variable degrees of cerebral damage may persist even in those patients who recover; variable confusion, slurring dysarthria, and ataxia are common in the recovery phase. The Purkinje cells of the cerebellum are particularly sensitive to heat injury and a severe cerebellar ataxia may be a permanent sequel.

Hypothermia

Accidental hypothermia is usually due to prolonged exposure to cold or immersion in cold water. Hypothermic coma, is, however, an occasional complication of myxoedema and can occur in elderly people living in unheated rooms in cold weather. Diagnosis depends upon careful measurement of rectal temperature which may be less than 90°F (34°C). Hypothermia is commonly used as an adjunct to anaesthesia; this too may have important complications and sequelae. Unduly prolonged hypothermia can lead to convulsions, irreversible coma, cardiac arrest and death, while less severe and prolonged hypothermia can give sequelae similar to those of cerebral anoxia. Semicoma, confusion and alternating rigidity of the limbs with coarse myoclonic jerking are sometimes seen during recovery. Immersion foot is a syndrome of local hypothermia involving the lower limbs; it occurred in shipwreck survivors and in soldiers living in trenches whose feet were cold and wet for a prolonged period. This condition caused extensive pathological changes in peripheral nerves, muscles and blood vessels and the neurological symptoms and signs were those of a severe peripheral neuropathy sometimes associated with gangrene. In frost-bite, by contrast, the principal pathological changes are in the blood vessels, and symptoms and signs of peripheral nerve injury are unobtrusive.

Disorders Due to Drugs and other Chemical Agents

Whereas many drugs will, in excess, produce manifestations of disordered nervous activity, those most often encountered in clinical practice as a cause of poisoning or intoxication are alcohol, either ethyl or methyl, barbiturates, psychotropic drugs, opiates, amphetamine and its derivatives, and heavy metals. Intoxication may result from excessive and prolonged indulgence or may be acute, as in a suicidal attempt. In the case of heavy metals, it is usually due to accidental ingestion, often in the course of the patient's occupation. Not only are there important specific symptoms induced by some of these drugs, but a characteristic clinical syndrome may follow their sudden withdrawal.

Alcoholism

Chronic alcoholism due to excessive ethyl alcohol consumption is one form of drug addiction and as a rule has potent psychological causes. It can develop insidiously in an individual who is at first merely a social drinker. Gradually his or her intake of alcohol increases so that any excuse or opportunity, however trivial, is regarded as a reason for having a drink, or another drink. It is when the patient begins to drink alone, when alcoholic beverages replace his meals, and when he has a compulsive and irresistible urge to drink, no matter the time of day, that he becomes an alcoholic. The individual who indulges in occasional episodes of excessive drinking with intervals of abstinence is not strictly an alcoholic, though he may become so if the intervals between the episodes shorten progressively, or if his debauches last for days rather than hours (a 'lost weekend'). Only occasionally does alcoholism develop quickly due to acute emotional stress and this usually implies a basically insecure personality. Even small quantities of alcohol impair significantly the performance of skilled motor activity as well as mental functions. Although the individual who has taken one or two drinks may be elated and may feel himself to be in a state of heightened perception, his reaction time is increased and his senses are dulled. Alcohol also increases renal water and electrolyte excretion and thus has a diuretic effect. Dehydration and gastrointestinal irritation are largely responsible for 'hangover' symptoms, including headache.

The symptoms of alcoholism are first gastrointestinal, and secondly nervous. The principal **gastrointestinal symptoms** are nausea, anorexia and diarrhoea, due to chronic gastritis and enteritis; these frequently contribute to malnutrition which in turn results in **polyneuropathy** and/or **Wernicke's encephalopathy** *(see above)*. Alcoholic liver cirrhosis, generally a sequel of long-continued alcoholism, is probably a result of nutritional deficiency combined with the toxic effects of alcohol. The **nervous symptoms** can be divided into those of acute intoxication and those which follow alcohol withdrawal. The symptoms and signs of acute intoxication are well known. The speech is slurred, the gait unsteady and the patient is either jocular and inattentive, noisy and aggressive, or dulled, confused and retarded. More severe intoxication results in stupor or coma; the diagnosis must be made not only upon the flushed face and alcohol-laden breath, but upon the absence of signs of nervous disease; it must always be remembered that subarachnoid haemorrhage, for instance, or head injury, can occur during an alcoholic debauch. Pure alcoholic coma, however, is rarely deep or prolonged, and there are no focal neurological signs. Although an estimation of blood-alcohol may indicate the amount of alcohol that the individual has consumed, this may not be closely related to the degree of clinical intoxication, as individual tolerance varies widely and depends to some extent upon habituation.

Many symptoms and physical signs may follow the **withdrawal of alcohol** after prolonged intoxication or after several days of heavy drinking. The commonest feature is a state of nervousness or **intense tremulousness** ('the shakes'), which is relieved by a further drink, but returns more severely when once again the patient abstains. He is alert, jumpy and easily startled, and has a marked tremor of the limbs. Sometimes these symptoms settle within a few days but occasionally there is a superadded **hallucinosis** in the form of visual experiences, or less commonly auditory hallucinations, such as voices, motor cars, radios and the like. Occasionally, too, a series of convulsions ('rum fits') occur either at the height of a drinking bout or on withdrawal. The most severe of all the syndromes of alcoholic withdrawal is **delirium tremens**. It commonly develops two to four days after the last drink, usually in individuals who have been excessive drinkers for several years. Often it is seen when the patient develops an intercurrent illness such as pneumonia or is admitted to hospital for an operation, or after an accident. He is typically restless, voluble and sleepless, living in a state of intense physical and mental activity both day and night. At the same time there are tremor of the limbs, intermittent muscular twitching, confusion and, as a rule, hallucinations. A fatal outcome, due to circulatory failure or even, in some cases, to exhaustion despite sedation, is not uncommon. Usually the illness lasts for three to four days, and the patient at last falls into a calm sleep and awakens lucid but amnesic, having no recollection of it.

Among the less common syndromes which result from alcoholism are **alcoholic cerebellar degeneration** (a progressive, symmetrical cerebellar ataxia of subacute type), and **degeneration of the corpus callosum** (Marchiafava–Bignami disease), a syndrome of progressive dementia with fits and eventual spastic paralysis, which develops almost exclusively in Italian wine-drinking males. Non-specific **alcoholic dementia** is more common; a rare manifestation is **central pontine myelinolysis** which gives pseudobulbar palsy and quadriparesis. Recently acute and chronic varieties of **alcoholic myopathy** have been described; the acute variety usually develops at the height of a debauch and may give myoglobinuria, while the subacute variety is more often progressive and resembles other metabolic varieties of muscle disease. Alcoholic polyneuropathy has already been considered (*see* p. 374).

The syndrome produced by the ingestion of **methyl alcohol,** which occurs in methylated-spirit drinkers and in others who consume home-made liquor containing wood alcohol, is characterised by an acute acidosis and by nausea, vomiting, visual loss, muscle pains and impairment of consciousness. If large quantities have been taken, death in coma is not infrequent. If recovery takes place, permanent visual loss due to optic nerve damage is common, some patients remain blind, while others show bilateral central scotomas.

Barbiturate Intoxication

Drugs of the barbiturate group have been prescribed so extensively by the medical profession that they have often been used in suicidal attempts by the depressed patient. Accidental excessive dosage is also seen, when a patient awakens during the night, and being bemused as a result of a tablet taken on retiring, then takes several more. It is important to note that alcohol can greatly potentiate the action of barbiturates. There are also some individuals to whom these drugs have been given as sedatives who have gradually increased their habitual dose and have thus developed a syndrome of chronic barbiturate intoxication.

Symptoms of **acute barbiturate poisoning** depend upon the dose taken. Mild intoxication results from taking about two or three times the maximum recommended dose; the patient is drowsy, but easily awakened and often shows nystagmus, dysarthria and ataxia. When the dose is five to 10 times normal, the patient is semicomatose and can only be awakened by vigorous stimulation, when he may mutter a few words and will then lapse again into unconsciousness. The patient who has taken from 15 to 20 times the usual dose or more is comatose with shallow respiration, absent reflexes and extensor plantar responses; sometimes blisters develop on the feet and legs. When the patient is in this condition, which can be fatal, treatment is urgent (*see* p. 441).

The clinical features of **chronic barbiturate intoxication** and those of withdrawal are similar to those of alcoholism. Increasing tolerance can be considerable, so that the patient who is habituated can take many times the recommended dose with comparatively little effect. Characteristically the addict is slow in his mental reactions, his perception is dulled and he is slovenly in dress and habits. The physical signs are nystagmus, dysarthria and cerebellar ataxia. Withdrawal of the drug is followed by a few hours of temporary improvement but later by tremulousness, nervousness, weakness and confusion. There may be a phase of delirium with hallucinations and delusions, and convulsions are very common after barbiturate withdrawal.

Other Sedative and Psychotropic Drugs

Since barbiturates, once used for diurnal and nocturnal sedation, have been gradually supplanted by other tranquillising drugs, many other drugs have been widely used, for example, in suicidal attempts. Anticonvulsant drugs such as phenytoin produce slurred speech, nystagmus, blurred vision and ataxia in moderate overdosage, symptoms and signs comparable to those produced by the barbiturates in higher dosage. The **benzodiazepines** are much safer and seldom cause more than prolonged but reversible coma except in patients with emphysema, when overdosage may be fatal. **Phenothiazines**, too, cause less respiratory depression and impairment of consciousness than other sedatives but may produce dystonic reactions in small doses, or hypotension, hypothermia, tachycardia, cardiac arrhythmia or fits when taken in larger quantities. The **tricyclic antidepressants** cause coma, a dry mouth, hypothermia, hyperreflexia, convulsions, pupillary dilatation, cardiac arrhythmia, respiratory failure and sometimes paralytic ileus or urinary retention.

Aspirin and other salicylates normally cause tinnitus, profuse perspiration and hyperventilation but rarely coma; the principal risk of **paracetamol** overdosage is liver damage and there are few if any neurological manifestations.

Amphetamine Intoxication

Amphetamines and related compounds were increasingly used in the recent past not only for their stimulant and antidepressive effects, but also in order to reduce appetite in patients who were attempting to lose weight. Such individuals often increased the dose up to a point where symptoms of intoxication or chronic addiction appeared. The principal symptoms of overdosage are restlessness and overactivity, dryness of the mouth, tremor, palpitations and tachycardia, hallucinations, irritability and profound insomnia. Very heavy dosage can give fits, hypertension and fatal ventricular arrhythmia. Withdrawal is followed by an acute delirious state with severe hallucinations and sometimes by a delusional psychosis which may last for days or weeks.

Marihuana (Cannabis)

This drug, used for many years in the Orient, was introduced more recently into Western countries, often being smoked in cigarettes. It produces a temporary sense of well-being and is a drug of habituation rather than of addiction. Its use is illegal; its principal danger is that it may introduce the habitué to more harmful narcotic drugs and recent work suggests that long-continued use in high dosage may produce dementia and cerebral atrophy.

Hallucinogenic Agents

The hallucinations induced by mescaline and lysergic acid (LSD) are often terrifying and rarely pleasurable; continued use may lead to irreversible psychosis. Addiction to these remedies is increasing.

Opiates

The drugs of the opiate group which occasionally cause symptoms of intoxication are opium itself and its tincture (laudanum), morphine, heroin (diacetylmorphine), dilaudid (dihydromorphine) and codeine (methylmorphine). Synthetic analgesics such as pethidine (demerol), methadone and dromoran are similar pharmacologically and can also be addictive; they can be considered together with the opiates.

Acute poisoning with these drugs is relatively uncommon except as a result of accidental ingestion, mistakes in dispensing or illicit use, as their issue is carefully controlled by law. The usual clinical features are stupor or coma, pin-point pupils, shallow respiration and bradycardia.

Chronic **opiate intoxication or addiction** is characterised by an initial phase of tolerance in which increasing doses of the drug are required to produce the desired effect, whether it be the pleasurable feeling of detachment which first encourages the eventual addict to use them, or the relief of symptoms for which they were initially prescribed. Prolonged therapeutic use of these drugs in illness is a potent cause of addiction, particularly in doctors and nurses. The phase of tolerance is followed by one of dependence, in which attempted withdrawal gives a series of characteristic symptoms. Some 12 hours or so after the last dose the patient begins to yawn repeatedly and there is lacrimation and running of the nose. This is followed by restlessness, insomnia, muscular twitching, generalised aching and shivering, and then by nausea, vomiting and diarrhoea. Commonly, these acute symptoms last for two or three days, but insomnia and weakness can persist for days or even weeks. Even when the stage of withdrawal and physical dependence has passed, emotional dependence or habituation remains and is an important cause of relapse. Physical, mental and moral dilapidation is invariable in the established addict, and most addicts will resort to any measure involving lying, feigning illness, stealing and many other subterfuges in order to obtain supplies.

Heavy Metals

Whereas poisoning with many heavy metals is accompanied by symptoms of involvement of the nervous system, the most important in clinical practice are arsenic, lead, manganese and mercury.

Arsenical Poisoning
The principal symptoms of acute arsenical poisoning are gastrointestinal, namely vomiting, diarrhoea and acute abdominal pain, though convulsions may occur. In chronic arsenical poisoning, however, whether resulting from criminal intent, from the excessive use of therapeutic arsenical preparations, or from contamination of food with arsenical insecticides, the main symptoms are neurological though hyperkeratosis, pigmentation and desquamation of the skin are also common. The nervous symptoms include headache, drowsiness, confusion and a symmetrical polyneuropathy which gives burning paraesthesiae in the extremities followed by muscular weakness and atrophy, distal sensory loss and absence of the tendon reflexes.

Lead Poisoning
In children, the principal symptom of lead poisoning, which sometimes

results from chewing painted objects covered with lead paint, is an encephalopathy giving somnolence, convulsions and coma. In adults, and particularly in painters using lead-containing paint, agonising colicky abdominal pain and anaemia are the commonest presenting symptoms. A peripheral neuropathy is also common, but is rarely symmetrical, and more often affects one limb. Thus a worker who is making batteries or accumulators may develop a unilateral wrist drop in the arm most often used, and the presence of a blue line on the gums and of punctate basophilia in the red blood cells will suggest that this is due to lead. Confirmation depends upon measurement of lead in the serum and in the urine. Sometimes lead in the bones gives a characteristic increased density in radiographs.

Manganese Poisoning

This industrial disease, seen almost exclusively in manganese miners, results from inhalation of dust and is observed particularly in Chile. It gives a clinical syndrome very similar to that of Parkinsonism but there is often associated lethargy and irritability. Marked improvement follows the use of levodopa (*see* p. 447).

Mercury Poisoning

Acute mercurial poisoning gives severe vomiting and diarrhoea followed by anuria and uraemia due to renal tubular necrosis. In infants, however, chronic mercurial poisoning due to excessive use of calomel teething powders probably caused most cases of pink disease (acrodynia). A syndrome of chronic mercurial poisoning in adults has been described, due either to the inhalation of mercury vapour in makers of thermometers, to the ingestion of fish which have fed on the effluent from a mercury factory (Minimata disease), or in police officers working with outdated mercurial finger-print powders. Sometimes this causes cerebellar ataxia, a syndrome characterised by excessive salivation, tremulousness, vertigo, irritability and depression or erethism (childish over-emotionalism) occurs.

An attempt has been made above to outline the symptoms of nervous dysfunction which can result from a variety of drugs and other poisons. There are many other poisons which give rise to neurological symptoms, but these are less often encountered in clinical practice. Thus atropine and related drugs in excess produce nervous excitation and confusion which may progress to mania; bromism, rarely observed nowadays, is character-ised by drowsiness, lethargy, dysarthria and sometimes by psychosis. Chloral hydrate has an effect similar to alcohol, and antihistamine drugs too may produce lethargy or coma and sometimes convulsions in children. Long-continued use of phenothiazines may give drug-induced Parkinson-ism or irreversible facial and limb dyskinesias (*see* p. 441). For a full description of the effects of these and of the many other drugs which affect the nervous system if taken to excess, the reader is referred to textbooks of clinical pharmacology and toxicology.

Neurological Complications of Endocrine Disease

It has been increasingly recognised that neurological symptoms and signs may be produced by hormonal abnormalities resulting from disease of the ductless glands. Thus in **hypopituitarism**, leaving aside the local effects of the pituitary tumours (chromophobe adenomas) which sometimes produce this syndrome, widespread muscular weakness and atrophy may develop. These improve when the hypopituitarism is treated. In **Cushing's disease**, which is usually due to hyperadrenalism, and much less often to a basophil adenoma of the pituitary (a tumour which is rarely, if ever, large enough to produce local symptoms), mental symptoms, including depression, paranoid ideas and confusional episodes are not uncommon, while occasionally there is evidence of increased intracranial pressure, with headache and papilloedema. A myopathy, often painful, and usually affecting thigh muscles predominantly to give weakness, atrophy and histological changes, has also been found in some patients with Cushing's disease, and resembles the steroid myopathy seen in some patients under treatment for long periods with steroid drugs (particularly triamcinolone). A subacute myopathy may also occur due to excess secretion of ACTH in patients who have undergone adrenalectomy for Cushing's disease, while a similar disorder accounts for muscular weakness in **acromegaly**.

The exact pathogenesis of **exophthalmic ophthalmoplegia or ophthalmic Graves' disease** remains in doubt, but it is thought to result from an excessive output of an exophthalmos-producing substance by the pituitary. Histologically there is striking oedema of the orbital muscles and connective tissue. The first symptom is usually pain in one eye followed by unilateral exophthalmos and diplopia. Often the superior rectus or superior oblique is the first muscle to become paretic. Although exophthalmos may be predominantly unilateral for some time, the other eye is eventually affected, and paresis of several extrinsic ocular muscles develops. Occasionally the exophthalmos is sufficiently severe for orbital decompression to be imperative but in less severe cases it can be reduced by steroids. The syndrome sometimes develops acutely after thyroidectomy. Often there are few if any symptoms of thyrotoxicosis.

Thyrotoxicosis (primary Graves' disease) is occasionally sufficiently acute to produce a severe confusional state, but this is uncommon. It is sometimes associated with myasthenia gravis and a rare syndrome of thyrotoxic periodic paralysis, which resolves when the thyrotoxicosis is relieved, has been described, especially in Orientals. A more common complication is a myopathy of girdle and proximal limb muscles (thyrotoxic myopathy). This condition improves, and generally recovers completely, when the thyrotoxicosis is adequately treated. In severe **myxoedema**, hypothermic coma is an occasional complication due to lowering of the body temperature, while acute psychotic episodes (myxoedematous madness) and even a reversible syndrome of depression and mild dementia may occur. More often there is muscular pain and aching, accentuated by exertion, with slowness of muscular contraction and relaxation (pseudomyotonia). These symptoms respond to treatment with thyroxin.

In **diabetes mellitus**, polyneuropathy is a well-recognised complication (*see* p. 375). Isolated cranial nerve palsies of the third and sixth cranial nerves are also common, but usually clear up spontaneously within a few weeks or months. They appear to result from focal infarction of cranial nerve trunks. **Diabetic coma** is usually associated with ketoacidosis, a blood sugar higher than 15 mmol/l and massive ketonuria. However, lactic acidosis is an occasional cause of metabolic acidosis in diabetic subjects, especially during treatment with hypoglycaemic agents, and must be distinguished from the lactic acidosis which can result from poisoning with methyl alcohol or paraldehyde. Hyperosmolality due to hyperglycaemia (hyperglycaemic non-ketotic diabetic coma) has also been described, and a similar syndrome has been observed in non-diabetic subjects with severe burns. The patient is wasted, pale and dehydrated, the rate and amplitude of respiration are increased, ocular tension is low, the pulse rapid and feeble and there is also hypotension.

An important complication, not of diabetes itself, but of its treatment, is **hypoglycaemia**, resulting from excessive insulin administration. Excessively low blood-sugar readings are also seen in some cases of hypopituitarism, in patients with hyperinsulinism due to an adenoma of the islets of Langerhans, and sometimes in liver disease. The first symptom of hypoglycaemia is often profuse sweating and light-headedness followed by confusion and sometimes abnormal behaviour. Such episodes usually occur several hours after a meal and thus are most commonly experienced during the night or early in the morning. Vertigo, diplopia and many other nervous symptoms occasionally occur. Gradually the patient lapses into coma and is found, sweating profusely, with flaccid limbs and extensor plantar responses. If the coma is severe, generalised convulsions may develop. Diagnosis depends upon obtaining a blood sugar estimation during an attack. In suspected cases of organic hyperinsulinism a 48 hour fast may be needed to produce an episode, while insulin tolerance tests and/or plasma insulin assay may be helpful. A deep hypoglycaemic coma which lasts more than a few hours can produce permanent cerebral damage, with clinical after-effects and histopathological changes resembling those of anoxia. Even after several hours of unconsciousness, however, complete recovery is still possible, but often takes several days. A rare complication of hyperinsulinism is a peripheral neuropathy of motor type.

Lassitude and asthenia are salient clinical features of **Addison's disease**, resulting from hypoadrenalism, but in addition, muscular weakness and wasting (Addisonian myopathy) occur in some cases, while papilloedema due to cerebral oedema has also been described. A myopathy, giving symptoms of generalised muscular weakness, is also an occasional feature of hypoparathyroidism, while paradoxically, muscular weakness, lassitude and polyuria can also be prominent in cases of **hyperparathyroidism** due to parathyroid adenoma. In both of these disorders of calcium metabolism, even when there is considerable evidence of proximal limb muscle weakness, the tendon reflexes usually remain brisk, a feature rarely seen in any other form of myopathy. In hypoparathyroidism following accidental operative removal of the parathyroid glands, or in **hypocalcaemia** due to any cause, there is excessive neuromuscular irritability, giving tetany and a positive Cvostek's sign. Idiopathic hypoparathyroidism is much less common, but in this condition, mental defect, recurrent major fits and calcification of the basal ganglia are constant features. The severity and frequency of the attacks of epilepsy are greatly reduced by treatment with calciferol or dihydrotachysterol.

Porphyria

The term porphyria embraces a group of diseases which have in common the excessive urinary excretion of uroporphyrin and coproporphyrin and of porphyrin precursors (porphobilinogen).

Congenital porphyria is a rare inherited disorder in which there is excessive photosensitivity from birth. Any exposure to sunlight results in blistering of the skin, and porphyrins are laid down in the affected area to give pigmentation; eventually extensive scarring takes place. When a similar disorder develops in adult life it is known as **porphyria cutanea tarda**.

It is, however, in **acute idiopathic porphyria** of the Swedish type, which is also the result of an inborn error of metabolism, that neurological manifestations occur. Attacks can be produced by the administration of drugs, particularly barbiturates and sulphonamides. They occur usually in early adult life and in either sex. The cardinal manifestations are attacks of abdominal pain which are often diagnosed initially as acute surgical emergencies, episodes of mental confusion, and a predominantly motor axonal polyneuropathy. Bulbar paralysis occasionally occurs. During latent periods between attacks there is generally excessive porphobilinogen G and excess δ-amino-laevulinic acid in the urine, but in the acute episodes the urine is port-wine coloured and contains large quantities of porphyrins. Remissions invariably occur and can last weeks, months or years, but many patients are seriously disabled by the polyneuropathy, even though this, too, may remit. The rare South African type is similar but the attacks are sometimes fatal and light sensitivity like that of the congenital type is sometimes seen.

Some Other Metabolic Encephalopathies

There are many **primary or endogenous metabolic encephalopathies**, most of which are inherited and which cause disorders of neuronal, glial or myelin structure whether due to storage of abnormal metabolites or abnormalities of development. Some of these are the leukodystrophies previously described, many others are associated with mental retardation and yet others give rise to the storage of abnormal lipids, proteins, amino acids, carbohydrates or mucopolysaccharides in the tissue of the nervous system. Some are due to identifiable single enzyme defects. To quote but one example not mentioned in this chapter or elsewhere, the X-linked **Lesch-Nyhan syndrome** of hyperuricaemia gives rise to severe mental retardation, self-mutilation, choreoathetosis and joint changes resembling those of gout. For details of the rare disorders not mentioned in this book the reader is referred to text-books of paediatric neurology. There remain to be considered, however, one of the more common of these disorders (hepatolenticular degeneration) and two types of **secondary or exogenous metabolic encephalopathy** in which an extracerebral disorder (such as uraemia or disorders of water and electrolyte metabolism) affect the brain only secondarily.

Disorders of Water and Electrolyte Metabolism

Hyponatraemia or water intoxication has been increasingly recognised as a cause of delirium, leading often to coma. It is most often due to inappropriate ADH secretion (as may occur in bronchial carcinoma) or to organic lesions (e.g. neoplasia) in the region of the hypothalamus and/or pituitary, but sometimes occurs without evident cause. Sometimes it results from compulsive water drinking in psychotic or alcoholic individuals or it may complicate renal failure.

Hypernatraemia may also cause delirium, less often coma; it is seen in children with severe diarrhoea, rarely in adults with diabetes insipidus, and can also be iatrogenic due to the administration of excessive quantities of intravenous saline. These causes of delirium, drowsiness or coma are recognised by measurement of the serum osmolality.

Uraemic Encephalopathy

The encephalopathy of chronic renal disease produces no specific neuro-pathological changes and is usually reversible by dialysis. Subacute delirium progressing to stupor or coma is usual and there is often multifocal myoclonus, while major convulsions are common. Acidosis and azotaemia are diagnostic but the picture may be complicated by concomitant hypertensive encephalopathy.

Hepatic Coma (Portal-Systemic Encephalopathy)

In patients with liver disease, whether acute hepatic necrosis, active chronic hepatitis, or chronic cirrhosis, certain characteristic neurological manifestations result from the fact that blood from the bowel, containing large amounts of nitrogenous substances, by-passes the liver through anastomoses between the portal and systemic arterial systems, and enters the systemic circulation. These nitrogenous substances, of which the level of blood ammonia is a useful index, can have a profound effect upon the brain. The early symptoms of 'hepatic coma' are confusion, apathy, difficulty in concentration and inappropriate behaviour. Gradually the patient may lapse into coma. In some cases the patients enter a chronic phase characterised by episodic confusion and abnormal behaviour; this may last for weeks or months and may be wrongly attributed to cerebral atherosclerosis or to presenile dementia, if clinical evidence of liver disease is unobtrusive. Although exaggeration of tendon reflexes is common, the most important neurological sign, which is almost pathognomonic, is a flapping tremor of the outstretched hands (asterixis), a movement reminiscent of the flapping of a bird's wings. The EEG in such cases reveals diffuse slow activity, often with typical triphasic waves. Less often an acute choreiform syndrome is seen and in some patients, particularly following portacaval shunt operations, a progressive myelopathy (spastic paraparesis) develops. A mild demyelinating peripheral neuropathy has also been described.

Clearly the mechanism by which these conditions are produced is enhanced by surgical procedures which create artificial anastomoses between the portal and systemic circulations. Episodes of encephalopathy can follow a high-protein meal, or a gastrointestinal haemorrhage (due to absorption of blood products). Treatment consists of a low-protein diet and the regular administration of intestinal antibiotics (e.g. neomycin) which destroy bacterial flora and so reduce the absorption of protein derivatives.

Hepatolenticular Degeneration (Wilson's Disease)

Hepatolenticular degeneration was first clearly defined by Kinnier Wilson in 1912, although similar cases were previously described by Westphal and Strumpell under the title pseudosclerosis. This condition, which affects either sex, is familial, being due to an autosomal recessive gene, so that it can affect several members of a sibship, but there is generally no history of the disease in previous generations. It usually begins in the first two decades and is characterised first by the appearance of symptoms indicating progressive degeneration of the basal ganglia, secondly by the development of liver cirrhosis, and thirdly by the presence of a ring of brown pigment around the margin of the cornea, the Kayser–Fleischer ring. The primary defect is one of copper metabolism and copper is deposited in the brain and liver as well as in the periphery of cornea. Characteristic biochemical features include amino-aciduria, an excessive output of copper in the urine (normal upper limit $70\,\mu g/24\,hr$), and a reduction of the serum copper level (normal range $75–100\,\mu g/100\,ml$); the serum copper oxidase is also reduced. The primary defect appears to be a congenital deficiency of caeruloplasmin, the copper-binding fraction of the serum proteins; as there is too little of this substance available to absorb ingested copper, the latter is either deposited in the tissues or excreted in the urine.

The principal clinical manifestations are usually neurological although occasionally symptoms of liver disease (jaundice, ascites, splenomegaly) predominate. The neurological manifestations, which generally begin in adolescence, include facial grimacing, tremor, dysarthria, ataxia and personality change. An alteration in the child's speech is often the first symptom. The tremor is usually of action type, but is sometimes present at rest, as in Parkinson's disease, or accentuated towards the end of move-ment, as in cerebellar ataxia. Sometimes there is a flapping or wing-beating movement of the outstretched hands, as in hepatic coma, and occasionally choreiform or athetoid posturing of the limbs, or plastic rigidity, are observed. Speech is invariably slurred, and facile euphoria or intellectual deterioration are frequent in the later stages. There are no changes in the reflexes or in sensation and the plantar responses are flexor. Often there is little clinical evidence of hepatic dysfunction, but spider naevi on the skin, 'liver palms', and splenomegaly are not infrequent, while gastrointestinal bleeding from oesophageal varices is an important complication, and liver function tests are usually grossly abnormal.

If untreated, the disease is usually fatal in five to 15 years from the onset; neurological disability is progressive, leading to immobility, emaciation and dementia, and death is usually due to intercurrent infection, gastroin-testinal haemorrhage, or hepatic failure. Treatment with chelating agents can modify the course of the disease, as these agents promote copper excretion. Dimercaprol and calcium EDTA, once used, have now been superseded by penicillamine (dimethylcysteine) which should be given continuously in a dose of 1–1.5 g daily. If treated early enough the disease is completely controlled and affected individuals become virtually normal, both mentally and physically, and remain so. Potassium sulphide in a dosage of 20 mg three times daily diminishes copper absorption and has been used as an adjuvant.

References

Adams, R. D. and Victor, M., *Principles of Neurology*, 2nd ed. (New York, McGraw-Hill, 1981).

Davies, D. M., *Textbook of Adverse Drug Reactions,* 2nd ed. (London, Oxford Medical Publications, 1981).

Goldensohn, E. S. and Appel, S. H. (Eds.), *Scientific Approaches to Clinical Neurology* (Philadelphia, Lea & Febiger, 1977).

Kennedy, A. 'Alcoholism', in *Early Diagnosis,* Ed. Miller, H. G. (Edinburgh, Livingstone, 1959).

Pallis, C. and Lewis, P. D., *The Neurology of Gastrointestinal Disease,* Major Problems in Neurology, No. 3 (London, Saunders, 1974).

Plum, F. (Ed.), *Brain Dysfunction in Metabolic Disorders* (New York, A.R.N.M.D. Vol. 53, 1974).

Plum, F. and Posner, J. B., The *Diagnosis of Stupor and Coma,* 3rd ed. (Oxford, Blackwell, 1980).

Spillane, J. D., *Tropical Neurology* (London, Oxford University Press, 1973).

Walshe, J. M., 'Neurological complications of liver disease and hepatolenticular degeneration', in *Diseases of the Nervous System,* Ed. Walshe, F. M. R., 11th ed., Chapters 12 and 13 (Edinburgh, Livingstone, 1958).

Walton, J. N., *Brain's Disease of the Nervous System,* 8th ed. (London, Oxford University Press, 1977).

Walton, J. N., Cerebral metabolism and its disorders, in Section X on Neurological pathophysiology, in *International Textbook of Medicine,* Ed. Smith, J. H. and Thier, S. (Philadelphia and London, Saunders, 1981).

20 Treatment in Neurology—An Outline

Whereas the preceding chapters have dealt with the foundations of neurological diagnosis and with descriptions of specific syndromes in which there is dysfunction of the nervous system, it is the treatment of the patient's disease and not diagnosis itself which is, or should be, the ultimate aim. While accurate diagnosis may be an essential first step before appropriate therapy can be recommended, this is not always the case and there are some patients suffering from nervous disease in whom the correct management is clearly apparent even though diagnosis remains obscure. In a case of progressive dementia arising in the presenium, for instance, there may be no certain means of deciding whether the illness is due to Alzheimer's disease or to atherosclerosis. Provided, however, that treatable conditions such as general paresis, vitamin B_{12} deficiency and frontal meningioma have been excluded, management then depends upon the patient's behaviour and social circumstances. If he is placid and manageable, despite his dementia and associated incontinence, and if he has a capable wife or other relatives, the situation should be explained to them and he should be nursed at home with suitable sedative drugs and nursing assistance. But if, on the other hand, he is violent or disturbed in his behaviour, if he lives alone, or if his relatives are frail or incompetent, there will generally be no alternative but to arrange his admission to a mental hospital.

Treatment, it must be remembered, is not merely a matter of prescribing drugs, and of seeing that they are properly administered (a problem sometimes much more difficult than the simple act of writing a prescription). It also involves management of the individual and of his relatives. When should the patient be treated and nursed at home and when in hospital? How far should special investigations be pursued, particularly if they are unpleasant or potentially dangerous? Are they to be carried out because of possible benefit to the patient, or merely to satisfy the doctor's curiosity? How much should he be told of the nature and prognosis of his illness, and how much information should be given to his family? When is it necessary to ask for a second opinion? These are questions which arise every day in clinical practice and which cannot easily be answered in the pages of a textbook. The ability to solve these problems with tact, patience and understanding stems not only from a knowledge of disease, but also from experience of patients as individuals and of their personalities, emotional reactions and family background. So diverse may be the personal and domestic circumstances of two patients suffering from identical illnesses, that although the correct pharmacological treatment is similar, the appropriate management when considered in more general terms may be totally different. The most important lesson that the student must learn is that his value as a doctor in the community does not depend merely upon his ability to diagnose illness and to prescribe appropriate drugs, but also upon the way in which he manages sick people and their relatives.

In considering specific disorders of the nervous system, it is clear that an increasing number of conditions can be cured or benefited by pharmacological or surgical methods of treatment. Even in the many neurological disorders in which the basic pathological process is relatively uninfluenced by any treatment at present available, substantial improvement in the patient's symptoms or in his attitude to his disease can often be achieved with drugs or physical methods. Often, too, it is of great value to the patient if the doctor can do no more than give an accurate forecast of the natural history and eventual outcome of the illness. In inherited conditions, it is also important to be able to give appropriate advice concerning the prospect of affection of other members of the family, if this information is sought, and particularly if the parents of an ill child are considering adding to their family. If, on the other hand, they already have other children, it may be wise to conceal this possibility until the parents become aware of it themselves. It is also wise in cases of progressively crippling illness, to keep some hope alive by referring to research which is being done in many parts of the world upon the chronic neurological diseases and by saying that these are not incurable conditions, but rather diseases for which the cure has not yet been found. It is, however, equally important to be sure that the hopes of the patient and his relatives should not be too lavishly encouraged, only to be shattered by subsequent events.

Although the treatment of some syndromes was touched upon briefly when they were described in the preceding chapters, this chapter will outline some of the principal methods of treatment of neurological disease and also methods which can be employed to relieve important symptoms of disordered nervous function.

The Relief of Pain

As mentioned in Chapter 4, pain is a common symptom of nervous disease, and the doctor is frequently called upon to choose an appropriate remedy for its relief. Much depends upon its severity, its situation and its cause. Musculoskeletal pain which is relatively mild and not due to serious organic disease can be relieved by the local application of heat, or by immobilisation, while the most appropriate remedy for tension headaches is not analgesic drugs but sedatives (*see below*) designed to relieve emotional stress. Indeed there is evidence that tricyclic antidepressant drugs and/or tranquillisers, such as the phenothiazines, may themselves possess analgesic properties. At least they have an adjuvant effect when given along with analgesic remedies, through relief of the overlay of tension, depression and anxiety which so often accompanies persistent pain.

Generally, however, if the cause of the pain cannot be eliminated immediately, analgesic remedies are indicated in order to produce symptomatic relief. Of these one often prescribed is aspirin (acetylsalicylic acid) in various forms, usually in a dosage of 600–900 mg three or four times daily in adults. Children may require a dosage of 60–600 mg depending upon their age. The irritative effect of this drug upon the gastrointestinal system, and the dangers of gastric haemorrhage, are reduced to some extent by utilising neutral soluble aspirin ('disprin', 'solprin', 'paynocil'). Other mild and useful remedies are paracetamol (500–1000 mg every four hours), fenoprofen (300 mg) and mefenamic acid (500 mg). When the relief obtained from aspirin is inadequate, owing to the severity of the pain, compound tablets containing a combination of aspirin, paracetamol and codeine or caffeine are often used. The usual dosage of these compound remedies in adults is two tablets, in children from five to 10 years of age, one tablet, and this dose can be repeated every four to six hours if necessary. Often headache, and pain of nerve of nerve-root compression of moderate severity is substantially relieved. A phenothiazine drug (e.g. chlorpromazine) may be added if relief of pain is incomplete. More severe and continuous pain may, however, require more powerful remedies; two such are codeine phosphate (15 mg) and dihydrocodeine (30–60 mg) and others are dextrapropoxyphene (60 mg) and pentazocine (25–50 mg).

All of the more powerful analgesics are drugs of addiction and should therefore be used sparingly. These powerful remedies are nevertheless appropriate when pain is a self-limiting illness in which analgesics are only required for a few days or at the most a few weeks. When the duration of the illness is likely to be measured in months, it is unwise to begin treatment with these remedies, unless the patient's expectation of life is short, either because of the nature of the disease, or on account of his age. In younger patients suffering chronic pain, it is important to persist with less powerful analgesics or to employ physical or surgical methods for its relief, for the patient may readily become addicted to the more powerful remedies. Of these powerful drugs, morphine and its derivatives remain the most satisfactory, except in patients with increased intracranial pressure or intrathoracic disease, in whom their depressant effect upon respiratory function can be dangerous. The average adult dose of morphine sulphate is 10 mg by injection, but for a maximum analgesic effect, up to 30 mg can be given, except in elderly patients. Levorphanol tartrate (dromoran) is more powerful than morphine but is similar in its side-effects and in its tendency to produce addiction. It is given in an oral dose of 1.5–3 mg or 2 mg by subcutaneous or intramuscular injection. Each may be given every four hours if necessary.

There are several synthetic analgesics which are comparable with morphine in their analgesic effect, but are less severe respiratory depressants. Of these, the most commonly employed is pethidine hydrochloride (Demerol) which is given by mouth or by intramuscular injection in a dosage of 25–100 mg. It is often used for the relief of intense headache resulting from subarachnoid haemorrhage or cerebral tumour; if there is associated vomiting, it is useful to give in addition chlorpromazine 25–50 mg every four to six hours, as this remedy may not only potentiate the action of pethidine but will also assist by reducing the frequency and severity of vomiting. Pethidine is also useful in the control of severe pain resulting from inflammation or compression of nerve roots. Pethilorfan, a combination of pethidine, 100 mg, with 1.25 mg of levorphan, is a valuable and powerful remedy for very severe pain. Naloxone 400 µg given intravenously will successfully counteract respiratory depression caused by morphine or pethidine. A less commonly-employed analgesic with a similar effect is methadone which is given in tablet form or by injection in a dosage of 5–10 mg. Other powerful synthetic remedies are phenazocine hydrobromide (5 mg), oxycodone (30 mg, given usually as a suppository) and two newer remedies, nefopam hydrochloride (30 mg) and buprenorphine (300 µg by injection) which are still being evaluated.

Also to be regarded as dangerous drugs which can be habit-forming but which are comparable to morphine in their effects are dipipanone (10 mg) and dextromoramide (5 mg) which can be given in tablet form. Another remedy occasionally employed with some success in patients suffering from pain of nerve-root origin, particularly when this is due to chronic degenerative changes in multiple intervertebral disks, is phenylbutazone (butazolidine) in a dosage of 100 mg three or four times daily, but this drug, which has important toxic effects upon the haemopoietic system and upon the kidneys in some cases, is more often used in cases of painful arthropathy. Even more successful as an analgesic and anti-inflammatory agent is indomethacin (25 mg capsules, 2–6 daily) but this drug, though on the whole less toxic than phenylbutazone, should also be used with care and is probably contraindicated if there is a past history of peptic ulcer. Other analgesics commonly used in musculoskeletal pain which also have anti-inflammatory effects less potent than those of phenylbutazone and indomethacin are, for example, naproxen (375–750 mg daily), ibuprofen (200 mg three times daily), diflunisal (250–500 mg) and their analogues. These and many other drugs are available commercially in a bewildering variety of combined tablets which may make the choice of remedy in any single case very difficult, but in general it is wise to begin with simple remedies, and only to employ the more powerful in resistant cases.

It should also be remembered that the pain (headache) caused by increased intracranial pressure can be relieved by measures which reduce this pressure. Lumbar puncture is not indicated because of the danger of tentorial or cerebellar herniation, but detensifying therapy (dehydration) is occasionally successful, at least temporarily. Remedies employed in the past to produce this effect were intravenous sucrose (100 ml of a 50 per cent solution every 12 hours) or rectal hypertonic magnesium sulphate (8 oz of a 25 per cent solution every six hours). An intravenous infusion of a 30 per cent solution of urea in a dosage of 1.0–1.5 g per kg body weight was even more effective but this remedy had a temporary effect only and was usually given for its immediate effect during a surgical operation. As it often produced a 'rebound oedema' within hours, urea soon lost favour. Steroid drugs (e.g. dexamethasone) are now the drugs of choice for reducing cerebral oedema due to the presence of a brain tumour or to some other cause, while the diuretic frusemide (40–120 mg) is also useful. Dexamethasone and betamethasone are now widely used to reduce brain swelling, however caused, and even patients with multiple intracranial metastases may show remarkable improvement for weeks or even months; large doses are necessary and it is usual to begin with 5 mg four-hourly and then gradually to reduce the dose once an effect has been achieved.

Whereas the pain of self-limiting or treatable diseases can be successfully relieved with the agents listed above, **intractable pain** which is resistant to the milder analgesics presents a more difficult problem of management. In some cases, local physical measures are effective. Thus in a patient with a painful phantom limb after amputation, repeated percussion of a neuroma in the stump several times daily with a rubber mallet or some other appropriate instrument may be helpful. Pain referred to a specific skin area is also relieved on occasion by repeated subcutaneous infiltration around the painful area either with local anaesthetic or even with saline. This method occasionally works in cases of persistent *post-herpetic neuralgia* (p. 91) which is particularly troublesome and long-lasting in the elderly. The pain of this condition and some other types of intractable cutaneous pain may also be relieved by the application, several times a day, of an electrical vibrator or of an ethyl chloride spray to the affected area of skin. This treatment is usually best given in hospital in the first instance so that the patient learns that persistence is necessary. Thus in post-herpetic neuralgia the period for which the vibrator is applied is gradually increased from two or three minutes to 20 minutes three times daily; appropriate analgesics are also usually necessary. More recently, percutaneous, low-intensity electrical stimulation carried out repeatedly through surface electrodes, using a small stimulator which can be carried in the clothing and activated at will, has been shown to be helpful in many cases. Electrical stimulation of the dorsal column of the spinal cord through implanted extradural electrodes can also be effective but carries much greater complications. Acupuncture has a vogue but both its action and its efficacy remain uncertain.

If local measures of this nature are ineffective, it may be necessary to resort to *surgical methods* of pain relief. First, however, it is worth trying chlorpromazine in gradually increasing dosage, up to 600 mg daily, if tolerated, as this drug reduces the patient's emotional reaction to his pain, and can almost be considered to produce a pharmacological leucotomy. There are, nevertheless, certain varieties of pain which regularly require surgical treatment. Causalgia, for instance, following peripheral nerve injury, is only relieved in most cases by sympathectomy. In tic douloureux, if the pain is strictly limited topographically, it is occasionally relieved by operative section of the appropriate peripheral nerve (supraorbital, infraorbital). As a rule, these measures give only temporary relief, and until comparatively recently it was usually necessary to divide the sensory pathways more centrally, either by alcohol injection of the Gasserian ganglion, or by surgical division of the sensory trigeminal root. Similarly, glossopharyngeal neuralgia often required intracranial section of the glossopharyngeal nerve. However, carbamazepine, given in a dosage of 100–200 mg two, three or four times daily has proved remarkably successful in relieving pain in most cases of both trigeminal and glossopharyngeal neuralgia, though it may have to be continued for many months until a spontaneous remission occurs. If pain is completely relieved, every few weeks an attempt should be made to reduce the dose or even to withdraw the drug until this is achieved successfully. Subsequently, in the event of relapse, treatment is recommenced and is usually just as successful as on the first occasion. Only patients who are unable to take this drug owing to side-effects or in whom pain relief is inadequate now require injection or surgical treatment. Alcohol or aqueous phenol injection of the Gasserian ganglion may have only a temporary effect, giving relief for one to two years in some cases, and is therefore the appropriate method to use in the elderly, but in patients under the age of 60, surgical division is more suitable. It is important to explain to patients undergoing these procedures that the affected side of the face will be rendered permanently numb, and one must always be certain that the pain is severe enough for this after-effect to be tolerated. Some patients in whom the pain was not particularly severe or disabling have complained of numbness and discomfort (anaesthesia dolorosa) after injection. It is also important that these procedures are only carried out in patients with true tic douloureux, as the pain of atypical facial neuralgia, which is often of emotional origin, is not relieved thereby.

When intractable pain is more extensive, measures which can be utilised, when other methods have failed, include epidural infusion of local anaesthetics, intrathecal injections of hot or ice-cold water, or of phenol in glycerine or oily contrast medium around appropriate nerve roots, surgical division of sensory roots or of the spinothalamic tract in the spinal cord (anterolateral cordotomy), percutaneous cordotomy using electrocoagulation, surgical destruction of appropriate thalamic nuclei, utilising stereotaxis, and, perhaps as a last resort, prefrontal leucotomy. Leucotomy, which must usually be performed bilaterally, with destruction or sectioning of the white matter in both frontal lobes, does not relieve pain, but by altering the patient's emotional responses, renders it more bearable. This method is now used very rarely. The selection of appropriate cases of intractable pain in which these skilled techniques are indicated, and the choice of the appropriate method, are matters which are the concern of specialist neurologists and neurosurgeons.

Sedation

Sedative and hypnotic drugs are required in patients with nervous disease not only in order to control agitation or violent and disturbed behaviour, but also in order to achieve restful sleep in patients whose illness produces sleeplessness. If pain is contributing to the patient's insomnia an analgesic as well as a sedative or hypnotic remedy may be needed. Drugs of this type are also of value in the relief of anxiety and emotional tension, but the tranquillising remedies will be considered below when the treatment of mental disease is considered.

In restless, disturbed or confused patients suffering from brain disease, chlorpromazine, given in an oral or intramuscular dose of 50 mg is most useful as are other phenothiazines such as haloperidol (10 mg by injection). In acutely delirious patients, paraldehyde is still occasionally employed, either 10 ml by mouth in orange juice or 5–10 ml given by deep intramuscular injection. This drug is safe and often effective, but it has an unpleasant smell, intramuscular injection may be painful, and occasionally an abscess may form at the site of injection. When mental disturbance is less severe chloral hydrate may still usefully be employed in an average dose of 1.3–2.0 g. It is often given in the form of a syrup of which the usual dose is 15 ml. Correspondingly lower doses are utilised in children, in whom this is a particularly useful hypnotic, as is promethazine (5–10 mg).

Until recently, the commonest sedative and hypnotic drugs in use were still the barbiturates, but these remedies are addictive and potentially dangerous, especially in suicidal attempts, and have been largely supplanted by the equally effective and much safer benzodiazepines. Long-acting barbiturates such as phenobarbitone (dosage 30–120 mg) are slow to have an effect; this remedy is of little value in promoting sleep but was used for long-continued mild sedation. When a rapid effect was desired, then drugs which act rapidly, such as quinalbarbitone (seconal, 50–200 mg) or cyclobarbitone (phanodorm, 200–400 mg) were more appropriate. However, since the effect of these remedies wears off in about four hours, those drugs which have an activity of medium duration were usually employed to give more prolonged sleep. In this category are butobarbitone (soneryl, 100–200 ml), pentobarbitone (nembutal, 100–200 mg) and amylobarbitone (sodium amytal, 65–200 mg). Many commercial preparations were used in which short and medium-acting barbiturates were combined to give both rapid action and a prolonged effect. If a barbiturate had be given parenterally, the drugs usually employed were sodium gardenal (soluble phenobarbitone, 200 mg) or somnifaine (aprobarbital and barbitone, 2–4 ml).

There are numerous other non-barbiturate remedies which also have a mild sedative effect. Among those in common use in the recent past were carbromal, 300–1,000 mg which is a derivative of urea, methaqualone (250 mg), dichloralphenazone (650 mg) and glutethimide (250–500 mg). Most of these have now been supplanted by benzodiazepines such as nitrazepam (5 mg) and flurazepam (15 mg) but these remedies, though effective and safe, tend to cause troublesome dreaming, especially in the elderly, and may produce an unacceptable 'hangover' effect the following morning because of their long half-lives. Shorter-acting drugs include temazepam (20 mg) and triazolam (125 mg) which have little or no hangover or cumulative effect but do not help patients who complain of early morning waking.

The Management of Epilepsy

There are now many drugs available for the treatment of epilepsy. But the doctor's responsibility does not end when he prescribes appropriate remedies for the control of seizures. There are also social and educational problems in which his help and advice are needed. Since the answer to many of these questions must depend upon the degree to which the attacks can be controlled by medication, and since the medication appropriate to the individual case depends upon the nature of the seizures, it is first important to consider some important points which arise in the investigation of patients who present with recurrent seizures. Brief 'blank spells' (absence seizures) occurring in childhood are usually correctly diagnosed as being the result of 'petit mal' epilepsy, a condition which generally responds to drugs of the succinimide group or to sodium valproate. On the other hand, attacks of major epilepsy and those of temporal lobe epilepsy are more appropriately treated by the hydantoinates or similar remedies. These have little effect upon true petit mal, while the succinimides sometimes make major attacks more severe and frequent. When clinical diagnosis is accurate, treatment is often comparatively straightforward, and there are many types of minor epileptic seizure which are difficult to classify according to clinical criteria, so that the correct choice of drug is not always easy. It is in this respect that the EEG can be of great help. Unfortunately this investigation gives negative findings all too often, despite the use of activating techniques, and in such cases treatment must be based upon clinical evidence alone. Probably, however, an EEG should, where practicable, be carried out in all patients who present for the first time with seizures which are presumed to be epileptic, as it sometimes gives findings of great value in deciding upon appropriate treatment. An important recent development has been the increasing use of measurement of blood levels of anticonvulsant drugs in order to monitor the effects of treatment. This method has given valuable information about the pharmacokinetics and about the half-lives of the individual remedies, allowing treatment to be planned much more logically and precisely.

In a child who is suffering from **petit mal** attacks alone, and who has never had a major seizure and whose EEG reveals symmetrical generalised spike-and-wave activity, it is reasonable to begin treatment with ethosuximide in an initial dosage of 250 mg once or twice daily, depending upon age. In a child over the age of three years, the dosage of this drug can be increased if necessary up to the maximum adult dose of 250 mg four times daily. Exceptionally some adolescent patients may require as much as 500 mg three times a day. A serum level of 300–700 μmol/l should be achieved. The only important side-effect of this drug is drowsiness. There is good evidence that even if the patient has had no major seizures it is wise from the beginning to give in addition phenytoin sodium 50 mg twice daily to prevent such attacks from developing. The other principal drug which is effective in absence seizures is sodium valproate, beginning with a dose of 200 mg two or three times daily depending upon age, and increasing up to a maximum daily dose of 2.0–2.6 g in an adult or to 30–50 mg/kg body weight in a child. This drug has the advantage that it may also control major seizures so that the addition of phenytoin may not be necessary. It has largely supplanted the methadiones such as troxidone and acetazolamide or chlortetracycline which were once used extensively in such cases. Side effects include nausea, thrombocytopenia, leucopenia and hepatic dysfunction; these are uncommon, but when they occur may demand withdrawal of the drug. Opinions differ as to whether in intractable cases valproate should be given along with or instead of ethosuximide but there is no objection to giving the two together. If major or focal attacks occur as well, then phenytoin in full dosage (*see below*) may have to be added. Despite the efficacy of these remedies, there are a few cases of petit mal which show virtually no response to any form of treatment, and in these individuals it is sometimes preferable to withdraw all medication.

It must be remembered that in some cases of major or focal epilepsy, including the temporal lobe type and particularly when the epileptic seizures begin in middle- or late-life, epilepsy is symptomatic of intracranial disease. It is often difficult to decide how far investigations should be pursued in cases of epilepsy of late onset. Some such cases eventually prove to be harbouring intracranial neoplasms, but there is a much greater number in which this is not the case. In some of the latter the lesion responsible is a scar in one or other temporal lobe, resulting from birth injury; in others it may be a cortical scar in another situation resulting from previous head injury or even from asymptomatic infarction. In cases of this type, the EEG is of value, as it may demonstrate a focus of spike or sharp-wave discharge, or of paroxysmal slow activity either in one or other temporal lobe or elsewhere, indicating that the patient's epilepsy is the result of a focal cerebral lesion. Or occasionally it will show focal slow activity of a type suggesting the presence of a cerebral tumour. In the past it was then necessary in such a case to decide how far invasive radiological studies such as angiography or air encephalography should be pursued, but now it is simply necessary to carry out a CAT scan in such cases and only to reserve the more invasive techniques for use in cases where a CAT scan is not possible or for those where it gives equivocal findings and when, for instance, the possibility of a vascular malformation arises. Only occasionally nowadays in intractable cases of focal epilepsy in which a consistent focus of spike discharge is demonstrated, say in one temporal lobe, and in which adequate anticonvulsant therapy has failed to control the attacks, is it necessary to consider surgical excision of the epileptogenic focus. Full radiological investigations and electrocorticography are usually indicated as a preliminary to this procedure.

In the treatment of **major** or **focal (including temporal lobe)** epilepsy in adult life it has been usual in the past to begin treatment with 30–60 mg of phenobarbitone twice daily and with phenytoin sodium (epanutin, dilantin) 100 mg twice daily. However, phenobarbitone and its analogues are being used much less often because of their side-effects and many authorities now prefer to give a single anticonvulsant such as phenytoin, making certain through the estimation of blood concentrations that a satisfactory therapeutic level is being achieved. This often requires no more than a single daily dose and it is rarely if ever necessary to give a drug more often than twice daily; however, this varies from patient to patient since different individuals metabolise these drugs at different rates. Children are given proportionately lower doses. An average dose in a child aged five years would be 30 mg of phenobarbitone and 50 mg phenytoin, each twice daily. Maximum doses for adults are usually 180 mg of phenobarbitone and 400 mg of phenytoin a day. Side-effects of phenobarbitone are skin rashes, drowsiness and ataxia, and hyperkinesis in childhood; these were sometimes avoided by substituting methylphenobarbitone (phemitone) in doses of up to 600 mg daily. Phenytoin in excessive dosage gives rise to sponginess and swelling of the gums, which must often be tolerated if the drug is effective in controlling the seizures; more troublesome are drowsiness, nystagmus and severe ataxia, symptoms which necessitate a reduction in dosage but not necessarily withdrawal, as the level of dosage producing toxic symptoms in the individual is often finely balanced. The usual therapeutic serum level which it is necessary to achieve is 40–80 μmol/l. Other side effects of this drug include skin rashes, macrocytic anaemia (which can be controlled by the administration of folic acid 5 mg twice daily), diffuse lymphadenopathy of immunological origin, osteomalacia (controllable with vitamin D), and even, in very occasional cases, mild sensory neuropathy and an irreversible cerebellar ataxia.

If phenytoin, alone or in combination with phenobarbitone, is insufficient to control the patient's attacks, whether these are of the major tonic-clonic or focal variety, it was often customary in the past to substitute primidone (250–500 mg three times daily) for phenobarbitone or even to add other anticonvulsant remedies such as methoin (300–400 mg daily), ethotoin (500–1500 mg daily), phenylethylacetylurea (600 mg daily), beclamide (1500–300 mg daily) or sulthiame (400–800 mg daily). These remedies are being used less and less often as it has been shown, for instance, that sulthiame, which, like primidone, often produces unacceptable side-effects, appears to act simply by increasing the serum concentration of phenytoin. However, carbamazepine (100–200 mg. three times daily) is a most effective anticonvulsant which can usefully be substituted for, or, as some would prefer, given along with, phenytoin in intractable cases. Similarly, sodium valproate, mentioned above as being effective in absence (petit mal) seizures, is a useful additional remedy in patients with tonic-clonic, myoclonic or focal seizures, when given along with phenytoin or carbamazepine. Clonazepam beginning with 1 mg at night and increasing slowly to 4–8 mg daily in adult patients, with proportionately smaller doses in children, is another remedy with significant anticonvulsant properties, either when given alone or in combination with other remedies, but often produces unacceptable sedation when given in dosage adequate to control epileptic attacks. However, it, along with sodium valproate, is probably the treatment of choice in myoclonic epilepsy.

The treatment of **status epilepticus** (recurrent major convulsions occurring without recovery between attacks) is a matter of considerable difficulty and the condition has a significant mortality. In the past, intramuscular phenytoin (100 mg six-hourly) and sodium gardenal (200 mg six-hourly) were often given but are now rarely if ever used. Paraldehyde (10 ml intramuscularly every four to six hours) may control the attacks but has been largely supplanted by diazepam (valium) which is given in an intravenous infusion in a dosage of 10 mg every 5 minutes until control is achieved or until 50–60 mg has been given. Other remedies sometimes used in intractable cases are chlormethiazole edisylate (40–100 ml of a 0.8 per cent solution given intravenously at 60–150 drops per minute) or lignocaine hydrochloride (200–300 mg/hr intravenously in a 0.2 per cent solution). A slow intravenous infusion of thiopentone has also been used but is only to be recommended if facilities for intubation and mechanical respiration are available. If these measures fail, intermittent positive pressure respiration with curarisation of the patient may be required for several days in addition to anticonvulsant therapy.

There are also many commercial preparations containing several anticonvulsant drugs in various combinations, but these are mentioned only to be condemned, as it is usually important to be able to adjust the dosage of the various remedies independently. There can be no condition more rewarding to treat than epilepsy, since with patience and repeated trial and error, provided the principles mentioned above are taken into account, over 50 per cent of epileptics can have their fits controlled by drugs. Some patients require several drugs in combination and a trial of different combinations is often required before success is achieved. It is also important to consider the question as to when treatment may be withdrawn. Usually, after three years of freedom from all attacks, a gradual reduction in the dosage of drugs over a three to six month period and eventual total withdrawal is justified. Patients should be warned that there is approximately a 50 per cent risk of relapse and that, if the attacks return, treatment must be reinstituted. Often, however, and particularly in children and adolescents, the attempt is worthwhile as the only alternative is to continue indefinitely.

Benign febrile convulsions, occurring only during febrile illnesses in children under the age of three years, usually carry a excellent prognosis and anticonvulsants can generally be withdrawn one year after the last attack or when the child is four years old. Infantile spasms, by contrast (*see* p. 127) may indicate underlying brain disease; they often show some response to ACTH but not to anticonvulsants.

Educational and social management must also be considered. Most epileptic children can attend ordinary schools and many lose their attacks (particularly if these are only petit mal) after puberty. Only a few whose attacks are impossible to control require prolonged institutional care or education in special residential schools. Restrictions to be imposed upon the activity of the child epileptic are largely dictated by common sense and depend to some extent upon the frequency and severity of his attacks. Thus it is reasonable to forbid cycling on the highway, rock climbing, and swimming except in company, but other restrictions are as a rule unnecessary and an over-protective attitude upon the part of the parents must be avoided. There is good evidence that attacks rarely occur during physical exertion, so that sport can usually be recommended.

In adult life, too, most epileptics can play a useful part in society, though there are some with mental handicap, frequent fits or behaviour changes or psychosis resulting from or associated with temporal lobe epilepsy, who require institutional care, usually in a mental hospital. The latter may also be true of some patients who have degenerative cerebral disease, of which epilepsy is merely a symptom. In other cases the guiding principle with regard to employment must be that the individual should not be placed in any situation in which he might injure himself or others if he had a fit. Thus he should not work at heights, with moving machines, and must not drive a mechanically-propelled vehicle. In Great Britain, up to 1 June 1970, no epileptic patient was legally entitled to drive a car or other mechanically propelled vehicle. Any patient receiving drugs for the treatment of epilepsy was, *ipso facto*, an epileptic and was not therefore entitled to hold a driving licence. In the past, therefore, it was usual to recommend gradual withdrawal of drugs after three years of freedom from attacks; then, if the patient remained attack-free for a further year it could perhaps be said that he no longer suffered from epilepsy and could be allowed to drive. In such circumstances there was, however, no legal obligation upon the licensing authority to restore a licence and many authorities held divergent views. It is now accepted in law that on medical advice a licence may be restored to an epileptic who has had no attacks, while awake, for two years but continues to take treatment, or to a patient certified as suffering only from attacks during sleep over at least a three-year period whether or not he is under treatment. If the patient prefers to attempt withdrawal of treatment, then one year of freedom from attacks after all drugs have been stopped, in addition to the previous three years of freedom, will still be necessary. A single isolated fit occurring under circumstances of exceptional provocation (e.g. during high fever, hypoglycaemia, after excessive alcohol intake or following a material head injury) need not necessarily carry a three-year ban, especially if the EEG is normal, but in such a case it is a wise precaution to wait at least six months before allowing the individual again to drive if the circumstances which precipitated the fit are unlikely to recur and if no further attacks take place. But a single fit occurring without obvious provocation, especially if the EEG shows focal or general epileptic discharge, should generally be regarded as epilepsy and should be treated and managed as such.

While it is the doctor's duty to impress upon the patient the danger to himself and others which may ensue if he continues to drive, he had, until recently, no obligation to report to the authorities the epileptic who continues to drive a car, but is now expected to do so.

Management of the Paraplegic Patient

The nursing and medical care of the patient who has paralysis of the lower limbs or of all four limbs can be considered under three principal headings. First proper care must be taken of the skin to prevent the development of pressure sores (bedsores); secondly, particular attention should be paid to the functioning of the bladder and bowels; and thirdly, contractures and deformities must be prevented as far as possible and physiotherapeutic measures must be utilised in order to make the best possible use of the voluntary activity, if any, which remains or returns in the weakened limbs. Pressure sores are due to prolonged pressure upon an area of skin which is at first reddened and then, as a result of ischaemia, it either becomes gangrenous or breaks down to form an ulcer. Loss of cutaneous sensibility and urinary or faecal incontinence leading to frequent wet or soiled beds are important contributory factors. The prevention of sores must depend first upon the posturing of the patient, with the assistance of special mattresses or foam-rubber cushions, secondly upon frequent turning, with a change of position every half-hour, and thirdly upon strict cleanliness of bed-linen with frequent washing and massaging of vulnerable skin areas. Various forms of skin protectives, such as barrier creams, may be helpful. Susceptible areas include the elbows, the skin over the scapulae, the sacrum and buttocks, the lateral aspect of the hips and the heels.

The patient with a total paraplegia, however caused, almost invariably develops retention of urine, though sometimes from the beginning there is retention with a dribbling overflow. Catheterisation is then essential. Authorities differ as to whether intermittent catheterisation with a strictly sterile 'no-touch' technique, or an indwelling catheter is preferable, but most now prefer the latter. If an indwelling catheter (polythene is preferred) is used, it should be changed every two or three days, and the technique of tidal drainage can usefully be employed at first if retention, either complete or partial, has been present for some time. Almost invariably urinary infection supervenes, and the urine must be examined microscopically for pus cells regularly.

When infection develops, the urine should be cultured and appropriate therapy with sulphonamides, urinary antiseptic drugs, or with antibiotics is given depending upon the infecting organism and its sensitivity to these drugs as revealed by microbiological tests. Regular bladder washouts with dilute chlorhexidine solution are also useful. Every few days, the catheter should be removed, or intermittent catheterisation delayed, to see whether satisfactory evacuation of the bladder can be achieved either by voluntary effort, with the aid of manual compression above the pubis, or following the oral administration of 10–30 mg of bethanechol or an intramuscular injection of 0.25 mg of carbamylcholine (carbachol) or distigmine (ubretid, 0.5 mg). If a single injection has no effect, it can be repeated half an hour later, but if there is still no evacuation, the catheter should be reinserted and the procedure attempted again a few days later. Eventually, in most cases of spastic paraplegia, automatic bladder action becomes established, even if the paraplegia remains complete, within a few weeks or months and the bladder is then evacuated automatically every few hours, whenever the intravesical pressure reaches a certain level. In some cases, surgical resection of the bladder neck is needed to facilitate this process, as the internal urethral sphincter becomes greatly hypertrophied. Once automatic bladder action is established, the male patient can be helped by the use of disposable urinals made of plastic which prevent inadvertent wetting of his garments. Incontinence pads may be used in the female but are much less satisfactory. Following lesions of the cauda equina, or permanent flaccid paraplegia due to cord infarction, the bladder remains permanently atonic and in many cases evacuation is only achieved by means of abdominal contraction or manual compression. Sometimes permanent catheter drainage or suprapubic cystostomy is then necessary.

Care of the bowels does not as a rule present as many problems as care of the bladder. Retention of faeces is usual in the initial stages and enemas are generally required every two or three days. Subsequently the patient usually regains some voluntary control over the act of defaecation, unless the cauda equina is damaged, when regular enemas may be needed indefinitely. Many paraplegic patients learn the technique of regular manual removal of faeces with a gloved hand, while others prefer a twice weekly enema. Sexual function is also totally lost, as a rule, in the paraplegic patient. Under exceptional circumstances when the male partner of a marriage is paraplegic and a child is greatly desired, the intrathecal injection of a small dose of neostigmine may produce ejaculation and artificial insemination of the wife will then be possible. A female paraplegic patient may be able to have a child though delivery by Caesarian section will often be needed.

The posture of the patient is all-important in preventing muscular contractures and consequent skeletal deformity. Thus a cage is usually required to take the weight of the bedclothes which would otherwise cause foot drop. Splinting of the legs is also required in some cases in order to prevent hamstring contractures. When flexor spasms at the hips and knee develop, 5–10 mg diazepam four times daily or baclofen (5 mg three times daily, increasing, if tolerated, to 60–80 mg daily) are sometimes of value. If these spasms are severe, surgical division of the obturator nerves or intrathecal injections of phenol in glycerin are sometimes necessary for their relief.

Management of the Comatose Patient

As in the paraplegic, so in the comatose patient, appropriate nursing care is essential if life is to be saved and undue disability avoided. The first essential is maintenance of an adequate airway. This is first achieved by turning the patient on to his side so that the tongue cannot fall back down the throat. Secretions and vomit, if present, should then be removed from the mouth, pharynx and upper respiratory passages, using suction if possible. If unconsciousness is at all prolonged it is wise to pass a nasal tube into the stomach and to aspirate the gastric contents so that the danger of inhalation of vomit can be avoided. If there is any difficulty in maintaining an airway, tracheal intubation is wise; if required for more than 24 hours a tracheotomy is then necessary. Despite these precautions, comatose patients are particularly liable to develop pulmonary collapse and/or consolidation.

Regular physiotherapy and the removal of secretions by suction through a tracheal catheter are therefore necessary. It is also usual to give prophylactic antibiotic therapy, usually at first with ampicillin, 250 mg every four hours, and the chest should be examined frequently. Care of the skin is equally as important as in paraplegic patients, and if there is retention of urine, catheterisation will be required. The urine should also be examined frequently, because of the danger of urinary infection, and the urinary output must be measured to be sure that renal function is being maintained. If faecal incontinence is troublesome it is often preferable to give daily enemas. It is also important to maintain an adequate intake of fluid and of food if unconsciousness is likely to be prolonged. No particular steps are necessary in this connexion as a rule if the patient is unconscious for 24 to 48 hours or less. Intravenous fluid may be necessary, but is best avoided initially because of the danger of pulmonary oedema. The serum electrolytes should, however, be estimated daily and may subsequently indicate the need for intravenous therapy with correction of electrolyte imbalance. Later, if there is no vomiting, an adequate fluid and food intake can be achieved by intragastric tube feeding, which can be continued indefinitely until the patient is capable of taking adequate nourishment by mouth. Milk and various protein hydrolysate preparations are the basis of most meals given by tube, but care should be taken to see that vitamin supplements and adequate quantities of sodium and potassium are added. Intravenous feeding may also be required if unconsciousness is prolonged.

Management of Respiratory Paralysis

There are many disorders of the nervous system which can cause paralysis of the muscles of respiration, with fatal results if assisted respiration is not employed. It is important that these methods of treatment should be started early, when the patient is showing symptoms merely of restlessness, anxiety, irritability and sleeplessness and before cyanosis or impairment of consciousness have resulted from respiratory insufficiency with hypoxia and carbon dioxide retention. Estimation of the arterial pO_2 and pCO_2 is helpful in indicating the need for artificial ventilation. The commonest conditions in which this is necessary are acute anterior poliomyelitis, postinfective polyradiculopathy (the Guillain–Barré syndrome), transverse myelitis, drug overdosage, myasthenia gravis and polymyositis or dermatomyositis, but there are many others in which respiration may cease while the heart continues to beat strongly. As a general rule, techniques of assisted respiration should only be used if the illness from which the patient is suffering is one in which some degree of recovery may be expected, for once a respirator has been started it is rarely justifiable to stop it. It is usually, for instance, a waste of medical and nursing skill to begin assisted respiration in a patient who has stopped breathing as a result of a massive intracerebral or pontine haemorrhage, unless surgical evacuation of the clot is proposed. In this context, the accepted criteria now employed in the diagnosis of brain death (p. 117) may be useful in reaching a decision.

Two principal methods of artificial respiration are available and when these are required, nursing in an appropriately staffed intensive care unit is indicated whenever possible. The first method, which utilises intermittent external pressure upon the thorax, is employed in the tank (iron lung) and cuirass respirators, and is applicable in cases in which the muscles of respiration are paralysed but those of swallowing are unaffected. In the alert and co-operative patient with chronic respiratory insufficiency (say due to bilateral diaphragmatic paralysis). a Bird-type respirator which inflates the lungs through a mouthpiece while the nasal passages are closed is sometimes helpful. When, however, the pharyngeal muscles are also paralysed, so that the patient cannot swallow food or secretions, intermittent positive-pressure respiration, in which the lungs are mechanically inflated and deflated through a cuffed tracheotomy tube, is needed. Each method requires a team of doctors and of nurses to give the patient constant supervision and to check continually that ventilation is adequate and that he is not developing hypoxia or carbon-dioxide retention. Many other nursing problems arise in relation to care of the patient's skin, bladder and bowels, quite apart from the physiotherapeutic and other treatment he requires for the primary condition which caused the respiratory paralysis.

Physiotherapy and Rehabilitation

Physiotherapy has an important part to play in the treatment of many neurological disorders. Thus when disease results in a partial or complete paralysis of a limb, or of more than one limb, appropriate physiotherapeutic treatment must be instituted as soon as possible. Its purpose is to help the patient to make the best possible use of the available power in the affected limb if the paralysis is partial, and to prevent muscular contractures, stiffening and deformity if it is complete. When paralysis is almost total, whether it be flaccid (a lower motor neurone lesion, or an upper motor neurone lesion during the stage of spinal shock) or spastic (upper motor neurone lesion), the first essential is that passive movements of the affected muscles should be carried out repeatedly through the maximum range at all affected joints. This action will maintain the elasticity of the muscles, will prevent the development of contractures and may, if spasticity is present, help in modifying the enhanced muscular tone. Later, once voluntary power begins to return, active movements are encouraged, first with support or positioning of the limb to nullify the effect of gravity and later against resistance. Repeated isometric contraction is particularly valuable. In a patient with a hemiplegia following cerebral thrombosis, for instance, this process may be very slow, requiring great patience and continual encouragement on the part of the physiotherapist and nurse, and confidence and determination from the patient. Nearly all hemiplegic patients can eventually be helped to walk, although in many, little useful function in the paralysed fingers is regained. The help of a physiotherapist is also essential in patients with respiratory paralysis, as skilful positioning will not only help the patient to expectorate secretion which might otherwise obstruct the bronchi, but will also help him to make the best possible use of ventilatory capacity which he regains.

Rehabilitation is important not only in restoring to useful activity those patients who are recovering from any illness causing paralysis, but may also be of inestimable value in some individuals suffering from chronic neurological diseases. Thus in patients with cerebellar ataxia, Fraenkel's walking exercises, in which the patient learns to walk along a line or to follow foot-prints drawn on the floor, may be beneficial. Similar exercises, if utilised with enthusiasm and persistence, and combined with vigorous passive movements, are also of value in the rehabilitation of the paraplegic, and in the education of children with cerebral palsy. They may even produce improvement in patients with diseases such as multiple sclerosis and Parkinsonism, in whom there is hope of remission or arrest. On the other hand, physiotherapeutic treatment of this type is not always indicated in other remorselessly progressive disorders such as motor neurone disease; it may be disappointing to the patient and frustrating for the physiotherapist, as the disease progresses rapidly enough to nullify any temporary benefit which may result from the treatment. On the other hand, in spinal muscular atrophy in childhood, in which the disease process often seems to arrest spontaneously, exercise plays an important role in maintaining or even improving power in those muscles which retain a nerve supply and in preventing or correcting contractures. Swimming is particularly helpful in such cases. Much the same is true in cases of muscular dystrophy, since, although the disease is progressive, regular moderate exercise may help to slow the rate of deterioration; it is also of benefit in such cases to demonstrate to the parents of affected children the passive movements (dorsiflexion of the ankle, extension of the knees) which they can employ to delay the onset of contractures and the attention to posture or the use of appliances which can prevent scoliosis.

There are many appliances which can compensate for disability and aid the physiotherapist. Thus in the patient who is beginning to walk after a disabling illness and even in some who are deteriorating slowly, walking machines, walking tripods, crutches, calipers and walking-sticks, may all be required at some stage to give the patient support and confidence. Night splints applied to a spastic or paralysed limb are often useful in preventing contractures, while in a patient with foot drop, a caliper and spring fitted to his shoe or a light plastic moulded splint to prevent the toe from dragging will improve his walking considerably. Similarly, a 'cock-up' forearm splint will be required in a patient with wrist drop. In obtaining for his disabled patients appropriate appliances and invalid aids, the neurologist is dependent upon the advice of his colleagues in physical medicine and upon the help of physiotherapists and occupational therapists.

Closely related to physiotherapy and rehabilitation are techniques of **manipulation** and **immobilisation**. Manipulation of muscles and joints is often required to overcome stiffness, or the adhesions and contractures which sometimes follow paralysis. An example is the painful 'frozen shoulder' which not uncommonly develops in the hemiplegic patient and which is often benefited also by an injection of 1 ml of hydrocortisone or an equivalent steroid into the capsule of the shoulder joint. Similar injections into the painful area are useful in cases of the 'tennis elbow syndrome', and, if given beneath the carpal ligament they may relieve, temporarily, at least, compression of the median nerve in cases of the carpal tunnel syndrome. The place of manipulation in spinal disorders and particularly in the treatment of intervertebral disk prolapse is a much more controversial matter, and one upon which there is singular lack of agreement amongst neurologists, physicians in rheumatology, orthopaedic surgeons and neurosurgeons. In a case of acute disk prolapse, whether lumbar or cervical, most neurologists would favour an initial period of bed rest for two to three weeks, with the aid (in cervical prolapse) of a collar made of soft 'gamgee' tissue.

In some cases of lumbar disk disease continuous traction applied through a suitable belt applied over the lower abdomen and attached to weights (15–30 lb) which are suspended over a pulley at the bottom of the bed relieves pain which is not relieved by bed rest alone. Continuous or intermittent traction of the neck is also helpful sometimes in cervical disk prolapse. If symptoms persist despite such treatment immobilisation in a plastic-moulded collar or in a plaster jacket or firm lumbar support (in lumbar disk disease) is then advised, usually with success. Should these measures fail, then manipulation in skilled hands has a place, although the risks of paraplegia following cervical manipulation or of a cauda equina lesion after lumbar manipulation must be borne in mind. Surgical exploration is usually indicated in relatively young patients in whom other measures tried over an adequate period have failed to relieve pain or when there are physical signs (paraparesis, lower motor neurone paralysis, sensory loss) indicating persisting compression of the spinal cord or of one or more spinal roots. Impairment of sphincter control, a 'cauda equina syndrome' or even foot-drop resulting from acute lumbar disk prolapse, are always indications for laminectomy, but minimal neurological signs (an absent ankle jerk or a small patch of sensory loss) may resolve with conservative treatment. In cases of chronic cervical spondylosis with spinal cord compression, immobilisation of the neck in a collar is rarely of benefit save for the relief of pain. The results of surgical decompression of the cervical spinal cord are variable but seem to be best in patients who are showing rapid deterioration and in whom there is myelographic evidence of severe compression of the spinal cord by one or two intervertebral disks.

Occupational Therapy

The occupational therapist plays an invaluable role in helping patients suffering from chronic progressive neurological diseases and those who are recovering slowly from disabling disorders of the nervous system (including head injury). As days and weeks of comparative monotony slip by, with improvement which may at first be imperceptible, particularly to the patient, it is essential that he or she should be kept occupied and interested. Not only does he require constant encouragement, but time spent in appropriate crafts is not only an antidote for despondency, but will also help to improve the power and co-ordination of his limbs. Occupational therapists are particularly skilled in performing detailed assessment of the effects which a particular disability may have upon the patient's daily life and in designing tasks and mechanical aids which may help him to overcome or compensate for his disability. This treatment is of especial value to the disabled housewife in assisting her to adjust to her disability in the performance of domestic tasks, but is also invaluable in the rehabilitation of the wage-earner as well as in the management of the seriously disabled. Television and organised sports (such as archery for the paraplegic) are also excellent for morale in appropriate long-stay hospitals. Even greater ingenuity may be demanded of the doctor who is supervising the slow recovery of a patient who has been ill in his own home.

Speech Therapy

The speech therapist is another important member of the team of individuals who are concerned in the treatment and rehabilitation of neurological cases. The greater part of her time is spent in the painstaking education of children who are born with defective speech or who begin to speak in an abnormal way. Two important categories are the deaf child and the child with severe cerebral palsy. While considerable improvement may be expected in these with patient training, complete recovery may be achieved within a few years in children with dyslalia. Stammering can also be improved in some cases, for example by teaching the use of syllabic speech. But speech therapy is also useful in patients suffering from dysarthria and more particularly aphasia as a result of disease of the brain (as after cerebral vascular accidents). With the aid of patient re-education, recovery can be accelerated and is in the end much more complete, provided the patient is capable of enthusiastic co-operation.

The Treatment of Infections

Whereas no specific therapy is yet available for many of the virus infections of the nervous system, bacterial infections of the brain and meninges, as elsewhere, are favourably influenced by chemotherapy and by antibiotics and it is important that treatment should be given in adequate dosage and by the most effective route.

Meningitis

General measures which are indicated in most cases include intensive nursing care and analgesics for the relief of headache; intravenous fluids are sometimes needed to correct dehydration or electrolyte imbalance, phenytoin to control or prevent seizures and intravenous mannitol (rather than steroids which may impair the host response to the organism) is sometimes needed to reduce intracranial pressure.

Pyogenic Meningitis

The prognosis of meningococcal meningitis, the commonest variety of pyogenic meningitis, was transformed first by the introduction of the sulphonamides and later by the antibiotics. Of the sulphonamides, sulpha-diazine in a dose of 1.5 g four hourly is the drug of choice, but so many organisms are now sulphonamide-resistant that this remedy is now little used. The most satisfactory of drugs for treatment of this condition is intramuscular benzyl penicillin G. Although very little penicillin normally penetrates the blood-brain barrier, substantial amounts of this drug cross the inflamed arachnoid to enter the subarachnoid space, so that intrathecal therapy is unnecessary. The usual adult dose is 600 mg of benzylpenicillin given intramuscularly every two hours at first and later six-hourly; the total daily dose in children is 10–20 mg/kg, in the neonate 30 mg/kg. Treatment should be continued for at least five to seven days and sometimes longer, depending on the clinical response.

The treatment of **other varieties of pyogenic meningitis** is similar, provided bacteriological tests reveal that the organism is penicillin-sensitive. Until a bacteriological diagnosis has been made, intramuscular benzylpenicillin is probably the most satisfactory initial treatment. Many authorities still suggest that the policy of giving 10,000 units (6 mg) of benzylpenicillin, well diluted in 10 ml of normal saline, by intrathecal injection as soon as turbid spinal fluid is found on lumbar puncture has much to commend it. Care must be taken not to exceed this dose in any single injection. The use of intrathecal treatment is steadily declining but many still hold the view that in pneumococcal, streptococcal, and staphylo-coccal meningitis, further intrathecal penicillin therapy is usually wise, at least for the first few days. Intrathecal injection should be repeated not more often than every 24 hours until a satisfactory reduction in the number of cells in the CSF is achieved and cultures become sterile. Often systemic penicillin must be continued for two or three weeks. If the organism, on culture, is found to be penicillin-resistant, then other antibiotics such as cephaloridine, streptomycin, chloramphenicol, or erythromycin will be required, again depending upon sensitivity. Indeed some evidence suggests that cephaloridine 1 g six-hourly in adults may even prove to be better than penicillin as the treatment of first choice and that newer cephalosporins (e.g. cefuroxime) could be still more effective. Erythromycin, of which the dose is 250–500 mg, six-hourly, is best reserved for staphylococcal infections which resist penicillin, while chloramphenicol (250 mg, six-hourly) is also useful as a wide-range antibiotic, and particularly in influenzal meningitis, but should only be used for relatively short periods as it is liable to produce blood dyscrasias. In influenzal meningitis, chloramphenicol is often combined with ampicillin or with sulphadiazine. Streptomycin was once used in some cases but has been largely supplanted by gentamicin which can be given intramuscularly in a dose of 2–5 mg/kg daily in eight-hourly divided doses; the intrathecal dose is 1 mg daily. Gentamicin, given along with ampicillin or sodium carbenicillin, is probably the treatment of choice for bacterial meningitis due to *E. coli*, to *Pseudomonas aeruginosa* or to other Gram-negative organisms. Antibiotic therapy may have to be continued for many weeks in influenzal meningitis before the spinal fluid returns to normal. In listerial meningitis, chloramphenicol or ampicillin (150 mg/kg daily in divided doses) are the most effective.

Systemic penicillin is also required, or other antibiotics depending upon the sensitivity of the infecting organism, if known, in cases of **extradural**, **subdural or cerebral abscess**. In each of these conditions, however, the most essential part of treatment is surgical drainage of the abscess, or sometimes, in cases of cerebral abscess, its total excision. Surgical drainage at an early stage is particularly imperative in cases of spinal extradural abscess.

Tuberculous Meningitis

The essential drugs in the treatment of tuberculous meningitis are streptomycin (1 g intramuscularly daily in adults, 200 mg–1 g in children), rifampicin (450–600 mg daily by mouth in adults and 10–20 mg/kg daily in children) and isoniazid (200–300 mg daily). Ethambutol (25 mg/kg body weight) is of little value in the treatment of meningitis. There is much controversy as to whether intramuscular streptomycin therapy in combination with rifampicin and isoniazid is sufficient, as many workers believe, or whether intrathecal streptomycin is also required. Some still favour the administration of 0.1 g streptomycin intrathecally, daily for six or seven days and thereafter twice weekly for three or four weeks, in adults. In children, a proportionately lower intrathecal dose (25–50 mg) is given. However, in general it is now believed that systemic treatment alone is sufficient in most cases and fewer patients are receiving intrathecal medication. Many authorities also give 20–30 mg of prednisone daily in addition, in an effort to prevent the development of adhesions in the subarachnoid space. In cases in which multiple subarachnoid adhesions and spinal block have developed despite treatment, it is sometimes necessary to give intrathecal streptomycin and 10–25 mg of hydrocortisone via cisternal puncture or even through burr holes in the lateral ventricles. Anticonvulsants may also be required, pyridoxine (10 mg daily) should be given to prevent isoniazid polyneuropathy and, if hydrocephalus develops, surgical treatment may be required. When the organism is resistant to the standard drugs mentioned above, ethionamide (10–15 mg/Kg daily) and cycloserine (15 mg/Kg daily) have been recommended but both are toxic and should be used only as a last resort.

Other Bacterial Infections

Leprosy is a disease which can be treated effectively with drugs of the sulphone group, of which the most effective is dapsone, which is given in a dosage of 25–50 mg twice weekly, increasing to a maximum of 400 mg twice weekly. It is now recommended that rifampicin should also be given for the first four weeks, clofazimine 100 mg three times weekly for a year, and dapsone indefinitely. The treatment of **tetanus** is complicated and difficult, particularly in the severe generalised cases and always requires skilled nursing in hospital. As the tetanus bacillus is penicillin-sensitive, benzyl-penicillin should be given in a total dosage of 2–4 g daily, preferably by six-hourly intramuscular injection or ampicillin (250 mg to 1 g four hourly) may be given, but this treatment does not modify the effects of the toxin. Hence human anti-tetanus immunoglobulin (HTIG or Humotet 30–300 IU/kg intramuscularly) should be given. The next essential is, if possible, to remove the source of exotoxin by excising the wound in which the bacteria are growing. It is also important to maintain adequate hydration, electrolyte balance and nutrition which must be achieved by appropriate tube-feeding and/or intravenous therapy. Most important and difficult of all, however, is the control of the tetanic spasms. The patient should be nursed in a quiet sound-proof room, preferably in an intensive care unit. While many drugs have been used in the past and diazepam in a dosage comparable to that used in status epilepticus, given along with chlorpromazine, may be sufficient when the illness is mild, the most effective treatment in severe cases is to perform a tracheotomy and to institute intermittent positive-pressure respiration, while keeping the patient's muscles continuously relaxed with tubocurarine, succinylcholine, or other relaxant drugs. The danger of hyperpyrexia may have to be averted by means of tepid sponging or other techniques of generalised cooling.

In cases of **botulism**, the only effective treatment available until recently was to give 5,000 units of botulinus antitoxin after tainted food had been ingested but before symptoms developed. When symptoms had developed, the appropriate dose was 20,000 units intravenously, and a daily dose was given intramuscularly for several days thereafter. It now appears that guanidine hydrochloride (20–50 mg/kg body weight daily) may be effective and even life-saving.

Virus Infections

Although some few of the larger viruses, such as that which may cause viral pneumonia, appear to be sensitive to the tetracyclines, unfortunately none of the dangerous neurotropic viruses is influenced by antibiotic therapy. In herpes simplex encephalitis, idoxuridine, given by intravenous infusion in a dosage of 200 mg/kg body weight daily, may be helpful though toxic, but dexamethasone (5 mg four times daily) often seemed just as effective in some cases because of its effect of reducing cerebral oedema. Adenine arabinoside (Vidarabine) (10–15 mg/kg daily for 10 days by intravenous infusion) has been shown to reduce mortality significantly in herpes simplex encephalitis and is also commonly used in herpes zoster. Other antiviral agents related to idoxuridine, amantadine, cytosine arabinoside and the interferons are likely to be used increasingly in the future. At present, treatment also involves the provision of adequate fluid and nourishment, the use of sedatives or analgesics as required, careful nursing including the institution of artificial respiration in appropriate cases (as in some patients with poliomyelitis), and the application of methods of physiotherapy and rehabilitation once the acute illness has subsided. In the acute stage of anterior poliomyelitis, physical exertion should be avoided as this may increase the severity of the paralysis.

Spirochaetal Infections

Although the leptospirae of **Weil's disease** and **canicola fever** are moderately sensitive to penicillin, and this antibiotic should certainly be given to such cases in appropriate dosage, it does not appear to have much influence upon the course of the illness in clinical cases, and treatment depends upon general principles of dietary and nursing care.

Penicillin is, however, the sheet-anchor of treatment for **neurosyphilis**, and is in the view of most neurologists the only drug required for cases of meningovascular syphilis, of general paresis, and of tabes dorsalis. This view is, however, contested by a few venereologists. Despite this difference of opinion there is no doubt that penicillin is effective. An average course of treatment is 600 mg of procaine penicillin given intramuscularly each day for twenty-one days. In patients allergic to penicillin, erythromycin, 500 mg four times daily for fifteen days, is probably the alternative drug of choice, but three courses of treatment should be given at monthly intervals. Alternatively cephaloridine 2 g daily for 21 days may be used. Often the course of treatment must be repeated at three-monthly intervals, on two or possibly three occasions until the CSF cell count and protein content revert to normal and the serological reactions become negative. It is not nowadays considered necessary to begin treatment with small doses of penicillin as Herxheimer reactions (exacerbation of symptoms at the commencement of treatment) are extremely rare. If such a reaction does occur it may be terminated rapidly by the use of prednisone or dexamethasone. Penicillin is almost invariably curative in meningovascular syphilis, but in general paresis and tabes dorsalis recovery is often incomplete. Few if any now favour fever therapy produced either by infecting the patient with benign tertian malaria, or by utilising a heating cabinet designed to produce hyperthermia. The use of bismuth and arsenical drugs in cases of syphilis has now been abandoned. Carbamazepine, phenytoin and steroids have all been tried in an attempt to relieve the lightning pains of tabes dorsalis, but none of these is universally effective.

Parasitic and Fungal Diseases

A long discussion of methods of treatment of parasitic and fungal disorders would be inappropriate in a textbook of neurology; many of those which affect the nervous system are relatively uninfluenced by treatment but torulosis (cryptococcosis) can be effectively treated with amphotericin B, while actinomycosis is sensitive to large doses of benzylpenicillin. It now appears that 5-fluorocytosine may be even more effective and less toxic in some cases of cryptococcosis than amphotericin *B. Malaria*, alone among the protozoa, can be effectively treated by means of a wide variety of agents, including quinine, chloroquine and primaquine.

Sydenham's Chorea

No single drug is effective in the treatment of rheumatic chorea. Salicylates have been abandoned and steroids are of no value. The movements, if troublesome, may be controlled by haloperidol 0.5–1.5 mg three times a day, depending upon the age of the patient. Rest, quiet surroundings and sedation, with diazepam 2–5 mg three or four times daily, are the most important additional measures in severe cases.

Allergic Disorders

There is now some evidence to suggest that many of the nervous diseases which appear to result from hypersensitivity, and particularly postinfective encephalomyelitis and polyneuritis, are favourably influenced by treatment with drugs of the steroid group (*see below*).

The Treatment of Mental Disorders

A detailed review of the innumerable methods of treatment for mental disease which are now available would be inappropriate in a volume devoted to neurology, but an outline will be given of some of the more important methods which are in current use. In cases of anxiety state or reactive depression, a willingness to listen to a description of the patient's symptoms and to his explanation of their probable cause, and an attitude of patience and understanding on the part of the doctor may be of more benefit than drugs. Indeed some individuals are cured by simple psychotherapy, particularly if the basic cause of their anxiety can be revealed and eradicated. Psychotherapy often requires little more than wise counselling and humanity and does not involve the more complex and time-consuming techniques of psychoanalysis. Often, however, the judicious use of drugs is of great benefit, though drug therapy without understanding, and without confidence of the patient in the doctor, will achieve little. Anxiety and tension can be substantially relieved by tranquillising drugs such as chlorpromazine (25–50 mg three times a day), meprobamate (200–400 mg three or four times a day), trifluoperazine, (2–6 mg daily), chlordiazepoxide (5–10 mg three times daily), thioridazine (25–50 mg three times daily), diazepam (2–5 mg three times daily), lorazepam (1–10 mg daily) and medazepam (15–30 mg daily). β-adrenergic blocking agents have also been used successfully in the treatment of anxiety, especially when associated with tremor, palpitations, tachycardia and anticipatory apprehension. Most successful in this respect have been propanolol 40 mg three times a day or taken before a stressful event, or oxprenolol 40–80 mg three times a day. Haloperidol (0.5–1.5 mg two or three times daily) is a particularly powerful tranquilliser which is especially useful in calming the manic patient or in agitated psychotic individuals. Chlormethiazole (500 mg two or three times daily) is of especial value in the treatment of delirious states and in drug addiction. Some powerful tranquillisers and particularly the phenothiazines may produce Parkinsonian features and in occasional cases unpleasant and irreversible dyskinesias of the limbs, face and tongue. If there is considerable weight loss and anorexia, as in cases of anorexia nervosa, 10–20 units of subcutaneous insulin and 50 g of glucose given before each meal was often used in the past to promote appetite, but chlorpromazine in increasing doses remains the most useful drug in the treatment of such cases. In the past tablets combining dextroamphetamine sulphate (5 mg) with amylobarbitone (50 mg), were often given for the treatment of reactive depression and anxiety but the use of these remedies must now be condemned as both barbiturates and amphetamines have been shown to be dangerous drugs of addiction. The forms of treatment referred to above are sometimes of benefit in cases of hysteria, but hysterical symptoms are often much more intractable unless their cause can be removed, and may require more sophisticated methods of treatment such as hypnosis or abreaction during light pentothal anaesthesia.

Many drugs are now available for the treatment of depression. Reactive depression or anxiety-depression, particularly in middle-aged women, often responds to a combination of phenelzine (15 mg three times daily) and trifluoperazine (1 mg three times daily). For severe endogenous depression, however, the drugs of choice are imipramine, desimipramine trimipramine or clomipramine (25 mg three times daily increasing up to 75 mg three times daily), amitriptyline (25–50 mg three times daily), dothiepin (25–75 mg daily) or nortriptyline (25–50 mg three times daily). Alternatively, trimipramine may be given in a single dose of 50, 75 or even 100 mg two hours before retiring to bed. Maintenance treatment may have to be continued for many months or even for years in some cases. The dangers of liver damage in patients receiving chlorpromazine and phenelzine or other aminoxidase inhibitors or toxic reactions due to the ingestion of tyramine-containing foods in those receiving the latter groups of drugs should be borne in mind. Patients taking amine oxidase inhibitors should be warned not to take cheese, broad beans, Marmite, and alcohol. Cases of severe depression which fail to respond to drugs may require electroconvulsion therapy (ECT) and may be cured by six to eight treatments given at intervals of two or three days.

The control of mania is essentially a problem of sedation, and paraldehyde, 10 ml intramuscularly, was often used in the past but haloperidol 5–10 mg intravenously is probably more successful.

Even more effective in the control of manic-depressive illness is lithium carbonate (300 mg tablets) given in a dose (usually 2–4 daily) sufficient to maintain a blood lithium level of 0.6–1.5 mEq/1. Remarkable benefit can be obtained in some cases of schizophrenia with reserpine in an initial dosage of 0.25 mg three times daily, increasing up to 1 mg or more three or four times a day, but this drug occasionally produces severe depression. It has also been used in senile psychoses but has been largely supplanted by newer drugs. Trifluoperazine is one, which given in a dosage of up to 5 mg three times a day is often useful in cases of paranoid psychosis or other delusional states. Chlorpromazine and its derivatives can also be of great benefit in some severely disturbed schizophrenic patients and may have to be given in a dosage of 200–300 mg three or four times daily. Newer remedies now commonly used in schizophrenia include benperidol (0.25–1.5 mg daily), chlorprothixene (up to 150 mg daily in elderly patients and up to 400 mg daily in severe schizophrenia), and flupenthixol hydrochloride (3–9 mg twice daily). It is in patients taking doses of chlorpromazine and related phenothiazine drugs of this magnitude that the risk of oro-facial dyskinesias (grimacing, lip-smacking, chewing, and protrusion of the tongue) and of drug-induced Parkinsonism is greatest. In some cases of schizophrenia, however, a satisfactory therapeutic response may also be obtained from electroconvulsion therapy given repeatedly over a long period.

Poisoning, Addiction and Drug Withdrawal

In all cases of accidental or suicidal poisoning it is first important whenever possible to determine the nature of the poisonous agent, in order that appropriate treatment may be given. For instance, in cases of carbon-monoxide poisoning, oxygen, and artificial respiration if need be, should be given. In cases of poisoning by drugs, unless the substance ingested has a strong corrosive effect, the stomach should be washed out immediately, and if, for instance, the patient has taken a strongly acid substance, an appropriate bland alkali (magnesium carbonate or sodium bicarbonate) should be given, while if the poison was a powerful alkali, vinegar in water is a suitable antidote. The commonest drugs which are now used for suicidal attempts are sedatives or antidepressive drugs. In such a case the first essential is to maintain adequate ventilation, by preservation of the airway and to use artificial respiration if required. Analeptic drugs, once widely used in such cases, are no longer recommended. Antibiotics (e.g. ampicillin 250–500 mg every four to six hours) should usually be given and many patients treated conservatively in this way recover completely.

In severe cases, intermittent positive pressure respiration is needed and a powerful diuretic such as frusemide (40–120 mg) may promote excretion of the drug via the kidneys. In occasional cases, if these measures fail, dialysis with the aid of an artificial kidney is successful in removing barbiturate, narcotic, or other sedative drugs from the body.

The treatment of acute **heavy metal poisoning** (arsenic, lead, copper) is similar to that of any form of acute poisoning. In chronic intoxication, the appropriate remedies are dimercaprol (BAL) or chelating agents such as calcium EDTA (versene). BAL is given by deep intramuscular injection in a 5 per cent solution; the dosage is 2 ml, four times on the first day, three times on the second, twice on the third and then daily for four days. Several courses of treatment may be required at intervals of a few weeks. The dosage of calcium EDTA is 0.5 mg given intravenously in 200 ml of saline over two hours; this should be repeated every eight to 12 hours for five days and another course may be required a few days later.

Drug addiction, whether to opiates, barbiturates, amphetamine or alcohol, is difficult to treat. There is hope of success if the underlying psychiatric disorder which caused the addiction can be treated effectively but more often there are basic defects in personality in the addict which are immutable. Some addicts, and particularly alcoholics, are salvaged through the interest and support they obtain from organisations such as Alcoholics Anonymous, whose members often attain a zeal for reform of almost religious intensity. In the addict who genuinely desires a cure, the process, though often painful and lengthy, is worthwhile, but many addicts undergo prolonged and distressing courses of treatment, only to relapse when once more they enter society. The cure of addiction almost always requires treatment in an appropriate hospital. The complicated steps required to treat the opiate addict are beyond the scope of this volume. In chronic barbiturate intoxication, withdrawal must be gradual in order to prevent psychosis and convulsions. Usually the patient is given 200–400 mg of pentobarbitone or a similar barbiturate three or four times daily, and the dosage is reduced by 100 mg daily. If severe withdrawal symptoms appear, a higher dosage is recommended for two or three days and then the process is repeated until complete withdrawal is achieved.

In chronic alcoholism, a similar regimen of gradual withdrawal is often effective, using progressively lower amounts of whisky or brandy. Sudden withdrawal may result in delirium tremens; intramuscular diazepam or chlorpromazine may be required to control excitement and/or convulsions, and intravenous fluid may be needeed to correct dehydration and electrolyte imbalance. There is some evidence that corticotrophin (ACTH), 100 units daily by intramuscular injection on the first two or three days, is beneficial, as some of the symptoms of delirium tremens are thought to be due to adrenal exhaustion. Chlorpromazine (50 mg six-hourly) or chlormethiazole (8–16 capsules, each of 500 mg, in each 24 hour period for the first few days) are particularly useful in the withdrawal period. Vitamins of the B group should also be given parenterally and are conveniently administered in the form of 'parentrovite'. Insulin (15 units) and glucose (50 g) three times daily have been used after the acute stage in order to promote appetite. Residual tremulousness is often relieved by chlordiazepoxide or diazepam. Vitamins in high dosage, including thiamine 200 mg or more should be given daily over a prolonged period, particularly if there is any evidence of polyneuropathy. Once withdrawal has been achieved, prolonged abstinence can be helped by the use of disulfiram ('Antabuse'). This drug is given in a dosage of from half to one tablet (0.15–0.5 g) daily. An alternative is citrated calcium carbimide ('Abstem', 50 mg twice daily). When a patient who is taking these drugs drinks alcohol, acetaldehyde is released into the circulation and gives rise to headache, palpitations, nausea and vomiting. Great care must be exercised in their use, as fatal reactions have been described following a large intake of alcohol; it is usually wise to begin administration in hospital and to give the patient a small glass of an alcoholic beverage during his stay, so that he may know what to expect if he drinks while receiving the drug. If he has no real desire to be cured, he has only to stop taking the tablets on leaving hospital; but these drugs are nevertheless of some value in strengthening the resolve of those who wish to overcome their addiction, and may help them to resist temptation.

Migraine and Related Disorders

Although migraine is a constitutional disorder which cannot be cured, it can be relieved considerably in most cases. The frequency and severity of attacks is increased by stress, fatigue and/or anxiety; adequate rest, relaxation, avoidance of stress, and the use of tranquillisers to relieve tension and anxiety are often helpful. In the patient who is suffering frequent severe attacks, prophylactic treatment is required to reduce both frequency and severity. Sometimes tablets of ergotamine tartrate, if taken regularly for short periods, have a prophylactic effect but prolonged treatment is dangerous because of the risk of ergotism. In children particularly, and in adults occasionally, prochlorperazine (Stemetil) given in a dosage of 5 mg three or four times daily may be useful. An increased frequency of migrainous attacks in women at about the time of the menopause is commonly due to an associated anxiety-depression which can usually be relieved by treatment with phenelzine, amitriptyline or dothiepin (*see above*) with dramatic improvement in the attacks of migraine. Even when there is no overt evidence of depression and anxiety, an antidepressive drug of this type given with a mild tranquilliser (*see below*) three times a day for several months may be remarkably beneficial. A notable advance in the prophylaxis of migraine was the introduction of methysergide (1–3 mg three times daily) which may reduce dramatically the frequency and severity of attacks and may have to be continued in diminishing dosage for several months. However, this drug carries the serious risk of causing retroperitoneal fibrosis and as this complication is dose-dependent it is unwise to give more than 6 mg daily for more than three months at a time, followed by a gap of at least three months before the remedy is reintroduced. More recently, dihydroergotamine (1–2 mg three times daily, pizotifen (500 µg–3 mg daily) and clonidine (0.025–0.075 mg twice daily) have also been shown to be effective prophylactically. Repeated trial and error with different remedies is often necessary to discover the most appropriate treatment in an individual case.

The actual attack of migraine, if it is mild, will often be greatly relieved by aspirin or by paracetamol. For more severe attacks, tablets containing ergotamine tartrate, and an antihistamine drug to combat nausea and vomiting are often effective, provided they are taken during the aura or the moment the attack begins. Examples of useful proprietary preparations are Cafergot (ergotamine tartrate 2 mg, caffeine 100 mg, belladonna alkaloids 0.25 mg, *iso*butylallylbarbituric acid 100 mg) and Migril (ergotamine tartrate 2 mg, caffeine 100 mg, cyclizine hydrochloride 50 mg) but there are many others; one or two tablets is the appropriate dose for a single attack. If these remedies prove ineffective, then dihydroergotamine mesylate 2–3 mg may be given or ergotamine tartrate in suppository form or inhaled as a fine powder should be tried, or else the more intelligent patients can be taught to give themselves a subcutaneous injection of ergotamine tartrate (0.5 mg) at the beginning of the aura. If the patient is then able to lie down for approximately 30 minutes, the attack may be aborted.

Ergotamine tartrate is also the most effective drug in the treatment of **periodic migrainous neuralgia**. Oral therapy should first be tried when a 'bout' begins; a tablet of Cafergot, Migril or dihydroergotamine or of a similar preparation should be given two or three times daily. If effective, this treatment is continued for several weeks, depending upon the duration of previous 'bouts', and repeated attempts to withdraw the tablets are then made until this is accomplished without the return of pain. Should these remedies be ineffective, then dimethysergide (1–2 mg three times daily) or dihydroergotamine (3–6 mg daily) should be given according to a similar programme. If oral therapy is ineffective injections of ergotamine tartrate, 0.5 mg subcutaneously, may be required once or twice daily during a bout. Treatment should not be continued indefinitely because of the danger of ergotism.

Narcolepsy and Related Disorders

In the past the drug of choice in treating narcolepsy and other conditions causing prolonged somnolence was amphetamine sulphate, or dextro-amphetamine, given in an initial dosage of 5 mg at 8 a.m. and 12 noon, and the dose was then increased if necessary depending upon the requirements of the individual patient. Some required as much as 40 mg daily to keep them awake, but this was exceptional. Gradually, however, because of the risk of amphetamine addiction, amphetamines are being used much less often. Methylphenidate 20–30 mg daily given at morning and midday is an alternative. Recently it has become apparent that many patients respond satisfactorily to desimipramine (25–75 mg three times daily).

Episodic Vertigo

Episodic vertigo of labyrinthine origin (e.g. Ménière's syndrome) can be very difficult to control. Phenobarbitone in a dosage of 30 mg two or three times daily was used for many years, but is of little value, and diuretics which were also widely employed are disappointing, even though the essential pathological change in Ménière's syndrome is a hydrops of the membranous labyrinth. Somewhat more effective are dimenhydrinate 50 mg three times daily, promethazine 25 mg three times daily, prochlor-perazine 5 mg three times daily and thiethylperazine 10 mg, also three times daily. Newer remedies for which even greater efficacy is claimed are cinnarizine 15 mg three times a day and betahistine 8 mg, also three times daily. These remedies all seem to reduce the severity of the attacks but not necessarily their frequency. They are also valuable in motion sickness and in vestibular neuronitis (epidemic vertigo) and have fewer side-effects than 0.5 mg hyoscine which is equally if not more effective. In some cases of Ménière's disease involving only one ear, if the attacks of vertigo are frequent and severe, labyrinthectomy is justifiable, despite the fact that the ear is rendered permanently deaf by this operation. In elderly patients, the ataxia which normally follows this operation, but is usually brief, can be very persistent and difficult to overcome. Some neurosurgeons still practise section of the labyrinthine division of the eighth nerve, but this must be done intracranially with all the risks of a posterior fossa exploration. The most satisfactory method, which is being used increasingly, is destruction of the membranous labyrinth by means of ultrasonic waves; this method is effective, carries little risk and leaves hearing intact.

Spasticity

Although many drugs have been advised for the relief of spasticity, none produces any dramatic improvement in the mobility of spastic limbs. Chlorpromazine in doses of up to 100 mg three times daily is occasionally of some benefit, if combined with physiotherapy. Mephenesin carbamate (Tolseram), given in an initial dose of 0.5 g four times daily, increasing gradually if tolerated up to 3–4 g four times a day, is costly and rarely produces sufficient clinical improvement to justify the expense of prolonged use; it is now rarely used. Chlordiazepoxide (10–20 mg three or four times daily) and diazepam (5 mg three times daily) are more effective and are often the drugs of choice. Occasionally, however, they so reduce extensor tone that the patient's lower limbs become almost flaccid so that he is unable to walk and hence treatment may have to be reduced or discontinued. Dantrolene sodium (25 mg daily in the adult, increasing slowly over several weeks to 100 mg four times daily, or 1 mg/kg in a child, increasing to 3 mg/kg four times daily) is a useful alternative but may have troublesome side-effects. Baclofen (5 mg three times daily, increasing up to 60–80 mg daily), a γ-amino-butyric acid derivative, is a useful recent addition, but also has many side-effects and some patients cannot tolerate it. When severe adductor spasms develop in the thighs, obturator neurectomy is occasionally necessary, while painful flexor spasms may be relieved in some cases by intrathecal injections of phenol in myodil or glycerine (described earlier for treatment of intractable pain) around the L1 and L2 roots. When spasm in the hamstrings is also troublesome as well as hip flexion, then the injection must be placed so as to affect the S1 roots. The danger of this method (particularly after bilateral injections) is that some of the phenol may diffuse around the S2 and S3 roots and will then cause temporary or even permanent bladder dysfunction. Rarely the pain of flexor spasms is sufficiently severe to justify intrathecal injections of alcohol, despite the certainty of producing bladder paralysis, or alternatively spinothalamic tractotomy may be considered. In most cases however, the judicious use of phenol injections is the most effective method and a surprising degree of voluntary power may be preserved in the affected limbs.

Parkinsonism

Many drugs are available for the partial relief of muscular rigidity in Parkinsonism and related conditions, and striking improvement can usually be produced when the optimum combination and dosage of drugs is achieved. This is an individual matter; drug tolerance varies widely from case to case; some patients respond to one drug, others to another, and often if a particular drug appears to be losing its effect, substitution of a different though similar remedy is successful.

It is now evident that in idiopathic paralysis agitans the principal symptoms and signs result from a deficiency of the inhibitory neurotransmitter dopamine in the degenerating pigmented cells of the substantia nigra. This deficiency can be overcome in part by the use of dopaminergic drugs such as bromocriptine (2.5 mg daily after a meal, increasing gradually to 40–100 mg daily, depending upon the clinical response and tolerance) which act by stimulating surviving dopamine receptors. However, this drug has little if any advantage over levodopa which, being a dopamine precursor, effectively represents a form of replacement therapy. Bromocriptine is therefore reserved at present for use in severely disabled, previously untreated patients, or more often for those who are intolerant of levodopa or in whom, after long-continued levodopa therapy, the so-called 'on-off' effect has become troublesome. Its side-effects are similar to those of levodopa. Amantidine (100 mg daily or twice daily) has mild dopaminergic properties and is a useful drug in mild Parkinsonism, being relatively free of side-effects.

Levodopa remains the mainstay of treatment in most cases, but is less helpful in post-encephalitic cases in which side-effects are often very troublesome. It improves akinesia, bradykinesia and rigidity more rapidly than tremor. It must not be given along with monoaminoxidase inhibitors or anti-psychotic drugs such as the phenothiazines, but tricyclic antidepressants are tolerated. Side-effects include nausea and vomiting (which are usually easily controlled by cyclizine or similar preparations) and involuntary movements which may variously consist of facial grimacing, 'foot-paddling', choreiform or athetotic movements. Confusion, disordered behaviour and postural hypotension are also sometimes seen. It is usual to begin with 125 mg daily, gradually increasing the dose to 125 mg four times daily and later still to as much as 4–6 g daily, depending upon the clinical response and upon dose-limiting side-effects, of which the involuntary movements are often the most troublesome. Nowadays levodopa is almost invariably given in combination with extra-cerebral dopa-decarboxylase inhibitors such as carbidopa (75–150 mg daily in divided doses) or benserazide (100–200 mg daily) which act by making more levodopa available to the brain so that a comparable clinical effect is achieved with less levodopa and hence side-effects are much reduced. Combined tablets in common use include Sinemet (125 mg levodopa with 125 mg carbidopa) and Madopar (100 mg levodopa with 25 mg benserazide). Improvement usually occurs initially over 6–18 months, after which slow deterioration may follow and the 'on-off' effect (improved performance during the 'on' period for 1–2 hours after a tablet and then 1–3 hours of akinesia and weakness in the 'off' period before the next dose) is troublesome and very difficult to control. Sometimes a change to another levodopa preparation or to bromocriptine is then necessary, or else treatment with anticholinergic drugs alone may have to be given for several months before reintroducing levodopa.

Anticholinergic drugs continue, therefore, to play an important part in treatment. They are believed to act by reducing the excessive cholinergic activity consequent upon the neurohumoral imbalance which results from dopamine deficiency. They may still be the drugs of choice for initial treatment in mild cases of paralysis agitans, more often in post-encephalitic Parkinsonism and drug-induced Parkinsonism, but are still widely and successfully used to complement treatment with levodopa preparations, especially when the side-effects of the latter restrict the tolerable dosage and consequentially the therapeutic effect. They can also be given safely along with anti-psychotic remedies. Most commonly used are benzhexol hydrochloride (2 mg twice or three times daily at first, increasing occasionally up to 10–20 mg daily), orphenadrine hydrochloride (50 mg tablets, three to eight daily), benztropine mesylate (500 μg–4 mg daily, taken at night or in divided doses), biperiden (1–2 mg once, twice or thrice daily), procyclidine hydrochloride (2.5 mg three times daily, increasing up to 60 mg daily) and methixine hydrochloride (2.5 mg three times daily, increasing to 15–60 mg daily); the latter drug is thought to be especially helpful in controlling tremor but this is uncertain. Two or rarely three of these drugs may be taken in combination. Side-effects include blurred vision (due to disordered ocular accommodation), dryness of the mouth, nausea, dizziness, mental confusion, visual hallucinations and urinary retention and may be severe enough, especially in elderly, atherosclerotic or demented patients to demand a substantial reduction in dosage. The oculogyric crises of post-encephalitic Parkinsonism are unfortunately resistant to most forms of treatment. The role of neurosurgery will be discussed below.

Myasthenia Gravis

Although edrophonium chloride (tensilon) is useful in the diagnosis of myasthenia, its transient effect means that it is not effective in treatment and the most important therapeutic agents are still neostigmine (prostigmine) and its derivatives. The remedy most often used is the long-acting pyridostigmine bromide of which the usual initial dose is 60 mg (in the adult, or 5–10 mg in neonates, 10 mg in young children) given two or three times daily and gradually increasing until maximum relief of weakness is achieved. Many patients require two or three tablets every four hours but individual requirements vary greatly. Atropine sulphate (0.5 mg twice daily) or propantheline hydrochloride (15 mg twice daily) are often given as well to overcome the muscarinic side-effects of the drug. Some authorities still use the shorter-acting and transiently more powerful neostigmine (15 mg tablets) while yet others prefer ambenonium chloride (5–25 mg three or four times a day) which is longer-acting even than pyridostigmine; however, atropine or propantheline should not be given along with the latter drug because of the possibility of masking cholinergic weakness.

Patients with this disease generally become skilled in adjusting the level and timing of their medication to suit their individual needs. It should be remembered that excessive dosage of neostigmine or its analogues may produce increased weakness (cholinergic crisis). If doubt exists as to whether weakness is due to under- or over-dosage, an intravenous injection of edrophonium will usually resolve the difficulty, since it will increase weakness in the patient suffering from overdosage, but will improve the patient who requires more pyridostigmine. Unfortunately there are some cases in which different muscles respond differentially and a dose adequate to improve strength in limb muscles may paralyse the diaphragm. Management in such cases may be very difficult; total temporary withdrawal of treatment may then be needed under observation in hospital, being certain, for example, that facilities for assisted ventilation are at hand. Cases of the myasthenic-myopathic syndrome complicating lung carcinoma are often extremely sensitive to neostigmine and readily pass into cholinergic crisis; in such cases guanidine hydrochloride (25–50 mg/kg body weight daily by mouth) produces striking improvement, but this drug is of no value in myasthenia gravis.

When steroids and corticotrophin were first introduced into the treatment of this condition, it was generally concluded that short intensive courses should be given, that these often caused temporary deterioration and then 'rebound' improvement in the condition. Now it is apparent that in all moderately severe and severe cases, continuous prednisone therapy, at first daily (60 mg at first, later 40, 30, 20, 15, 10 mg, depending upon the response) and later on alternate days should be tried. Some patients (often younger individuals without thymomas) respond dramatically, others not at all, and the response is quite unpredictable. There are even some patients who are not improved by prednisone but who do well with six to twelve months of treatment with azathioprine or cyclophosphamide. Plasmapheresis (a technique of washing the circulating AChR antibodies out of the circulation) may be dramatically successful in producing temporary improvement, especially in a crisis situation, and some believe that regular monthly or bimonthly treatments may produce sustained long-term improvement. In general, however, it is felt that this method is of no long-term benefit.

In very occasional cases of myasthenia gravis, severe respiratory weakness develops despite treatment and artificial respiration is needed. The place of thymectomy remains controversial. Certainly, it must always be considered in severe cases. Some believe that it should be carried out in all cases, even those with the restricted ocular form, others that it is most effective in young women who have suffered from the condition in a relatively severe form for a short period of time, but most neurologists would now advise that it be done in all patients with generalised myasthenia unless their symptoms are rapidly and totally controlled by pharmacological means. If X-rays reveal the presence of a thymic tumour, some believe that this should be treated first by radiotherapy and later the thymus should certainly be removed, as many thymomas become malignant. In some few cases of myasthenia, particularly those in which the external eye muscles are primarily affected, the muscular weakness eventually becomes unresponsive to treatment and permanent structural changes develop in the muscles. Once this has happened, the condition cannot be significantly influenced by any form of treatment though ptosis frames may be needed to support the drooping upper eyelids. In other cases, however, spontaneous remissions occur from time to time and are usually heralded by decreasing pyridostigmine requirements.

Metabolic and Deficiency Disorders

The appropriate treatment of **deficiency disorders** is to correct the deficiency. In cases of alcoholic polyneuropathy, Wernicke's disease and other varieties of vitamin B_1 deficiency, thiamine 100 mg three times daily should be given, while pellagra is treated with nicotinamide 200 mg three times daily. Since most deficiencies are multiple, it is often more satisfactory to give multiple vitamin therapy, provided it is adequate. A useful preparation is 'parentrovite', which contains thiamine, nicotinamide, riboflavine, pyridoxine and ascorbic acid and which can be given intravenously or intramuscularly. It is normal to begin treatment with one of each of the high-potency ampoules, given twice daily for the first two or three days, and then to give one of each of the 'maintenance' ampoules daily. After a week it is generally possible to change over to oral treatment, say, with one or two tablets of 'orovite' (50 mg thiamine, 5 mg riboflavine, 200 mg nicotinamide, 5 mg pyridoxine) or a similar combined tablet, three times daily.

In patients with vitamin B_{12} deficiency, the anaemia is satisfactorily corrected as a rule by means of intramuscular injections of hydroxocobalamin (vitamin B_{12}), 250 μg given daily or on alternate days at first and thereafter weekly or twice weekly. When neurological symptoms or signs are prominent, however (as in cases of subacute combined degeneration of the spinal cord), a substantially higher dosage is required and it is usual to begin treatment with 1 mg daily, reducing later to 1 mg weekly. When maximum benefit has been obtained (usually within three to six months) the maintenance dose can often be reduced to 1 mg every two months. Cyanocobalamin should no longer be used since, unlike hydroxocobalamin, it contains cyanide and is thus ineffective in tobacco amblyopia or in other optic neuropathies which may sometimes be associated with pernicious anaemia.

Neurological complications of endocrine disease are treated by controlling the primary endocrine disorder, and the detailed treatment of these diseases is beyond the scope of this volume. Cases of hypopituitarism usually require about 25 mg of cortisone daily and often thyroxin and testosterone as well, while Cushing's syndrome resulting from adrenal hyperactivity may necessitate bilateral adrenalectomy followed by steroid maintenance therapy. The nervous complications of diabetes mellitus are improved when the diabetes is satisfactorily controlled with diet and insulin, and cases of hypoglycaemia due to an adenoma or to hyperplasia of the islets of Langerhans usually demand surgical removal of the tumour or subtotal pancreatectomy. Hypoglycaemia following gastric operations is best treated by glucose, while reactive hypoglycaemia paradoxically responds best to a high-protein, low-carbohydrate diet. Similarly, the neurological complications of Addison's disease improve when the hypoadrenal syndrome is treated with appropriate steroids, while thyrotoxic myopathy is also improved when the thyrotoxicosis is treated with carbimazole, radioactive iodine or by surgery. The myopathy and the mental disturbances which occasionally complicate myxoedema can be corrected immediately by the administration of tri-iodothyronine, followed by maintenance therapy with thyroxin. The treatment of exophthalmic ophthalmoplegia is often very difficult. A thiouracil preparation or carbimazole should be given if there are signs of associated thyroid over-activity but thyroidectomy is not indicated in the acute stage as this may increase the exophthalmos. Prednisone or dexamethasone should be given to reduce orbital oedema but if the condition is progressive and severe, radiotherapy to the orbit or surgical decompression may be required. In cases of idiopathic hypoparathyroidism, the associated epileptic seizures require anticonvulsant therapy, but additional benefit is also obtained from the use of dihydrotachysterol 0.5–2 mg daily. When symptoms and signs of hypoparathyroidism follow thyroidectomy, symptoms can usually be controlled by the regular administration of vitamin D with calcium in the form of lactate or gluconate.

The most important measure in controlling symptoms of **hepatic coma** (portal-systemic encephalopathy) is restriction of the amount of protein to not more than 20–40 g daily in the diet. The absorption of protein derivatives can also be reduced significantly by the oral administration of neomycin, 4–10 g daily. However, since prolonged use of neomycin may lead to opportunistic infections, say with *Candida*, its use is best reserved for cases of acute encephalopathy. Lactulose, 10–20 ml of a 50 per cent solution given three times daily by nasogastric tube acidifies gastric contents and also reduces ammonia production. Recent evidence also suggests that levodopa is beneficial in reducing confusion and in promoting arousal, while bromocriptine (p. 447) may be even more effective.

In cases of **hepatolenticular degeneration** (Wilson's disease), treatment with potassium sulphide, 20 mg three times daily, is useful as a long-term measure, as this preparation reduces the absorption of copper. Repeated courses of BAL or calcium EDTA (*see above* under 'heavy metal poisoning') have been shown to promote excretion of copper and to produce limited clinical improvement. The most effective agent, however, is penicillamine (dimethylcysteine) which is relatively non-toxic and can be given continuously in a dosage of 0.5–1.5 g daily; it is expensive, but if treatment is begun sufficiently early the affected children develop normally and may show no sign of disease. Pyridoxine 50 mg daily should be given in addition. Unfortunately penicillamine may sometimes cause nephropathy, a lupus-like syndrome, ageusia, thrombocytopenia and granulocytopenia in some cases and even drug-induced myasthenia. When such reactions, which are fortunately relatively uncommon, occur, tri-ethylene tetramine hydrochloride may ultimately prove to be a satisfactory alternative or else one may have to revert to BAL.

Drugs in Some Degenerative Diseases of the Nervous System

Recent work demonstrating that there may be a reduction of the number of functioning cholinergic neurones in the central nervous system in patients with various forms of hereditary ataxia and in Alzheimer's disease has led to the experimental use of choline and lecithin, each acetylcholine precursors, in such cases. Some objective evidence of temporary improvement in cerebellar ataxia has been observed but this treatment is still under trial. Similarly, the slight improvement thought to have been demonstrated in some demented patients under treatment with drugs such as cyclandelate (400 mg three times daily) or naftidrofuryl (100 mg three times daily) remains somewhat speculative, though such treatment can do little if any harm.

Steroid Drugs and Corticotrophin in Neurology

The principal neurological disorders in which steroids are of value are acute postinfective encephalomyelitis and its variants, some forms of demyelinating polyneuropathy (especially subacute relapsing cases), polymyositis and dermatomyositis, myasthenia gravis, temporal arteritis, cerebral sarcoidosis, and the neurological complications of 'collagen' or 'connective-tissue' disease. Recent controlled trials have suggested that such treatment is of no value in acute cases of the Guillain–Barré syndrome. There is also some evidence that intermittent administration of corticotrophin (ACTH) may possibly reduce the severity of relapse in multiple sclerosis. Prednisone will also reduce or abolish myotonia, but is inferior in this respect to procaine amide and phenytoin, while injections of hydrocortisone beneath the carpal ligament will relieve symptoms in some cases of median nerve compression in the carpal tunnel. Steroid drugs are also useful in preventing or delaying the development of adhesions in the subarachnoid space in tuberculous meningitis. The newer synthetic steroids (dexamethasone, betamethasone) in a dosage of 5 mg four times daily have been shown to be remarkably successful in reducing cerebral oedema in cases of head injury, brain tumour or abscess or massive infarction and especially in patients with cerebral metastases in whom there is some evidence to suggest that growth of the metastases may also be retarded. In benign intracranial hypertension treatment with such remedies may have to be continued, in diminishing dosage, for several months.

For routine use prednisone or prednisolone are the preferred drugs. There is no certain evidence that corticotrophin, which must be given by injection, is superior to oral treatment with prednisone, though 80 units of corticotrophin may be given daily for two or three days or longer when long-continued steroid therapy is being withdrawn, in order to help re-establish spontaneous adrenal function. There is, however, a suggestion from clinical trials that corticotrophin is preferable to cortisone in cases of multiple sclerosis and an initial course of 80 units daily may be followed by 80 units every other day and later twice weekly for up to six weeks.

Recent evidence suggests that there is little advantage in continuing treatment for more than six weeks in cases of multiple sclerosis and long-term maintenance therapy is of no value. In subacute and chronic forms of steroid-responsive demyelinating polyneuropathy, however, relapse may follow the premature reduction and withdrawal of treatment. In normal clinical practice prednisone and prednisolone, of which the initial dosage is 60 mg daily, and the maintenance dose 10–20 mg daily are usually given. Some workers prefer to use double these doses on alternate days. This may help a little to prevent the inevitable growth retardation which occurs whenever it is necessary to give prolonged steroid treatment in children. Methyl-prednisolone and triamcinolone, of which 4 mg are approximately equal in their effects to 5 mg of prednisone, are also effective remedies, but triamcinolone should not be given over a prolonged period as it produces severe steroid myopathy. Similar objections apply with lesser force to betamethasone (1 mg three times daily at first, later reducing to 0.5–1 mg daily) and to dexamethasone (4.5 mg daily reducing to 1–1.5 mg daily) but in some cases these drugs are apparently superior to prednisone or appear to be effective when the latter seems to be losing its effect. It is impossible to define an appropriate course of treatment applicable to each of the neurological conditions mentioned above, as the dosage must be varied in individual cases, depending upon clinical response, but it is usual to give 60 mg prednisone daily for two or three days, 40 mg daily for one or two weeks, 30 mg daily for another two weeks or more, and the dose should then be progressively reduced to 20, 10 or even 5 mg daily provided the patient's disease is kept under control. In cases of encephalomyelitis, treatment can be discontinued within two to three months, but in patients with steroid–responsive polyneuropathy, and in temporal arteritis maintenance therapy may need to be continued for six months to one year or even longer. In polymyositis, myasthenia gravis and in cases of cerebral sarcoidosis maintenance doses of treatment may be required for several years. Sometimes potassium supplements are necessary and it is wise to give calcium or small doses of fluoride, in order to prevent osteoporosis, to patients receiving these drugs over long periods. Apart from the systemic side-effects (moon-face, fluid retention, hirsutes) of these remedies, peptic ulceration is an occasional troublesome complication and may require the simultaneous administration of cimetidine. Some degree of myopathy (steroid myopathy) almost invariably develops in patients receiving high doses of any steroid over a long period but usually resolves when the drug is withdrawn. This complication may be particularly difficult to recognise in cases of polymyositis. Steroid-induced diabetes may be permanent and requires the standard treatment for diabetes.

Immunosuppressant Drugs

This group of remedies (cyclophosphamide, azathioprine, and methotrexate as well as vincristine and lomustine have been used to treat intracranial neoplasia. They may be combined with steroids and/or radiotherapy but the choice of drug, the dosage and the best combination to be used in an individual case is a matter for the expert. These remedies are also being used increasingly in patients with polymyositis, myasthenia gravis and other auto-immune disorders. There is, however, no evidence that they are of value in multiple sclerosis. In polymyositis and myasthenia it is nowadays common to give azathioprine or cyclophosphamide along with prednisone and it is often possible in consequence to reduce the dose of prednisone more rapidly, thus reducing side-effects. Both azathioprine (1–5 mg/kg daily) and cyclophosphamide (25–100 mg daily) are effective in many cases but a careful watch must be kept for signs of bone-marrow suppression and in general azathioprine is preferred as cyclophosphamide may cause infertility, alopecia and other troublesome side-effects. In the adult an average course of azathioprine would be 100 mg daily for six months and then 50 mg daily for six months.

Anticoagulant Therapy

The value of anticoagulant therapy in cerebral vascular disease is still uncertain. One serious difficulty in the past was that differential diagnosis between cerebral infarction on the one hand and haemorrhage on the other could not usually be established with certainty by any method, whether clinical or investigative. This situation has been greatly improved by the CAT scan. Evidence collected to date, however, suggests that this treatment is of no value in cases of established cerebral 'thrombosis', particularly if the resultant hemiplegia is complete. The role of these drugs in cortical thrombophlebitis is also dubious, partly because the latter condition is difficult to diagnose with certainty and partly because it is often complicated by haemorrhagic venous infarction. It has been shown, however, that in patients suffering from cerebral embolism, particularly when there is a known source of emboli, long-term anticoagulant therapy will reduce the frequency and severity of subsequent episodes. There is also evidence that in carotid or basilar insufficiency, particularly when recurrent ischaemic attacks are occurring and when arterial stenosis, if present, is not surgically accessible, the episodes can be abolished or reduced by this form of treatment, if continued for up to two years. Much depends upon whether the micro-emboli responsible for the ischaemic attacks are made up of platelets or cholesterol; in the former case anticoagulants might be expected to help, in the latter they would not. Anticoagulants are of no value in patients with a slowly-evolving 'stroke' due to cerebral infarction, or in those in whom weakness is increasing episodically. Indeed while anticoagulant therapy had a considerable vogue up until about 10 years ago, its use in cerebral vascular disease has declined sharply in recent years. However, there has been an increasing tendency to use instead, especially in patients with transient ischaemic attacks, whether in carotid or vertebro-basilar territory, drugs which inhibit the aggregation of platelets. Dipyridamole (50 mg three times a day) and sulphinpyrazone (200 mg four times daily) have been used but are of uncertain value. Much the most successful remedy appears to be aspirin (300 mg daily) which has been shown to reduce the frequency of ischaemic attacks as well as the incidence of subsequent stroke in such patients, especially in males. If more conventional anticoagulant drugs are to be used, and this is now rare, the usual regimen is to begin with intravenous heparin, 10,000 units every eight hours for 36 to 48 hours and with phenindione (dindevan) 200 mg on the first day, 150 mg on the second day, and a dosage which thereafter is varied according to the plasma prothrombin level, which should be estimated daily at first. Warfarin sodium (1 to 5 mg tablets) may be used similarly. The aim should be to reduce the prothrombin concentration to a consistent level of between 10 and 20 per cent of normal. This can generally be achieved with 25–75 mg of phenindione or 1 mg of warfarin daily, but individual tolerance varies widely. After two weeks it is usually possible to find a level of maintenance dosage which produces adequate and consistent lowering of the prothrombin and it may then be possible to carry out the estimation twice weekly, once weekly and later even fortnightly. Many patients become skilled at assessing the dosage they require, depending upon the prothrombin level, in much the same way as the intelligent diabetic works out his own insulin requirements. Complications are few, but haemorrhage from any site, unless scanty, generally necessitates immediate withdrawal of the drug and the administration of menaphthone (vitamin K).

Surgical Treatment

A detailed discussion of the indications for and techniques of neuro-surgical treatment would be inappropriate in this volume and the brief commentary given below is included in order to draw attention to some of those neurological disorders in which judicious surgical treatment may be of benefit.

Head Injury

In cases of concussion and cerebral contusion, the essential aims of treatment are: to maintain an airway, to ensure that pulmonary ventilation is adequate and that hypoxia and carbon dioxide retention are avoided; to sedate the noisy or disturbed patient; and to give adequate fluid and nutrition while partial or complete restoration of cerebral function is gradually being achieved through natural reparative processes. In severe cases, particularly those in coma, tracheotomy is required, and if hyper-pyrexia develops it may be necessary to reduce the body temperature, either by surface cooling, or by the administration of chlorpromazine and pethidine, 25–50 mg of each every four to six hours. Routine antibiotic therapy, generally with penicillin, should be given in all severe cases because of the danger of respiratory infection. An associated linear skull fracture does not as a rule necessitate any immediate surgical treatment, but if there has been bleeding or leakage of CSF from the ears or nose, subsequent operation may be required to close the tear in the dura, since there is a serious risk of meningitis developing as a result of the spread of infection from the middle ear or paranasal sinuses. If the fracture is not linear, but there is actual depression of skull fragments, early operative treatment is generally indicated in order to raise or excise the depressed portions of bone, and subsequently it may be necessary to close the skull defect with a tantalum plate or some similar prosthesis.

The most imperative indications for surgical treatment in cases of head injury are, however, **extradural haemorrhage** and **subdural haematoma**. In cases of extradural haematoma the haemorrhage must be evacuated and the middle meningeal artery is plugged or coagulated. A subdural haema-toma can usually be evacuated satisfactorily through one or more burr holes; in acute cases where the haematoma develops rapidly after the injury the prognosis is often poor but most subacute or chronic cases do well after operation. Only rarely in longstanding cases is it necessary to excise the membrane which has formed as a lining of the subdural space.

Cerebral and Spinal Abscess

The appropriate surgical treatment for an extradural intracranial abscess is systemic treatment with the appropriate antibiotics, and drainage of the abscess. A subdural empyema can also be evacuated successfully through burr holes in many cases and it is often necessary then to irrigate the subdural space with a weak antibiotic solution. Occasionally a wider exposure is needed and a bone flap must be turned in order to achieve complete evacuation of the subdural space. Early surgical drainage of the spinal extradural space is imperative in cases of spinal extradural abscess and the laminae of two or three adjacent vertebrae must sometimes be removed to allow adequate exposure and drainage, although occasionally drainage is satisfactory without laminectomy. A cerebral or cerebellar abscess should not be approached surgically until it seems likely that the infection has become reasonably confined as a result of systemic antibiotic therapy. However, all such cases should be under neurosurgical observation in case a sudden rise in intracranial pressure should result in tentorial or cerebellar herniation with consequent brain-stem compression, when urgent decompression may be required. Certain abscesses in 'silent' areas of the brain can be excised completely, including the capsule. More often it is necessary to aspirate the abscess and to instil into the cavity antibiotic with a radio-opaque substance and thereafter to aspirate and inject antibiotic daily until the cavity is seen to shrink.

Intracranial Tumour

The steps required in the diagnosis of intracranial tumour and the principles governing investigation of the tumour suspect in order to identify the location and nature of the growth, if present, were outlined on pp. 326–328.

Many meningiomas can be excised completely, except for some of those in the cerebellopontine angle or in the region of the sphenoidal ridge; these often envelop important structures such as cranial nerves and major cerebral arteries. In some such cases the surgeon may have to be content with incomplete removal. The same difficulty may arise in cases of acoustic neuroma, but many of these tumours, if diagnosed sufficiently early, can be removed completely, although there may be residual facial weakness and some facial anaesthesia on the side of the lesion. It is virtually impossible to remove gliomas of the cerebral hemisphere completely; if such a tumour is confined to one frontal lobe, say, it may be advisable to carry out a frontal lobectomy in order to create an internal decompression which may prolong life. Often it is necessary to turn a bone flap and to take a biopsy from the tumour (sometimes this can be done via a trephine hole) as its histological characteristics will be of value in assessing prognosis, but radical surgery, and decompression achieved by removing areas of the skull vault, are generally contra-indicated in such cases as these measures merely prolong and accentuate suffering. The situation with regard to gliomas (particularly cystic astrocytomas) of the cerebellar hemisphere is, however, different, as these can sometimes be completely excised, particularly in children, with excellent results and sometimes without recurrence. The same is true of cerebellar haemangioblastomas. Also relatively benign and slow-growing, and occasionally completely removable, are oligodendrogliomas, particularly if lying in one frontal or temporal lobe. Gliomas of the brain stem and of the spinal cord are also comparatively benign in some cases and considerable and prolonged improvement may be achieved with radiotherapy.

Radiotherapy, even with newer improved techniques, is not invariably indicated in cases of cerebral hemisphere glioma since the duration and quality of survival of the patient may be little improved thereby. However, in some patients with slowly-growing gliomas a course of radiation treatment is undoubtedly worthwhile but it has little value in patients with highly malignant and rapidly growing tumours. Circumstances vary so much from one patient to another that each deserves individual considera-tion in this respect. In most patients with cerebral metastases this treat-ment certainly deserves consideration. Cases have been described in which a primary bronchial carcinoma and a single cerebral metastasis have been removed successfully but this is exceptional as most metastases are multiple. Often, however, it is a single large metastasis which produces the patient's symptoms and even if a primary growth is demonstrated in the lung or elsewhere the intracranial growth usually takes precedence with respect to treatment. Partial or complete removal may be fully justified in such cases followed by radiotherapy if histological examination demon-strates that the neoplasm is likely to be radiosensitive, as improvement may follow for several months or occasionally even longer. Even when metastases are multiple and inoperable (particularly when the primary tumour is in the lung or breast) remarkable and sustained improvement, at least for a time, can often be achieved by the use of steroids. Cytotoxic drugs given systemically have also been shown to have a markedly beneficial though temporary effect in some patients with gliomas and metastases and particularly in children with medulloblastomas. The aim must always be not just to prolong life but to relieve suffering and improve the quality of life.

Colloid cysts of the third ventricle can also be removed completely in many cases, though the technical approach is difficult, but medullo-blastomas, ependymomas and craniopharyngiomas are often inoperable. However, the drainage of a cyst in cases of craniopharyngiomas is sometimes of considerable, though temporary, benefit, while children with medulloblastomas can usually be greatly improved, again temporarily, by radiotherapy. Some pedunculated ependymomas of the fourth ventricle can also be removed in their entirety. Radiotherapy is also a useful adjuvant in cases of pituitary adenoma, but in most cases, particularly when the tumour is a chromophobe adenoma, surgical removal is indicated. Sometimes when a relatively benign but inoperable neoplasm is present in the posterior fossa and is causing internal hydrocephalus through blockage of the aqueduct, an appropriate palliative measure is to insert a Spitz–Holter valve by means of which CSF from one lateral ventricle is allowed to drain through a tube into the venous circulation. Such a procedure is also of great benefit in cases of communicating hydrocephalus, however caused.

Finally it is important to mention the intracranial and spinal arteriovenous angioma; a small proportion of these malformations which are small and lie in relatively silent areas of the brain (e.g. the frontal lobe) can be excised completely, but there are many which are too large or are situated too close to important areas of cortex for this measure to be considered. Some few cases of this type are benefited temporarily by the ligation of major superficial vessels which enter the malformation. A similar procedure, or occasionally total removal, is also possible in some angiomas of the spinal cord.

Parkinsonism and Other Involuntary Movements

Stereotaxic surgery, a technique through which, with radiological aid, an instrument can be inserted into individual nuclei in the depths of the brain, has been widely used in the surgical treatment of Parkinsonism. It had been shown earlier that severe unilateral tremor can be abolished by dividing the crossed pyramidal tract in the cervical spinal cord, but destruction of the globus pallidus or more often of a part of the ventrolateral thalamic nucleus, by the passage of a coagulating current, by injecting alcohol, or by the use of a freezing (cryogenic) probe, not only abolishes contralateral tremor in many cases but also reduces rigidity. The operation has usually been done in patients with Parkinson's disease who are physically fit, mentally alert, and who are considerably disabled by tremor and/or mainly unilateral rigidity. Advanced age and bilateral signs are not necessarily a contraindication, but the risks are greater when the operation must be done on both sides.

Operation is contraindicated in patients with severe akinesia or dementia. Since the introduction of levodopa there has been a dramatic and progressive reduction in the number of patients subjected to surgery. Probably in the future, operation will be reserved for those patients who are unable to tolerate this or related drugs or those who are disabled by severe tremor which drug treatment does not relieve. Stereotaxic surgery has also been utilised for the abolition of involuntary movements in patients with hemiballismus, spasmodic torticollis, dystonia and Huntington's chorea, but with limited success and it has also been applied in the treatment of intractable pain. It is unsuccessful in the treatment of athetosis. The procedure is time-consuming and carries certain risks so that the selection of appropriate cases for this form of treatment is a matter for the specialist.

Epilepsy

Surgical treatment can only be utilised in cases of epilepsy when clinical and EEG evidence indicates that the epileptic seizures are the result of focal epileptic discharge arising in a localised and accessible area of the brain. It is only indicated when adequate treatment with anticonvulsant drugs has been given over a prolonged period and has failed to control the patient's seizures. The primary aim of procedure is to localise by means of electrocorticography and then to excise the diseased area of the cerebral cortex and/or the subcortical structures in which the epileptic discharge is arising. Clearly, therefore, surgical treatment is not appropriate if the focus is found in the primary motor or sensory area. Surgical treatment is particularly applicable in the treatment of intractable cases of temporal lobe epilepsy, in which excision of the anterior portion of the affected temporal lobe sometimes relieves the patient's attacks and also improves his temperament and behaviour. In some cases of infantile hemiplegia in which epilepsy and behaviour disorders are intractable, surgical removal of the entire diseased cerebral hemisphere, with the exception of the basal ganglia (hemispherectomy) was shown to result in abrupt cessation of the attacks, without significant worsening of the hemiplegia; this operation was found to be particularly helpful in some cases of the Sturge–Weber syndrome. Unfortunately, follow-up of cases subjected to this operation has shown that the long-term results are disappointing. Haemorrhage into the cavity from which the affected hemisphere was removed followed by cerebral haemosiderosis proved to be a major complication and the operation has been largely abandoned.

Cerebral Vascular Disease

Surgical treatment is being utilised increasingly in cases of intracranial haemorrhage. Evacuation of a subdural haematoma is essential once the diagnosis is made, and some relatively young patients who develop a primary cerebral haemorrhage due to hypertension or some other cause can be improved if the haemorrhage is localised by arteriography or ventriculography and then drained through a burrhole. The results of this procedure have not, however, been shown to improve the prognosis greatly in cases of haemorrhage into one cerebral hemisphere, whatever the age of the patient. However, in cases of spontaneous intracerebellar haemorrhage, whatever the age, surgical evacuation of the clot is well worth considering; diagnosis of this condition has become much easier with the CAT scan. Surgical treatment is even more appropriate in cases of subarachnoid haemorrhage resulting from rupture of an intracranial aneurysm or angioma. Everything depends upon the results of arteriography, which should ideally be performed within the first few days after the haemorrhage. If it reveals an intracranial or subdural extension of the bleeding this may require evacuation, but the essential problem is to deal with the primary cause. Some aneurysms can be excised, their parent arteries can sometimes be ligated, they can be trapped between ligatures, opened and packed with muscle, or coated with a layer of acrylic resin. The use of hypothermia as an aid to anaesthesia has greatly reduced the risks of operation. The appropriate technique to be utilised and the timing of the operation is a matter for the expert, but all cases of subarachnoid haemorrhage should now be considered as possible candidates for surgery.

It is also evident that in some patients suffering recurrent cerebral ischaemic attacks, particularly in the distribution of one internal carotid artery, angiography demonstrates a localised stenosis of the artery in the neck. In such cases and in certain others in which aortic arch angiography demonstrates local stenosis of major vessels, thrombo-endarterectomy is effective in curing transient ischaemic attacks and may prevent a major stroke. As yet intracranial arterial stenosis cannot be treated surgically, in a direct sense, but surgical anastomosis between one external temporal branch of the external carotid through a trephine hole in the skull with the middle cerebral artery on the same side (extracranial-intracranial anastomosis or ECIC) has proved of benefit in some patients with severe intracranial stenosis or even occlusion of the internal carotid artery. The long-term benefits of this operation are now being studied.

Spinal Cord and Root Compression

In every case in which myelography suggests the presence of a benign intraspinal neoplasm, laminectomy should be performed, as most of these neoplasms can be totally removed, with excellent results. Surgical treatment is not, however, indicated as a rule in traumatic paraplegia due to fracture-dislocation of the spine, as damage to the spinal cord is generally at its maximum immediately after the injury. Laminectomy is, nevertheless, indicated urgently as a rule, in any other case in which there is evidence of localised spinal cord compression resulting in a progressive paraplegia. Even if the lesion compressing the cord is known to be malignant (e.g. metastasis or myeloma) laminectomy and decompression may be needed to avoid total paralysis before radiotherapy or chemotherapy can be effective.

The place of surgery in treating cases of cervical spondylosis with myelopathy remains controversial. Any attempt to remove the prolapsed intervertebral disks or the bony ridges into which they have often been converted, is almost certain to result in severe damage to the spinal cord. Simple laminectomy of two or three vertebrae, with division of the denticulate ligaments in order to produce a decompression, is indicated in those cases in which neurological disability is advancing despite other forms of treatment and in which myelography indicates the presence of central disk protrusions at one, two or rarely three levels. This operation is the procedure of choice when infolding of the ligamentum subflavum is causing pressure upon the posterior columns of the cord and when there is also an anterior ridge. In some cases when there are one or several chronic disk protrusions anterior to the cord an anterior approach to the affected intervertebral disks through the neck (the Cloward operation) may be more appropriate. Surgical treatment is also indicated sometimes when there are symptoms and signs of long standing compression of one or two spinal roots, either in the cervical or in the lumbar region, and particularly if the myelogram shows that the root-sleeve or sleeves at the appropriate levels fail to fill with contrast medium. The root canal should be opened and it may be necessary to divide fibrous adhesions. It should also be remembered that occasionally a large lumbar disk prolapse into the extradural space can compress multiple roots of the cauda equina giving a clinical picture like that of a cauda equina tumour; in such a case, too, surgical removal of the prolapsed portion of disk is imperative.

Peripheral Nerve Disorders

The surgical management of lesions of the peripheral nerves is often regarded as being the province of the orthopaedic, plastic or general surgeon, but many neurosurgeons do operate upon such cases. In this category one must include operations such as removal of a cervical rib or fibrous band which is compressing the inner cord of the brachial plexus, or removal of a neurofibroma growing from the sheath of a peripheral nerve. Section of the carpal ligament to relieve median nerve compression is an operation which is done by orthopaedic, general and neurological surgeons; the operation can be done 'blind', using an instrument known as a retinaculotome which is inserted through a small incision, or else an open exposure of the carpal tunnel can be made. Both methods are successful. In peripheral nerve injuries it is now generally agreed that if a nerve has been divided, the results are usually better if secondary suture is performed some weeks after the original injury, rather than immediately when the primary laceration of the skin is sutured. The results of ulnar nerve suture are much better than those achieved after suture of the median nerve. If the results of peripheral nerve suture are unsatisfactory, it is often possible to carry out various operations involving muscle or tendon transplants to compensate for residual disability, but these do not require detailed discussion here. Transplantation of the ulnar nerve to lie in front of the elbow is, however, often required in a progressive ulnar nerve lesion due to compression and irritation of the nerve trunk as it lies behind the medial epicondyle of the humerus and various other operations are sometimes indicated in other entrapment syndromes (*see* pp. 270–276).

The Management of the 'Incurable' Case

So many of the chronic neurological disorders are relatively uninfluenced by any form of treatment that patients suffering from them often present difficult problems in management. The specialist and more particularly the general practitioner will often need to mobilise all his reserves of patience, tact and human understanding in dealing with these problems. As already mentioned, physiotherapy is often of temporary benefit in some such cases and many appliances and invalid aids are available to assist patients in compensating for and adjusting to their disabilities. But when the patient, despite his efforts and those of his doctors, sees himself deteriorating it is not surprising that he often becomes despondent. To strike the right note of encouragement, of sympathy combined with firmness, to offer a glimmer of hope without unjustifiable optimism, and to think of something new to say to the patient and his relatives at each weekly visit; these are the problems which often strain the doctor's resources to the utmost. When to tell the patient the truth about his condition? When to encourage his desire for yet another opinion and when to dissuade him? What to tell his relatives and what to withhold? These are questions which cannot be answered in any text-book, as so much depends upon the patient's personality, his responsibilities and his domestic circumstances.

The correct path to follow can only be chosen in the light of experience and there can be few circumstances in which the doctor's judgement is more important. Some patients demand and deserve to be told the truth and their resolve and resistance is strengthened by knowing the facts of the situation, however gloomy, while others prefer ignorance and seem curiously lacking in insight to the end. Some are helped by sedative or antidepressive remedies when despair deepens, others regard their illness as a challenge, and triumph in every minor victory over disability. It is only to be expected that some patients will resort to unorthodox forms of treatment when orthodox medicine has failed. While it is the doctor's duty in such a case to advise his patients against accepting potentially dangerous or inappropriate remedial measures, particularly if this involves a financial outlay he can ill afford, the physician who regards this deviation upon the part of his patients as being a personal affront or evidence of loss of faith in his ability shows lack of understanding.

When it becomes clear that the illness is drawing towards its close, management must be guided by a few simple principles. The most important are that pain and suffering should be relieved, and emotional distress alleviated by all available means, so that the patient is made as comfortable as possible. The question as to whether he should be nursed at home or in hospital during this terminal period depends upon many variables, including the efficiency and devotion of his relatives and the nature of his illness. If there is no reason to suppose that the nursing and medical care which the patient would receive in hospital would be in any way superior to that he is obtaining at home, it is better that he should remain in familiar surroundings. But even in the best circumstances there are occasions when, because of confused or irrational behaviour, incontinence and the like, admission to the hospital cannot be avoided.

Of the drugs which are available for the relief of pain and suffering in a terminal illness, morphine and its analogues are unquestionably the best, but sedatives such as chloral or benzodiazepines are often required in addition, while phenothiazines too are often helpful, as they not only potentiate the action of many other drugs but also help to relieve the nausea and vomiting which are often troublesome features. If the patient dies peacefully in reasonable comfort, and his relatives have been well-informed and know that everything possible, from both the medical and nursing standpoint has been carried out, the doctor can be satisfied that his duty has been done.

References

Ashworth, B. and Saunders, M., *Management of Neurological Disorders* (London, Pitman Books, 1977).

British National Formulary (London, British Medical Association and The Pharmaceutical Society of Great Britain, 1981).

Calne, D. B., *Therapeutics in Neurology*, 2nd ed. (Oxford, Blackwell, 1980).

Conn, H. F., *Current Therapy, Nineteen Eighty*, (Philadelphia and London, Saunders, 1980).

Davidson, D. L. W. and Lenman, J. A. R., *Neurological Therapeutics* (London, Pitman Books, 1981).

Davies, D. M., *Textbook of Adverse Drug Reactions*, 2nd ed. (Oxford, New York, Toronto, Oxford University Press, 1981).

Goodman, L. S. and Gilman, A., *The Pharmacological Basis of Therapeutics*, 5th ed. (New York, Macmillan, 1975).

Marshall, J. and Mair, J., *Neurological Nursing*, 2nd ed. (Oxford, Blackwell, 1967).

Northfield, D. W. C., *The Surgery of the Central Nervous System* (Oxford, Blackwell, 1973).

Sutherland, J. M. and Eadie, M. J. *The Epilepsies: Modern Diagnosis and Management*, 3rd ed. (Edinburgh and London, Churchill Livingstone, 1980).

Index